To Gust

With best wishes
from

John [illegible]

CANCER HANDBOOK
OF EPIDEMIOLOGY AND PROGNOSIS

CANCER HANDBOOK OF EPIDEMIOLOGY AND PROGNOSIS

J. A. H. WATERHOUSE

Reader in Medical Statistics, University of Birmingham
Director, Birmingham Regional Cancer Registry

With a foreword by SIR RICHARD DOLL,
Regius Professor of Medicine, University of Oxford

CHURCHILL LIVINGSTONE EDINBURGH AND LONDON 1974

Heidelberg, Dezember 1975

CHURCHILL LIVINGSTONE
Medical Division of Longman Group Limited

Represented in the United States of America by Longman Inc., New York, and by associated companies, branches and representatives throughout the world.

First Published 1974

ISBN 0 443 00938 4

Library of Congress Catalog Card Number 73-91454

Printed in Great Britain

FOREWORD

When, ten years ago, General de Gaulle invited governments to contribute half of one per cent of their defence budgets in a concerted effort to discover the causes of cancer and the means by which it could be prevented or cured, the response was cool. His proposal was symptomatic, however, of a growing realisation that cancer had become not only one of the main causes of suffering and mortality, but that it might be possible so to improve treatment as to cure a large proportion of cases or to prevent the disease altogether. With these objectives in mind, information about changes in the incidence and fatality of cancer became of greater interest and an increasing effort was put into the collection of statistics that would provide reliable figures for whole areas.

Notification of cancer to a central authority was begun in Britain in the 1930s under the auspices of the Radium Commission, which made such notification a condition for the supply of radium. At that time the expectation was that detailed clinical reports about individual cases would provide insight both into the causes of the disease and into the efficacy of different methods of treatment, irrespective of the fact that only a small proportion of cases were registered and these all from selected hospitals. This hope proved illusory, and it is now realised that advances in treatment are more likely to be made by detailed study in a single Institute or by means of specifically designed and controlled trials.

The value of cancer registration depends on the ability to secure notification of the vast majority of cases that occur within a given area. Detailed information about each case is not needed, apart from the sex, age, and ethnic group of the patient, his place of residence and place of work, the site and histology of the tumour, the date of diagnosis and the general intention and outcome of treatment. With these data, we can monitor the incidence of different tumours in different parts of the country, detect clusters that might be due (for example) to occupational hazards, detect changes in incidence that give warning of new hazards, demonstrate the effect (or lack of effect) of preventive measures, compare incidence rates in different parts of the country or in different countries, and monitor the extent to which the benefits of a new treatment are made available to the whole population.

In the last decade cancer registration has been developed extensively in Britain, with the encouragement of the Department of Health and Social Security and the Registrar General. The responsibility for collecting data, however, rests with the Regions and the completeness of the data collected has varied greatly from one to another.

Figures for the whole country have been published from time to time by the Registrar General, but their value has been diminished by the knowledge that registration has been far from complete in some parts of the country. Incidence rates for a limited number of sites have been published by sex and age for five regions (U.I.C.C., 1966 and 1970) and other selected data have been published privately by some of the Regional registries. There has, however, been no comprehensive compilation like that now reported by Dr Waterhouse from Birmingham, and all students of cancer will be grateful to him for the immense amount of careful and detailed work that has gone into the preparation of the figures. The epidemiologist will appreciate particularly the detailed breakdown by site, the separate inclusion of bladder papilloma and cervix carcinoma-in-situ, and the extension of the five-year age groups up to 95 years of age. No one will believe that the rates in extreme old age are reliable (because of incomplete investigation), but the extension is a beginning which will encourage the collection of better data in the future. The clinician will be particularly grateful for the analysis of survival rates by age at diagnosis and for the calculation of "corrected" survival rates which eliminate the effect of non-cancer mortality with age and so allow an indication to be obtained of the frequency of cure. Comparison of the corrected survival rates at 5 and 10 years following radical treatment suggests that cure may occur far more commonly than is often supposed.

RICHARD DOLL

PREFACE

The varieties of cancer, whether of anatomical site or of histological type, are so diverse in their behaviour, in their response to different forms of therapy, in their patterns of survival, as well as in their manifestation in the community, and in their changing trends, that it is impossible simultaneously to comprehend them all. To be able to refer rapidly and conveniently to some of the salient quantitative features of the disease, set out by site in a standard form, could be of service to the student, to the practising clinician, and to the research worker. It is the aim of this book, therefore, to provide information on the incidence and on the survival rates of malignant disease classified by age, sex and site.

Information of this kind to be of value must necessarily be both reliable and representative. The source of the data presented here is a large area in the midlands of England with a population of five million which in its make-up happens to be remarkably typical of the country as a whole. Because the efficiency of registration has exceeded 95 per cent for more than a dozen years it is virtually free from selective bias, and sufficient in numbers for all but the rarest conditions. In giving a general picture of the pattern of cancer morbidity by relative incidence rates it is therefore of wide application. In finer comparisons it must naturally portray primarily the features of the region from which it is taken. Some idea of the degree of variation in incidence both internally within a country and between countries can be obtained from the volumes of "*Cancer Incidence in Five Continents*".

This book also sets out for each site of cancer the survival data, by sex and age and treatment policy. Again the data refer to the totality of cases in a large region, forming a completely unselective series. For this reason the overall rates of survival will often appear low, since both treated and untreated cases are included. A number of different survival indices are given, from the traditional five- and ten-year survival rates, crude and age-adjusted, and the survival rate by successive years from diagnosis, to the median survival time, with its quartiles. The method of age adjustment by means of the life table throws into relief the relative disadvantage of the cancer patient to his fellow in the general population, a disadvantage which can diminish to negligible proportions for a number of sites. Such facts are not as well known as they should be, not only among the public at large but among medical men, and among actuaries: for a diagnosis of cancer should not necessarily deprive a man of the benefit of insurance. Although it was not written primarily with this end in view, if the book can help to dispel some of the cancerphobia which is grounded on ignorance it will have achieved a useful purpose.

1974 J. A. H. WATERHOUSE

Acknowledgments

Many people have contributed to the preparation of this book. I am indebted to Sir Richard Doll for his Foreword; to Miss J. M. Levi, to whose untiring energy and devotion the Registry owes its birth and continued nurture; to Dr. G. M. Holme for continual interest and encouragement; to Miss Jean Powell, to whose organisational and analytic abilities in the preparation of the material for the book I am greatly indebted. I would like to thank Dr. Deryk Darlington for the anatomical diagrams, which convey all the detail that is required and combine art with simplicity. Miss Barbara Cornes has drawn the originals for each of the many graphs, and to her and to Mrs. U. Howe, as also to Miss Joan Cowley and Mrs. D. Oxley, I am most grateful for painstaking thoroughness in checking the accuracy of all the figures. Mrs. W. Morris and Mrs. F. Trow-Poole were responsible for most of the punch-card analysis and together with many other members of the staff of the Registry, past and present, provided an invaluable contribution. Mrs. Ann Kirkpatrick and Miss Beryl Wridgway have read the final proofs with exemplary skill and diligence, which it is a pleasure to acknowledge. Finally I would like to thank Mr. A. D. Lewis, Production Director of Churchill Livingstone, for his helpful advice and unending patience.

CONTENTS

PART I

INTRODUCTORY NOTES

INTRODUCTORY NOTES

(i) General

This book is designed to provide information about cancer in convenient form for easy reference. Its concern with diagnosis and treatment extends only to the statistical aspects of these topics, though it should not thereby be too hastily dismissed as of no practical relevance. The process of diagnosis is essentially a matter of weighing the relative likelihoods of several possible choices, when a knowledge of the incidence rates by age may well be of importance in differential diagnosis. Moreover, the results of treatment, in relation to its type, the age of the patient, and the survival rate, is also statistical in form, showing a measure of stability in large groups, but almost impossible to predict for the individual. In these respects of course the kind of information available resembles what in a Life Table is known as the *expectation of life*. In much the same way as Life Tables are used to provide the basis for the calculation of premiums and annuities in the field of insurance for the population at large, the information herein can be used to compute similar indices for the cancer patient. Though its accuracy of prediction in the narrower field of a single disease cannot approach that of tables which are based on the risks of the totality of disease, it is capable of providing a reasonable estimation for a diagnostic group otherwise virtually disfranchised from the use of insurance.

Mortality rates for malignant disease have been available in various degrees of specificity by sex, age, site of tumour, district of residence, occupation, etc., for many years and for many countries. The quality of certification of death, both in terms of its accuracy and amount of detail, has improved consistently in most countries of the world. Although there are still many exceptions, they are for the most part now reasonably comprehensive, and in combination with improvements in census data they can provide a good overall picture of the pattern of cancer mortality, and its relation to mortality in general.

In sharp contrast to that situation, data about the *incidence* of cancer—i.e. the distribution by site, sex and age at the time of diagnosis rather than at the time of death—has for long been available only from hospital series, which have been published seldom for epidemiological reasons but to demonstrate the results of treatment. Such series inevitably reflect the modes of selection for admission to the hospital, which variously may depend upon social factors, wealth, occupation, district of residence, or individual preferences of doctor or patient. In consequence they cannot properly be regarded as representative, whether in terms of the pattern at diagnosis, or of survival in general. Morbidity information therefore, in this field as in many others, has trailed well behind that of mortality in both reliability and comprehensiveness.

The concept of the cancer register, or registry, has in many ways transformed this situation. The registry can take many forms, from a simple notification bureau to a central file of detailed clinical and other data for each patient, and it may be confined to including only the patients attending one or any of a small group of hospitals, or it may attempt to cover an entire administrative area. They are frequently distinguished as "hospital-based registries" and "population-based registries". In several instances—in Scandinavia, for example—the population base of the registry may be that of the whole country.

Two problems are of particular importance for all such registries: first, to ensure that as few as possible cases of cancer escape registration; and secondly, that duplications of registration are minimal. The latter problem is usually the more readily soluble, but depends essentially upon suitable precision of identification. As a problem it tends also to be enhanced by the demands of the first, since in order to maximise the likelihood of registration it is generally necessary to encourage notification from a variety of sources, with the probable consequence of multiple notification. Given good identification data, however, it is usually preferable to attempt to ensure that multiple notification leads to only one entry on the register than to run the risk of missing a case that should have been included.

The extent to which a population-based registry contrives to include the cancer cases that occur in its territory determines its value from the viewpoint of epidemiology. The higher the degree of efficiency of registration, the more representative the data are of the pattern of malignant disease in that area. They can thence be used, in a manner analogous to that for mortality rates, to provide rates of morbidity from cancer of specific sites, by sex and age. Such rates can be used to typify the incidence of the disease, for purposes of comparison with rates obtained in a similar way from other areas. Data of this kind have been collected from a number of cancer registries throughout the world at the instigation of the UICC (Union Internationale Contre le Cancer), processed and tabulated in standard form, and published under the title "Cancer Incidence in Five Continents".* Though there are some variations in standards and in registration efficiency between the registries included, these volumes constitute a serious attempt to provide morbidity data on a worldwide scale. The geographical comparisons they enable to be made are often of more relevance in determining the aetiology of the disease than are those based on mortality alone.

Birmingham Regional Cancer Registry

The data which are the source of the material in this book come from the Birmingham Regional Cancer Registry. Though its origins go back in unbroken sequence to 1936, when it was based on a single hospital, it was not until the 1960's that its registration efficiency exceeded 95 per cent. Its territorial base is the Birmingham hospital region, consisting of the five counties surrounding and including the city of Birmingham: Herefordshire, Shropshire, Staffordshire, Warwickshire and Worcestershire. Its population slightly exceeds five million, and is representative in its make-up of the country as a whole, possessing industrial, commercial and agricultural occupational groups in proportions similar to the national. It is well suited therefore to serve as a basis for epidemiological studies and furthermore to typify prognosis at an average level for patients treated throughout the region, rather than for a selected hospital series. In providing indices of prognosis, separately for all types of treatment and for radical, it exceeds what is available in "Cancer Incidence in Five Continents", as it does also in the amount of site detail recorded, especially in the subdivision by systems of the body. Its lesser range of geographical and climatic variation however is balanced by its much extended range of clinical information.

All these topics fall well within the confines of epidemiological studies as they are comprehended today. Much of the methodology which was developed as a result of preoccupation either with the patterns of spread of epidemics, or in the analysis of rates of mortality, has been adapted and applied in a wider field. Epidemiology now can properly be said to be concerned with the interaction of disease and community in the widest sense. In the impact made by a disease on a community, it is the collective features which form the subject of study, in contrast to the pattern exhibited by its course in the individual. Among others, these features include the proportion of people affected by the disease, specified separately by sex, age, etc.; its natural history and aetiology; the types of treatment and their relative efficacy; its overall contribution to sickness in the population and to mortality. But it is equally pertinent to inquire into the impact made by the community on the disease, as an aspect of epidemiological study. Variations of habit and custom, dietary and occupational differences, climate and geography, can all influence the pattern of disease in a community. It is the description and investigation of such variation, in its relation to environmental and other factors, which constitute the subject matter of the science of epidemiology.

In so far as they refer to a particular region at a particular time, the data assembled here must reflect the specific epidemiological features which characterise that region. In their narrowest interpretation they can present only an historical description of a situation now past. Changes however, do not occur so rapidly in this field as to invalidate their relevance —lung cancer, for instance, in males increased from 27 per cent. of all cancers to 30 per cent. in ten years—and moreover the data from successive years have been grouped together, both for greater reliability and to avoid the random fluctuations of

* Cancer Incidence in Five Continents, vol. I (1966) ed. Doll, Payne and Waterhouse
Cancer Incidence in Five Continents, vol. II (1970) ed. Doll, Muir and Waterhouse
Published by UICC and Springer-Verlag, Berlin

small numbers of cases. Indeed there are some purposes for which the data may be said to typify not the Midlands alone but the whole of Britain, although this would be to ignore certain variations in geographical distribution which, though relatively minor in degree, are of importance in internal comparisons. Where there are differences in incidence which are regional in origin and atypical of the country at large, they have been noted in the relevant sections. An example of this kind is epithelioma of the scrotum which, although small in numbers of cases, occurs with disproportionate frequency due probably to the concentration of light engineering works in the area. Otherwise the credentials of the data are good in that they can be said to be representative and reasonably free of bias or artefact.

The data are not of course collected primarily for epidemiological purposes. The Birmingham Registry, in common with most others, exists first to maintain records of good quality for each cancer patient, and to collate those records in a single file from their various sources. The Registry may, and in Birmingham does, play an important part in the follow-up of patients, both in its organisation and again in maintaining adequate records, up to and including the death of the patient. Procedures for follow-up differ from those used in initial registration, but need also the same high standards. A patient lost to follow-up, even though he cannot be traced in the death register, is by convention regarded as dead. The proportion of patients of whom there is no trace is less than 1 per cent. and often less than ½ per cent. The principal purpose both of registration and of follow-up is therefore to maintain a high standard of records for each patient, first in the interests of patient-care, and secondly by the analysis of these clinical records to provide more general information on the management of the disease. Epidemiological study is thus superimposed upon the basic structure of data collected by a Registry, and its quality must depend upon that of the primary data. Many Registries today however, have also in mind the subsequent epidemiological analysis of the data when designing their basic record forms. In fact much of the methodology of recording clinical and other data for cancer patients, which has been worked out and advanced under the stimulus of expanding epidemiological investigations, could serve as a model for similar work in other fields of medicine.

(ii) Arrangement of Material

In the preparation of this book it has been envisaged that its use would be primarily as a work of reference. For this reason the general site data have been presented in a standard layout on a pair of facing pages, and likewise the information arranged by systems is presented in a basically similar form and includes in each case the page-pair layout in addition. The two most important quantitative features are those of incidence and of prognosis. Summarised as "Risk" and "Fate", they form the subject matter of the page-pair. The left-hand page (Risk) includes a table of incidence expressed as the rate per 100,000 population, by sex and five-year age-group; a few indices to describe certain salient features of the disease, and three graphs. The right-hand page (Fate) presents several aspects of the pattern of survival for each sex, both in tabular form and as graphs. For purposes of broad comparison a transparent "bookmark" is provided on which are printed certain graphs for "All Sites". They can show how an individual site compares in its curve of incidence with that for all cancers—on a logarithmic scale, which permits the legitimate comparison of slopes—or in its survival for successive years after treatment.

In general the intention has been to present the data variously in tabular or graphical form, but with a minimum of comment or discussion. Notes are included in order to clarify the definition, or to explain conventions used in the mode of presentation, but not otherwise to comment on features characteristic of the data. Certain comments of a general kind occur in the more detailed discussion of the methodology which is included after the Site section.

To avoid unnecessary duplication, numbers of cases as well as rates have not been given. It is of course essential to know the number of cases (denominator) on which any calculated rate has been based, and these numbers have always been provided. The number of cases of disease, whether of a particular site or of All Sites, is not the same for all the parameters quoted. In round figures, distributions by anatomical site detail are based on a grand total of 130,000 cases, incidence rates on 80,000 cases, five-year survival rates on 40,000 cases and ten-year rates on 27,000 cases.

(iii) Definitions of Terms and Indices Used

Malignant disease

All conditions classified under rubrics 140–209 (inclusive) of the eighth revision of the ICD (International Classification of Diseases—see *Manual of the International Statistical Classification of Diseases, Injuries, and Causes of Death:* W.H.O., Geneva, 1967). This includes solid tumours classified by site (nos. 140–199), and neoplasms of the lymphatic and haemopoietic tissues (nos. 200–209). Also included are benign (no. 225) and unspecified (no. 238) tumours of the central nervous system. *Papilloma of bladder* (no. 223.3) and *carcinoma-in-situ of cervix* (no. 234.0) are excluded, as of "benign" or "unspecified" malignancy respectively. Each of these diseases is presented in page-pair form after the main section on Systems.

Classification by site: Although the main basis of classification of disease has been made according to the eighth revision of the ICD, classification according to the seventh revision has also been included, and is noted on the second ("Fate") page of each page-pair, while the eighth revision rubrics appear on the first ("Risk") page. A list of three-digit categories of Neoplasms for the seventh and the eighth revisions appears on page 9.

Incidence Rate

The quantity obtained as a result of dividing the number of cases of disease in a given sex and age-group by the number in the population of the same sex and age-group, and multiplying by 100,000 to produce the rate per 100,000. For most of the incidence rates in this book, the numbers of cases are drawn from six consecutive years and averaged, while the population is that for the Birmingham region at the time of the 1961 Census (see Table opposite).

Graphs

The incidence rates by sex and age are shown in two graphs, one with a standard scale which is logarithmic, and the second on an arithmetic scale. The latter is generally more familiar, but has the disadvantage that a common vertical scale will not accommodate all the wide range of rates. For this reason, a scale suitable for each site has been selected, so as just to include conveniently the greatest rate for that site. The logarithmic scale can remain the same for each site and yet display the shape of its incidence curve equally well. It has the further advantage of permitting the comparison of slopes or shapes of one curve with another although differently situated in absolute measure (see Section on Methods for fuller discussion of this attribute). In particular, the shape can be compared with that for All Sites which is printed on the plastic card bookmark.

TABLE

Population by sex and age: Birmingham Region (1961 Census)

Age	*Males*	*Females*
0—	197,503	186,117
5—	178,969	169,599
10—	202,284	192,481
15—	184,530	174,739
20—	156,434	153,019
25—	157,459	148,001
30—	168,437	157,978
35—	177,925	172,734
40—	165,040	163,243
45—	170,271	165,531
50—	160,698	159,293
55—	140,234	144,231
60—	105,608	126,437
65—	74,420	103,551
70—	52,717	80,945
75—	33,306	57,846
80—	17,795	33,571
85—	6,256	13,374
90—	1,084	3,045
95 +	123	518
Total	2,351,093	2,406,253

Indices of distributions by sex and age

Mean age (*years*): this is the arithmetic mean of the ages of all cases of the disease, separately by sex. It is an "exact age" mean because half a year has been added, to allow for the fact that a quoted age (x) refers on average to an exact age midway between x and $(x+1)$.

Ninety-five per cent. between ages: this gives the central 95 per cent. range of ages, such that $2\frac{1}{2}$ per cent. of all cases (for each sex) are below the lower point, and $2\frac{1}{2}$ per cent. above the upper point. If the age-distribution were symmetrical and close to the Gaussian ("normal") form it would be equivalent to the range of two standard deviations above and below the mean.

Children under 15 (*per cent.*): a self-explanatory proportion, separately by sex, of those aged under

15 years in relation to the total number of cases of the disease.

Median age (*years*): the median is the "middle value" of the age when the cases are arranged in order of age; it is such that there are as many cases below that age as there are above it. In a symmetrical distribution of age, the median coincides with the mean; when the distribution is not symmetrical, the difference between the median and the mean gives an indication of the degree of asymmetry.

Proportion by sex (per cent.): this index gives the percentage, out of the total number of cases (both sexes) of the disease, of male cases, and then of female cases. Together the two add to 100 per cent.

Proportion of all cancers by sex (per cent.): this index quotes, for each sex, the percentage which the total cases of a particular cancer are of the total of all cancers of the same sex.

Trend: to give a general idea of whether a particular cancer is increasing or decreasing relatively to the totality of cancers, separately by sex. It is the "proportion of all cancers by sex" which has been used, but calculated separately for each of ten consecutive years. The direction of the trend is indicated by "+" if it is increasing in proportion to all cancers, or "−" if it is decreasing; when the + or − is enclosed in brackets the trend has not attained to statistical significance, but if not in brackets, a single sign (+ or −) denotes the 5 per cent. level of statistical significance ($P<.05$), a double sign (+ + or − −) the 1 per cent. level ($P<.01$), and a triple sign (+ + + or − − −) the 0.1 per cent. level ($P<.001$).

Graph

The separate distributions of the cases of a particular disease by age and sex are shown on a single graph, for purposes of comparison; they can also be compared with the corresponding distributions for All Sites which are printed on the plastic card bookmark.

Survival rates

Survival rates, whether at 5 years or 10, when described as "crude" are merely the percentage of cases still living at the time of their fifth, or tenth, anniversary date. The *anniversary date* used here is the date on which definitive treatment of the malignant condition began, or in the case where no treatment was given, the date of diagnosis of malignancy. The crude rates have been "*corrected*", or adjusted, to allow for the increase of general mortality rates with age ("natural" mortality) by a life table method. The object of the correction is to relate mortality from cancer to the general impact of mortality at the same age, to avoid the use otherwise of inappropriate comparisons which could be grossly distorted by differences in the ages of the patients treated. A corrected survival rate of 100 per cent. for instance indicates, not that no patients have died, but that no more than the number expected to have died, from all causes of mortality, for patients of that age-group; in such an example the cancer might properly be regarded as "cured", or at least no longer to place the patients at a mortality disadvantage in relation to their contemporaries of the same age.

Graphs

Survival rates are displayed in six graphs, three for each sex. The first pair shows the rates, both crude and corrected, by age-group for All Cases of the disease, whether treated or not; the second pair includes only those given Radical treatment. *Radical treatment* refers to any form of treatment at the end of which it was considered the growth had been eradicated. The proportion of cases so treated is quoted, also by sex. The last two graphs show the survival rates (crude) in successive years up to the fifth for All Cases, and for those given Radical treatment.

Indices of survival

The Five Year Survival Rate (per cent.) and the Ten Year Survival Rate (per cent.): these give, respectively for five and ten years, the percentage of cases alive on those anniversaries, separately by sex, for All Cases and for those given Radical treatment. The rates quoted are first the crude rate, described above, for all ages, and secondly the *Corrected* rate, also described above, where the correction has been made for each five-year age-group and represents therefore an appropriately weighted age-adjusted index. The Total Cases on which the rates have been based are also quoted. Sometimes the ten year survival rate exceeds the five year rate, more often in the *corrected* than in the crude rate. This is primarily due to the fact that the ten year rates are based on earlier figures, when registrations for the whole of the region were not complete. They were also more weighted towards hospital cases, because patients dying without attending hospital were not at that time all included. The survival rates in consequence were rendered slightly more favourable; the same effect appears when comparing the five year rates for that period with those quoted here.

Survival Time (*months*): the Median (50 per cent. S.R.) is that time, in months, at which half (50 per cent.) of the patients treated (or diagnosed—see definition of *anniversary date* above) have died, and half remain alive; it is thus the time at which the crude survival rate is 50 per cent. Although the five year survival rate has been used as an index of survival for many years, its range of variation for different sites of the disease is very great. An alternative measure, expressed as the Median Survival Time provides a more striking basis of comparison, especially taken in conjunction with the quartiles. The First and the Third quartiles are defined in a similar way, as the time at which, for the *First quartile*, one quarter have died and three quarters (75 per cent.) are alive, and for the *Third quartile*, the time at which three quarters of the original cases have died and one quarter (25 per cent.) survive. The median is of course identical with the second quartile.

(iv) Notes on Part II: Systematic Epidemiology of Malignant Disease

In this section data are presented in relation to certain major groupings of cases of malignant disease, rather than by the specific sites which appear in Part III. For each group there is a first page-pair showing the Incidence (Risk) and Prognosis (Fate) in the same layout as in Part III. Following these pages is a table giving a breakdown in percentage form by detailed anatomical site for each sex, quoting also the five-year survival rate for each site. An anatomical diagram (an outline drawing) is also included for many of the divisions to illustrate more conveniently the distribution by individual sites and the survival rates. The section begins with All Sites, and under this heading the anatomical breakdown is into Systems or site groupings used subsequently in the section. It also includes a table giving for the principal sites the mean age by sex, and the percentage of children, again by sex. Following All Sites are thirteen site groupings, usually but not always corresponding to one of the systems of the body, in accordance with their order in the ICD. The last of these groupings is "Unknown Primary", when the analysis by anatomical site relates to the site of the secondary.

The next two sub-sections refer to conditions not properly described as malignant disease, though they may in some cases anticipate malignant disease at the same sites. The first is Bladder Papilloma, and the second is Carcinoma-in-situ of the Cervix ("Stage 0"). Both sub-sections include only page-pair information. They are followed by an analysis of Childhood Malignancy, included here because of its intrinsic interest, and because of its contrast to the pattern of cancer in the adult. The analysis is based on nearly 2,000 cases taken from the whole of the region, thus representing an unselected series, both for the comparison by sites and for survival rates.

The distributions by detailed anatomical site which are included in this section are based on a total of more than 130,000 cases. This total differs from that on which the incidence tables for individual sites have been based and they may therefore show occasionally minor divergences. When allocating a tumour to a site an advanced tumour involving more than one site, where it is not possible clinically to identify the site of origin, or where the information available is inadequate to specify the site, has been put into "unspecified" (e.g. "Oropharynx, site not further specified"). Usually such "unspecified" sites have been excluded from those shown on the anatomical diagrams, though of course they appear in the tables.

Frequently it is only possible to obtain information on detailed subdivisions of an organ if the patient was treated surgically. Apart from exploratory surgery, the mere fact that surgical treatment was possible is likely to imply better survival rates than for the organ as a whole, for instance where localisation of diagnosis to this degree may have been possible while surgical treatment was not. Occasionally site detail becomes available from autopsy reports, but may not correspond well with the situation at time of diagnosis. Interpretations and inferences based on the localisation of tumours to detailed sites should be made with these *caveats* in mind. Comparisons of the distributions by sex for individual sites may be made more, or indeed less appropriate by using the proportional figures quoted in the tables; it is in any case a simple matter to recover the actual numbers of cases by sex from the totals in the tables whenever it is considered to be more useful to contrast absolute numbers.

(v) Notes on Part III: General Site Data

This section consists entirely of page-pairs, one for each of fifty sites (see list p. ix) in the order of the eighth revision of the ICD. The first page ("Risk") presents data on the incidence of the disease, the second ("Fate") on the pattern of survival (see also above, for definitions of terms used). Exclusions from this section of some of the eighth revision three-digit categories are primarily due to small numbers of cases, for instance, rubric 158, peritoneum, yielded only eight cases in ten years), but are also due to grouping together. Leukaemia, allocated four rubrics in the eighth revision for the various cell-types, is here presented only as *Acute* or *Other*; and rubrics 195–199 inclusive are almost all included in the category *Unknown Primary*, for which anatomical localisation of the secondary is given in Part II. Certain other categories have been subdivided: 182 for example into *Endometrium*, and *Uterus, other;* and 184 into *Vulva*, and *Other female genitalia*; furthermore, *Scrotum* has been extracted from the *Skin* rubrics (190, 191) for presentation separately. Finally, in common with the practice of many cancer registries throughout the world, benign (rubric 225) and unspecified (rubric 238) tumours of the central nervous system have been included with the malignant tumours.

Tumours of the skin included in this section are distinguished by site of occurrence as of *Face and head* or *Trunk and limbs.* The histological breakdown into Melanoma and Other of the ICD classification is provided in Part II, where further histological subdivisions are also given.

Because of the differences, deceptively minor but often of considerable significance, between the classifications of the seventh and the eighth revisions of the ICD, all page-pairs in this section quote the references separately to each revision's rubrics. The arrangement of sites is in the order of the eighth revision in the Notes.

(vi) List of three-digit categories in malignant neoplasm section of eighth revision of ICD

140 Lip
1 Tongue
2 Salivary gland
3 Gum
4 Floor of mouth
5 Mouth, other and unspecified
6 Oropharynx
7 Nasopharynx
8 Hypopharynx
9 Pharynx, unspecified
150 Oesophagus
1 Stomach
2 Small intestine, including duodenum
3 Large intestine, except rectum
4 Rectum and rectosigmoid junction
5 Liver and intrahepatic bile ducts, specified as primary
6 Gall bladder and bile ducts
7 Pancreas
8 Peritoneum
9 Unspecified digestive organs
160 Nose, nasal cavities, middle ear and accessory sinuses
1 Larynx
2 Trachea, bronchus and lung
3 Other and unspecified respiratory organs
170 Bone
1 Connective and other soft tissue
2 Malignant melanoma of skin
3 Other malignant neoplasm of skin
4 Breast
180 Cervix uteri
1 Chorionepithelioma
2 Uterus, other
3 Ovary, fallopian tube, and broad ligament
4 Other and unspecified female genital organs
5 Prostate
6 Testis
7 Other and unspecified male genital organs
8 Bladder
9 Other and unspecified urinary organs
190 Eye
1 Brain
2 Other parts of nervous system
3 Thyroid gland
4 Other endocrine glands
5 Ill-defined sites
6 Lymph nodes, secondary and unspecified
7 Respiratory and digestive systems, secondary
8 Other secondary
9 Without specification of site
200 Lymphosarcoma and reticulum-cell sarcoma
1 Hodgkin's disease
2 Lymphoid tissue, other
3 Multiple myeloma
4 Lymphatic leukaemia

5 Myeloid leukaemia
6 Monocytic leukaemia
7 Other and unspecified leukaemia
8 Polycythaemia vera
9 Myelofibrosis
Also:—
225 Benign neoplasm of brain and other parts of nervous system
238 Neoplasm of unspecified nature of eye, brain and other parts of nervous system

(vii) List of three-digit categories in malignant neoplasm section of seventh revision of ICD

140 Lip
1 Tongue
2 Salivary gland
3 Floor of mouth
4 Mouth, other and unspecified
5 Oral mesopharynx
6 Nasopharynx
7 Hypopharynx
8 Pharynx, unspecified
150 Oesophagus
1 Stomach
2 Small intestine, including duodenum
3 Large intestine, except rectum
4 Rectum
5 Biliary passages of liver (stated as primary)
6 Liver (secondary and unspecified)
7 Pancreas
8 Peritoneum
9 Unspecified digestive organs
160 Nose, nasal cavities, middle ear and accessory sinuses
1 Larynx
2 Bronchus and trachea, and lung primary
3 Lung, not specified whether primary or secondary
4 Mediastinum
5 Thoracic organs, secondary
170 Breast
1 Cervix uteri
2 Corpus uteri
3 Uterus, other (including chorionepithelioma)
4 Uterus, unspecified
5 Ovary, fallopian tube and broad ligament
6 Other and unspecified female genital organs
7 Prostate
8 Testis
9 Other and unspecified male genital organs
180 Kidney
1 Bladder and other urinary organs
190 Malignant melanoma of skin
1 Other malignant neoplasm of skin
2 Eye
3 Brain and other parts of nervous system
4 Thyroid gland
5 Other endocrine glands
6 Bone (including jaw bone)
7 Connective tissue
8 Lymph nodes, secondary and unspecified
9 Other and unspecified sites
200 Lymphosarcoma and reticulosarcoma
1 Hodgkin's disease
2 Other lymphoma (reticulosis)
3 Multiple myeloma (plasmacytoma)
4 Leukaemia and aleukaemia
5 Mycosis fungoides
Also:—
223 Benign neoplasm of brain and other parts of nervous system
237 Neoplasm of unspecified nature of brain and other parts of nervous system

PART II

SYSTEMATIC EPIDEMIOLOGY OF MALIGNANT DISEASE

INCIDENCE RATE (per 100,000)

Male —— *Female* - - - -

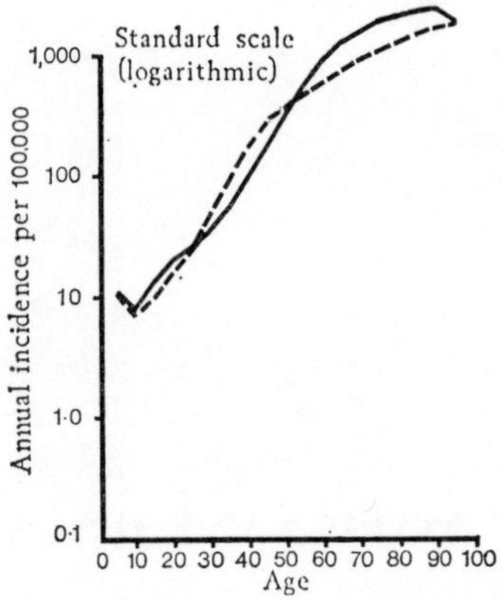

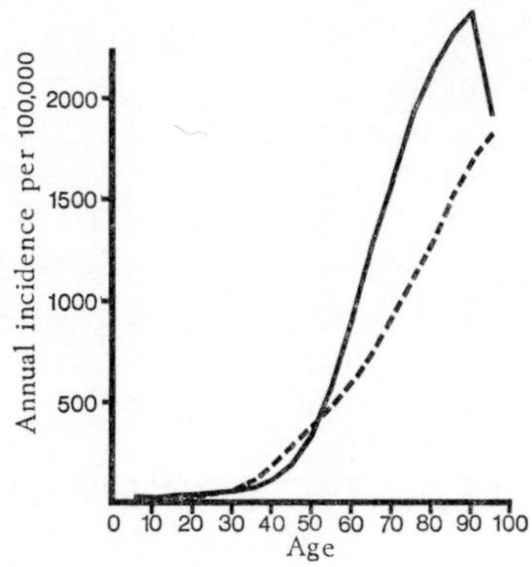

INCIDENCE RATES (per 100,000) by Age

Total cases 43107 *males*; 40613 *females* (of which age not stated for 75 *males* and 86 *females*)

Age	M	F	Age	M	F	Age	M	F
0–4	15.3	13.5	*35–39*	69·2	120·9	*70–74*	1809·0	1012·8
5–9	7·0	6·9	*40–44*	132·6	235·5	*75–79*	2098·2	1185·0
10–14	9·0	7·3	*45–49*	219·2	318·4	*80–84*	2238·5	1439·2
15–19	18·1	12·5	*50–54*	432·1	412·3	*85–89*	2509·6	1664·9
20–24	22·8	20·0	*55–59*	704·2	531·1	*90–94*	1906·5	1795·3
25–29	28·5	29·6	*60–64*	1166·7	653·2	*95+*	1897·0	1866·2
30–34	41·4	64·4	*65–69*	1434·7	831·6	*All ages*	305·6	281·3

SEX AND AGE DISTRIBUTION

	Male	*Female*
Mean age (*years*)	62·9	62·4
95% between ages	30 & 85	31 & 88
Children under 15(%)	0·9	0·8
Median age (*years*)	63·8	63·5
Proportion by sex (%)	51·5	48·5
Proportion of all cancers by sex (%)	100·0	100·0

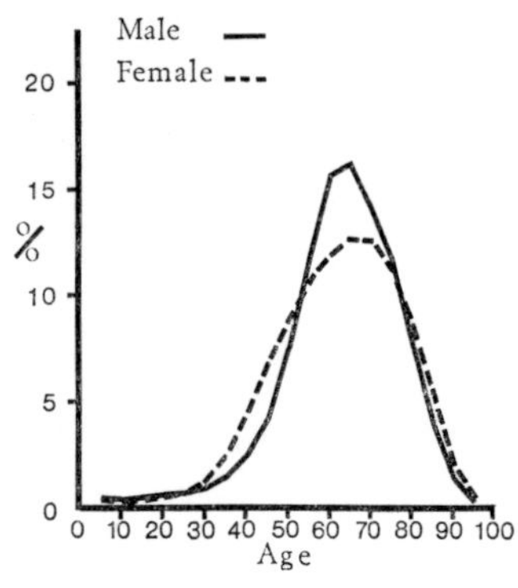

5-YEAR SURVIVAL RATES BY AGE

Crude —— *Corrected* ----

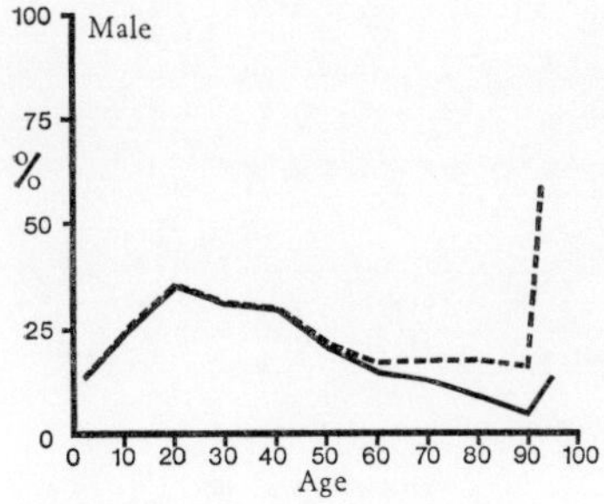

ALL CASES

Total 41236
Male 20898
Female 20338

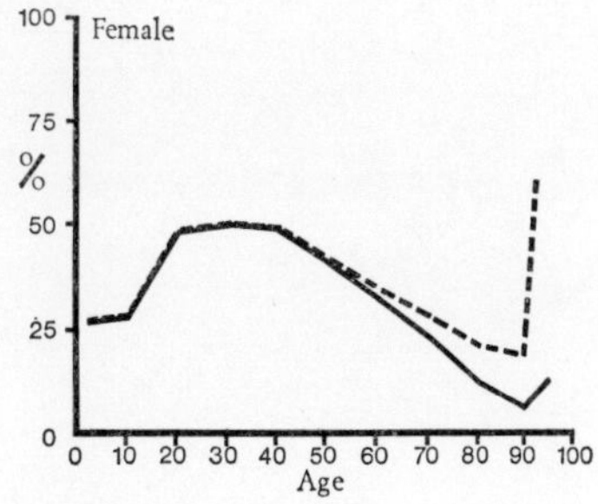

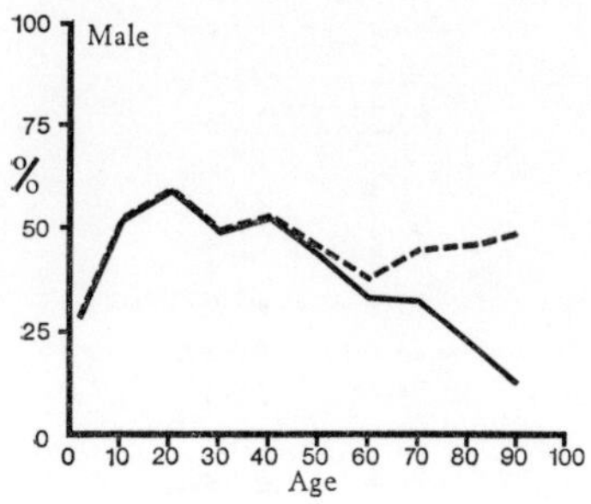

RADICAL TREATMENT

(44·7% of total)
33·8% *male*
56·0% *female*

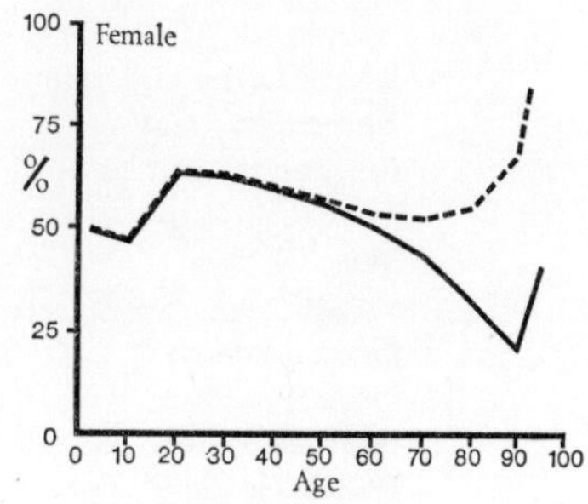

INDICES OF SURVIVAL

	All cases *Male*	All cases *Female*	Radical Treatment *Male*	Radical Treatment *Female*
FIVE YEAR SURVIVAL RATE (%)				
Crude	14·4	29·2	35·0	49·3
Corrected	*18·5*	*34·5*	*42·9*	*55·1*
Total cases†	20898	20338	7056	11394
TEN YEAR SURVIVAL RATE (%)				
Crude	11·4	23·4	26·3	36·4
Corrected	*18·7*	*31·9*	*41·0*	*46·9*
Total cases†	13057	13977	5081	8654

†Number of cases on which survival rate is based

SURVIVAL TIME (*months*)	All cases *Male*	All cases *Female*	Radical Treatment *Male*	Radical Treatment *Female*
First quartile (75% S.R.)	1·2	2·9	8·2	17·6
Median (50% S.R.)	**5·3**	**15·3**	**26·4**	**57·7**
Third quartile (25% S.R.)	22·6	>60	>60	>60

ANNUAL SURVIVAL RATES

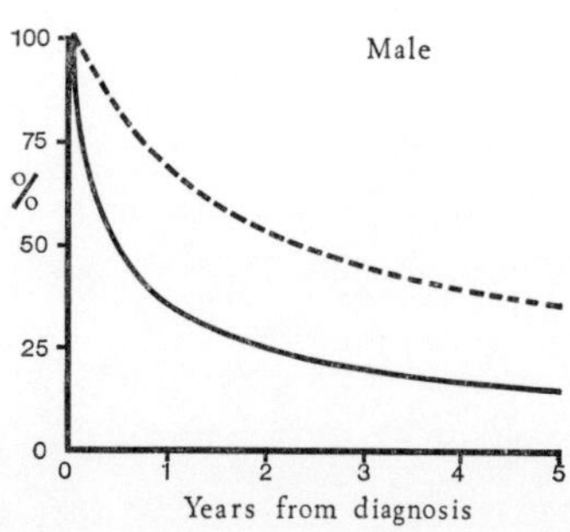

All cases ——
Radical treatment ----

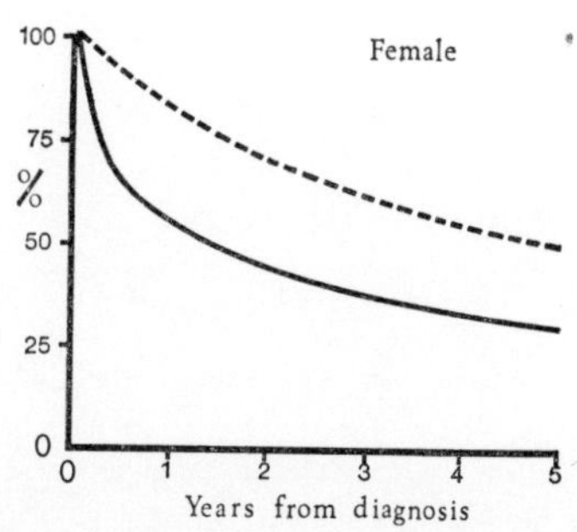

ALL CASES OF MALIGNANT DISEASE*

Survival rates and proportional distribution by system and sex

	Distribution (%) of total		5-year survival rate (%)	
	Male	*Female*	*Male*	*Female*
Buccal cavity and pharynx	3·5	1·9	30·8	45·6
Alimentary tract	28·8	26·6	10·7	12·8
Respiratory system	30·8	4·6	6·5	7·1
Bone, connective tissue, muscle, etc.	0·9	0·8	25·9	32·7
Skin	10·9	10·0	54·8†	56·2†
Breast	0·2	25·1	44·9	42·6
Genital system	8·5	17·9	22·2	39·7
Urinary system	5·9	2·5	24·4	23·3
Nervous system, etc.	2·3	2·1	17·5	30·6
Endocrine glands, etc.	0·5	0·9	31·9	47·4
Malignant lymphomas	3·0	2·4	20·2	22·7
Leukaemias, etc.	2·0	1·9	10·8	10·3
Unknown primary	2·7	3·3	2·8	2·1
All sites	100·0	100·0	14·4	29·2
Total cases	66,907	63,770	20,898	20,338

* Includes also benign and unspecified tumours of the central nervous system, but excludes carcinoma-in-situ of cervix (and of other sites), and papilloma of bladder.

† Survival rates quoted for *Skin* apply only to those cases where the histology is *melanoma* or *squamous cell carcinoma*. (see p. 46)

5-Year Crude Survival Rates (%) by system

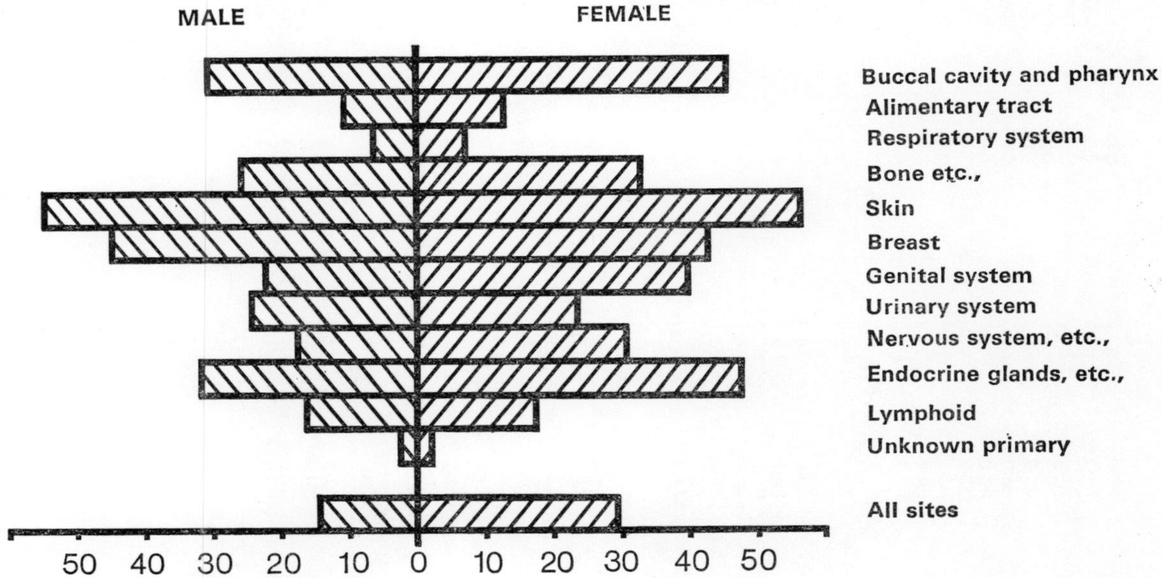

Distribution of Systems as % of all Sites by Sex

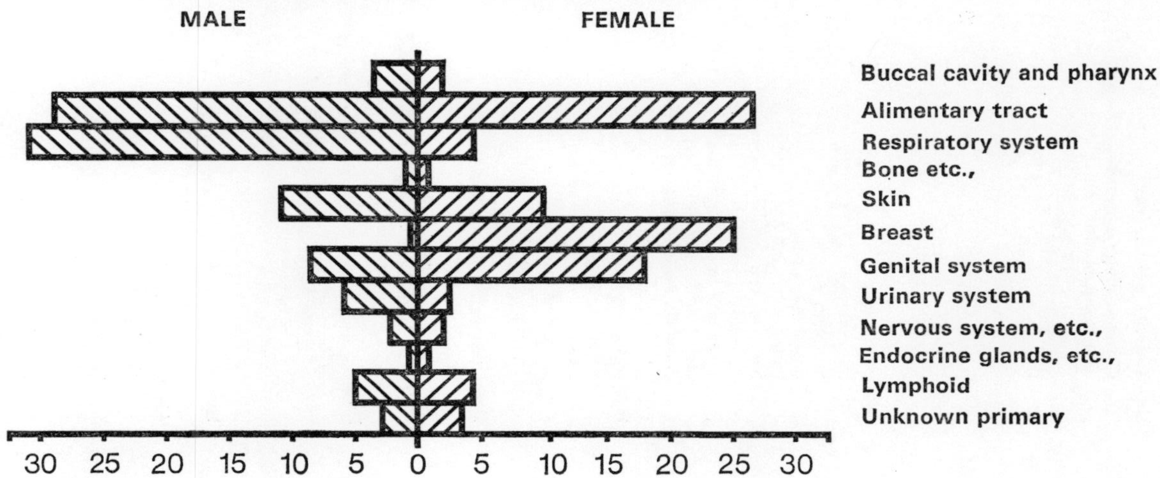

MEAN AGE AND PROPORTION OF CHILDREN (UNDER 15), BY SYSTEM, SITE DETAIL AND SEX

	Mean Age		Children (%)	
	Male	*Female*	*Male*	*Female*
ALL SITES	**62·9**	**62·4**	**0·9**	**0·8**
Buccal cavity and pharynx	**63·5**	**60·6**	**0·4**	**0·3**
Lip vermilion (squamous-cell ca.)	64·9	69·1	0·0	0·0
Tongue, posterior third	67·4	64·6	0·0	0·0
Tongue, other and unspecified	67·3	68·5	0·5	0·0
Salivary glands	50·8	52·2	0·5	0·8
Floor of mouth	65·9	64·0	0·0	0·0
Mouth, other	66·0	67·6	0·6	0·0
Fauces	68·0	62·8	0·0	0·0
Nasopharynx	55·2	60·8	2·3	0·0
Hypopharynx	66·9	60·8	0·0	0·0
Other pharynx	66·6	64·9	0·0	0·0
Alimentary tract	**65·3**	**68·6**	**0·1**	**0·1**
Oesophagus	67·9	68·2	0·0	0·0
Stomach	64·5	69·8	0·0	0·0
Small intestine	60·6	66·4	0·0	0·0
Colon	66·1	68·2	0·0	0·0
Rectum, etc.	66·3	67·4	0·0	0·0
Appendix	40·0	36·1	10·0	12·2
Liver and intrahepatic ducts	58·0	62·1	6·3	3·4
Gall bladder and bile ducts	64·8	70·0	0·0	0·0
Pancreas and ampulla of Vater	65·3	70·0	0·0	0·0
Respiratory system	**62·3**	**63·1**	**0·0**	**0·3**
Nasal sinuses	62·6	64·2	0·0	1·0
Larynx	62·6	63·0	0·0	0·0
Lung and trachea	62·3	63·1	0·0	0·0
Mediastinum and pleura	56·4	58·1	0·0	7·4
Bone, connective tissue, muscle, etc.	**48·9**	**51·7**	**2·0**	**0·9**
Bone	44·6	49·4	10·6	9·8
Connective tissue, etc.	51·6	52·6	3·9	3·9
Peritoneum and retroperitoneal tissue	—	72·5	0·0	0·0
Skin	**62·9**	**64·6**	**0·0**	**0·1**
Skin—(melanoma)	52·1	52·7	1·2	1·0
—(squamous-cell ca.)	68·3	69·9	0·0	0·4
—(basal-cell ca.)	61.9	64.9	0·0	0·1
—(other)	59·9	64·2	0·6	0·4
Breast	**63·9**	**59·6**	**0·0**	**0·0**
Genital System				
Female		**58·5**		**0·0**
Cervix		55·0		0·0
Endometrium		60·9		0·0
Other uterus		59·8		0·0
Ovary		57·9		0·1
Vulva		67·2		0·0
Other female genital organs		63·7		0·6
Male	**69·0**		**0·1**	
Prostate	72·9		0·0	
Testis	37·6		2·2	
Penis	64·8		0·0	
Scrotum	58·4		0·0	
Other male genital organs	82·5		0·0	

	Mean Age		Children (%)	
	Male	*Female*	*Male*	*Female*
Urinary system	**64·7**	**66·6**	**0·9**	**1·9**
Bladder (carcinoma)	66·6	69·6	0·1	0·0
Kidney, etc.	59·3	62·1	3·2	4·8
Nervous system, etc.	**45·6**	**46·9**	**6·9**	**7·7**
Central nervous system	46·2	46·7	8·8	11·2
Peripheral nervous system	29·3	41·2	41·0	23·4
Eye and orbit	51·0	51·7	12·0	13·8
Ear	59·7	61·7	0·0	0·0
Endocrine glands, etc.	**53·9**	**56·6**	**3·0**	**1·8**
Thyroid	59·9	59·1	0·0	0·7
Other endocrine glands	50·4	53·2	4·4	0·0
Developmental tumours	42.2	31·9	11·2	29·4
Malignant lymphomas	**50·5**	**56·3**	**4·8**	**3·0**
Reticulosarcoma	53·0	58·7	5·5	3·3
Lymphosarcoma	54·8	59·6	7·5	3·5
Hodgkin's disease	41·7	46·4	5·1	5·0
Other reticuloses	47·9	55·9	5·7	3·1
Myelomatosis	61·3	62·5	0·0	0·0
Leukaemias, etc.	**51·6**	**53·9**	**11·9**	**12·6**
Leukaemia, acute	43·0	47·0	21·1	20·3
Other leukaemias	62·0	64·0	1·2	1·2
Polycythaemia, etc.	58·4	65·1	0·0	0·0
Unknown primary	**64·5**	**66·6**	**0·4**	**0·2**

Rates printed in italics are based on less than ten cases

0·0* means (with*) that the number of cases is *not* actually zero, but only to the degree of accuracy quoted, i.e. it is less than 0·05.

0·0 means (without*) that there were in fact *no cases.*

BUCCAL CAVITY AND PHARYNX ICD (8th) **140–149**

INCIDENCE RATE (per 100,000)

Male —— *Female* ----

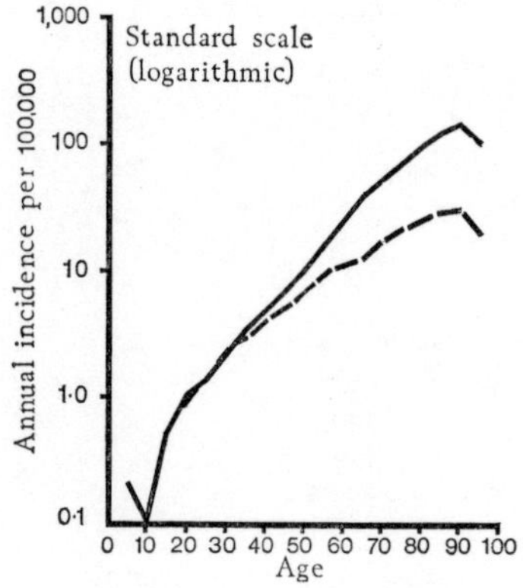

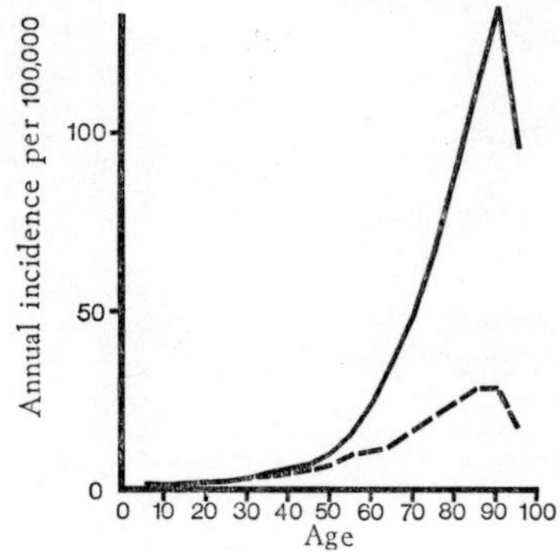

INCIDENCE RATES (per 100,000) by Age

Total cases 1416 *males*; 770 *females* (of which age not stated for 2 *males* and 2 *females*)

Age	M	F	Age	M	F	Age	M	F
0–4	0·3	0·0	*35–39*	3·7	3·0	*70–74*	57·9	19·6
5–9	0·1	0·0	*40–44*	5·9	4·9	*75–79*	82·6	21·6
10–14	0·1	0·2	*45–49*	6·9	4·8	*80–84*	104·9	27·3
15–19	1·0	0·9	*50–54*	12·0	7·7	*85–89*	141·2	31·2
20–24	1·1	0·9	*55–59*	17·7	10·7	*90–94*	107·6	16·4
25–29	1·5	1·9	*60–64*	31·7	9·8	*95+*	0·0	32·2
30–34	2·8	2·6	*65–69*	43·0	13·7	*All ages*	10·0	5·3

SEX AND AGE DISTRIBUTION

	Male	*Female*
Mean age (*years*)	63·5	60·6
95% between ages	28 & 87	25 & 87
Children under 15(%)	0·4	0·3
Median age (*years*)	65·1	62·0
Proportion by sex (%)	64·8	35·2
Proportion of all cancers by sex (%)	3·3	1·9
Trend over 10 years	— — —	(-)

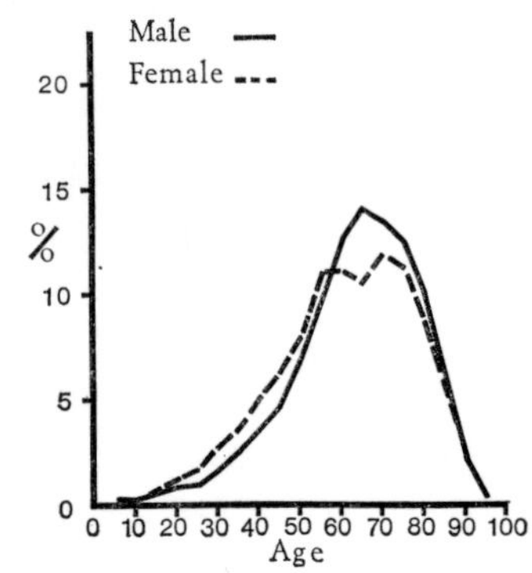

5-YEAR SURVIVAL RATES BY AGE

Crude ——— *Corrected* - - - -

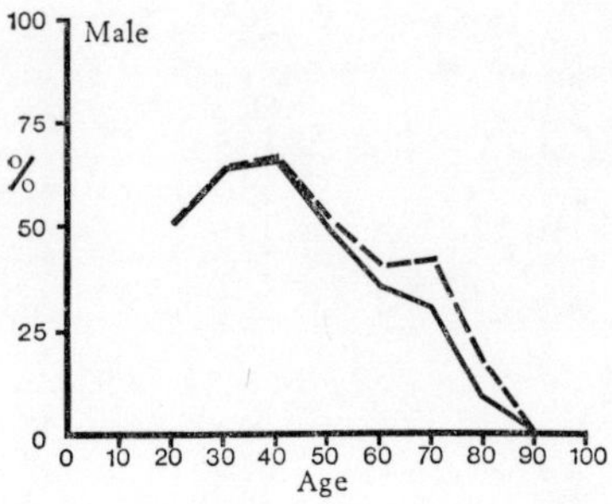

ALL CASES

Total 1406
Male 952
Female 454

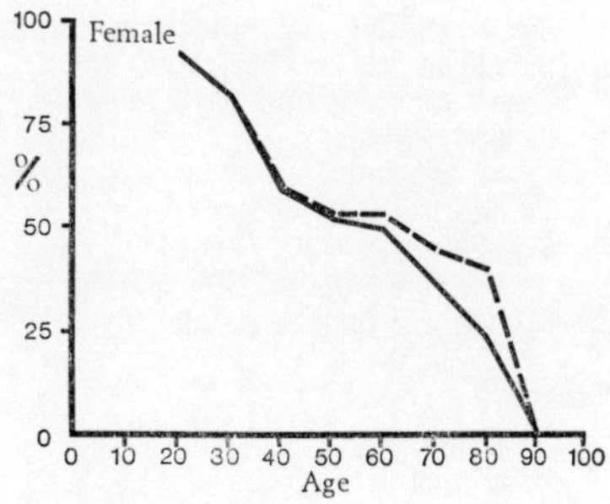

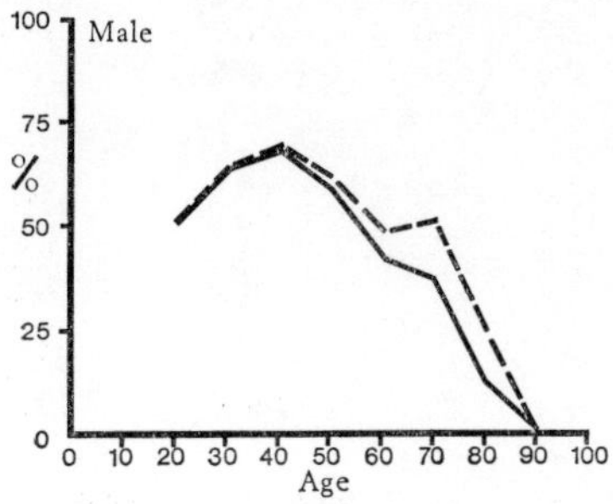

RADICAL TREATMENT

78·4%of total)
8·0% *male*
79·3% *female*

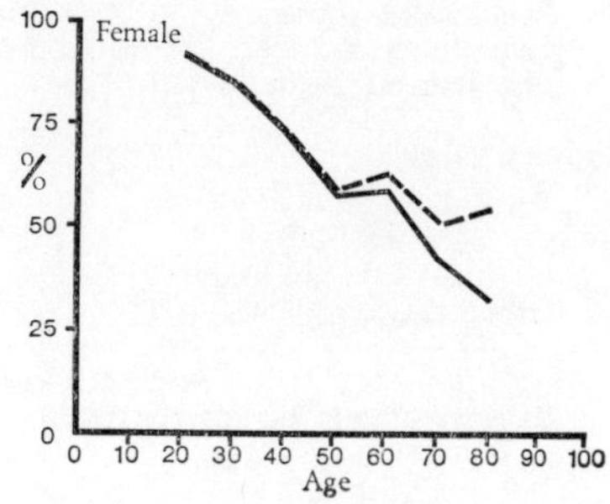

INDICES OF SURVIVAL

	All cases		Radical Treatment	
	Male	*Female*	*Male*	*Female*
FIVE YEAR SURVIVAL RATE (%)				
Crude	30·8	45·6	38·2	54·7
Corrected	*41·7*	*52·9*	*50·3*	*62·0*
Total cases†	952	454	743	360
TEN YEAR SURVIVAL RATE (%)				
Crude	19·3	28·8	28·3	42·6
Corrected	*39·1*	*41·6*	*52·7*	*58·1*
Total cases†	999	385	674	272

†Number of cases on which survival rate is based

SURVIVAL TIME (*months*)				
First quartile (75% S.R.)	6·5	6·7	13·2	7·3
Median (50% S.R.)	**18·2**	**37·5**	**>60**	**24·2**
Third quartile (25% S.R.)	>60	>60	>60	>60

ANNUAL SURVIVAL RATES

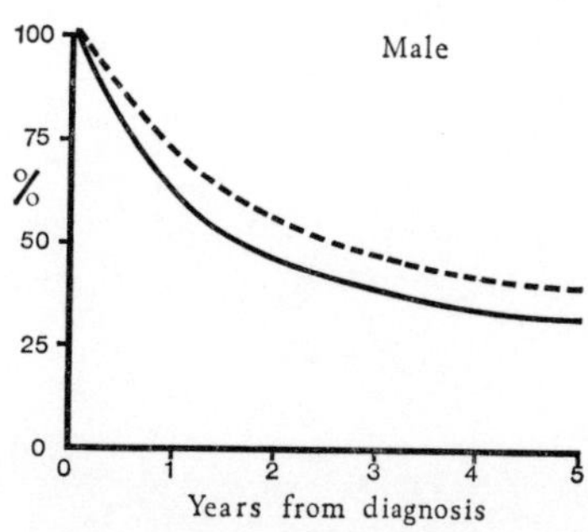

All cases ———
Radical treatment - - - -

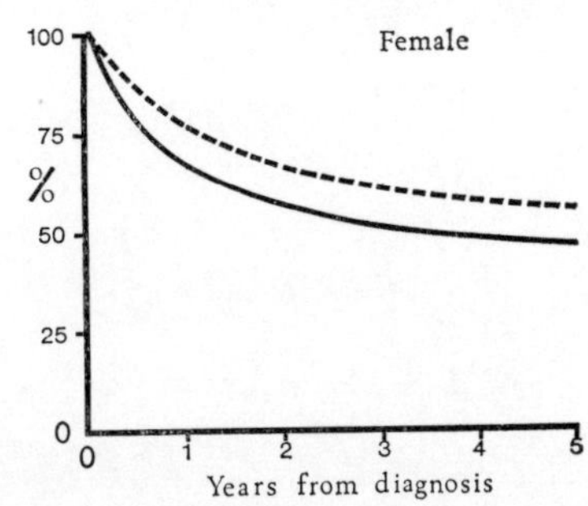

BUCCAL CAVITY AND PHARYNX

	Distribution (%) of System		5-Year Survival Rate (%)	
	Male	*Female*	*Male*	*Female*
Mouth	**67·8**	**40·5**	**30·3**	**38·4**
Lip vermilion—squamous carcinoma	18·5	3·6	66·9	53·3
Buccal aspect of cheek and lips	3·5	4·9	36·1	47·4
Upper alveolus and hard palate	3·2	4·1	21·4	50·0
Lower alveolus	3·5	3·9	21·9	47·6
Floor of mouth	7·6	3·2	17·1	18·8
Tonsil, pillar of fauces	12·4	5·0	15·7	42·9
Tongue—posterior third	5·0	1·5	10·0	42·9
—other and unspecified	13·6	13·8	21·2	25·9
Mouth, no further detail	0·5	0·5	*25·0*	*50·0*
Pharynx	**18·6**	**28·5**	**7·2**	**15·7**
Nasopharynx	6·0	6·1	9·6	34·5
Oropharynx	1·0	0·5	*14·3*	*0·0*
Pyriform fossa	6·9	4·7	6·7	5·6
Postcricoid region	2·1	14·1	3·8	11·0
Hypopharynx, other, and no further detail	1·4	2·7	6·7	18·2
Pharynx, no further detail	1·2	0·4	*0·0*	—
Salivary glands	**13·6**	**31·0**	**65·3**	**82·5**
Parotid—right	4·9	11·9	69·2	82·7
—left	5·3	11·5	79·6	86·0
—side not known	0·9	2·9	*75·0*	75·0
Other salivary glands—right	0·8	1·5	*28·6*	*100·0*
—left	0·7	1·8	*33·3*	87·5
—side not known	0·1	0·2	—	*100·0*
Salivary glands, no further detail	0·9	1·2	100·0	100·0
Whole system	**100·0**	**100·0**	**30·8**	**45·6**
Total cases	2,365	1,233	952	454

Rates printed in italics are based on less than ten cases

0·0* means (with*) that the number of cases is *not* actually zero, but only to the degree of accuracy quoted, i.e. it is less than 0·05.

0·0 means (without*) that there were in fact *no cases.*

— in the Survival Rate column means that no survival rate can be calculated because there were no cases in that category. This might not accord with the figure given in the Distribution column, which may indicate a non-zero number of cases; the reason for such apparent discrepancies is that the survival rates are based on a fewer number of years than that used as the base of the Distribution figures.

No separate diagram is included for salivary glands.

BUCCAL CAVITY

Distribution by detailed site of tumour
(5 Year Survival Rates in parenthesis)

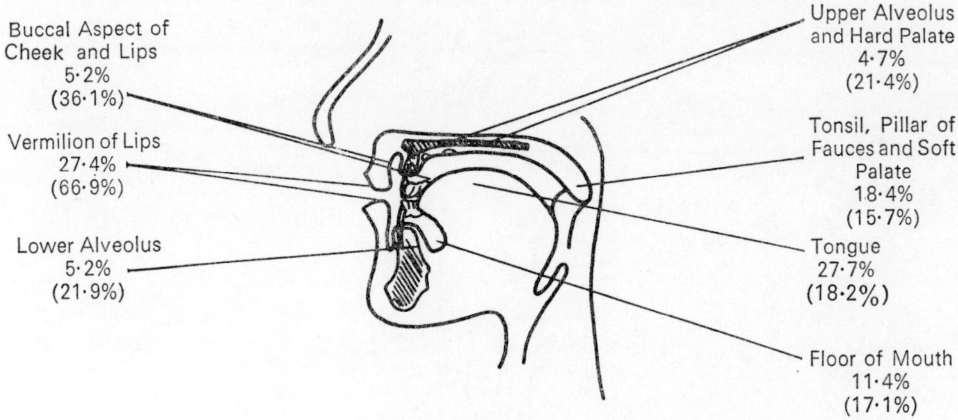

Males

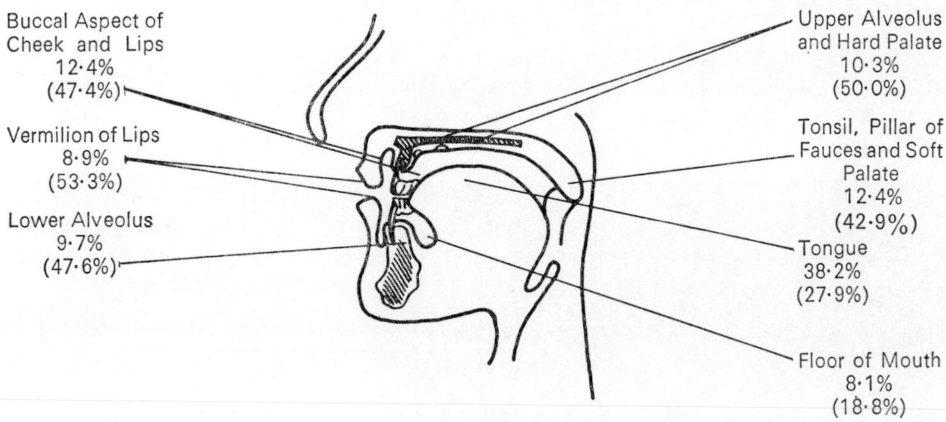

Females

BASES OF DISTRIBUTIONS

Anatomical only: 1592 cases (Males); 494 cases (Females)
5 Year Survival Rates: 662 cases (Males); 175 cases (Females)

5 Year Survival Rates for cases without further specification of site detail:

Males (4 cases): *25·0%*
Females (2 cases): *50·0%*

PHARYNX

Distribution by detailed site of tumour
(5 Year Survival Rates in parenthesis)

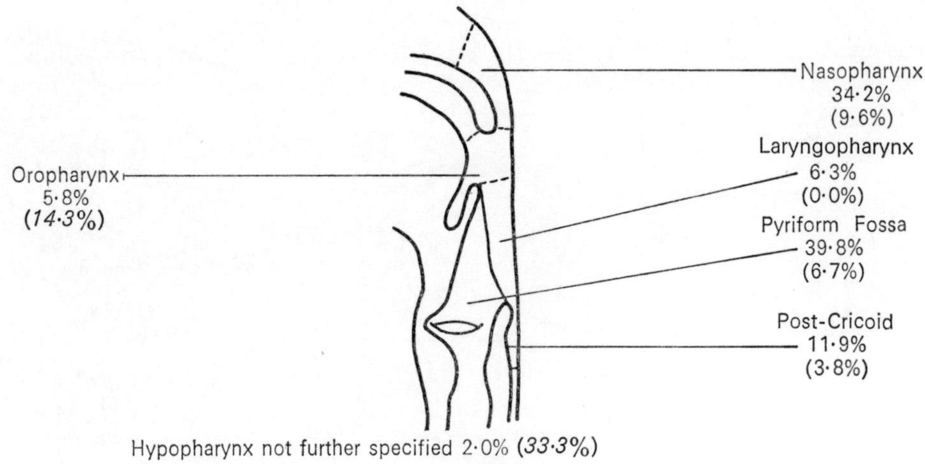

Males

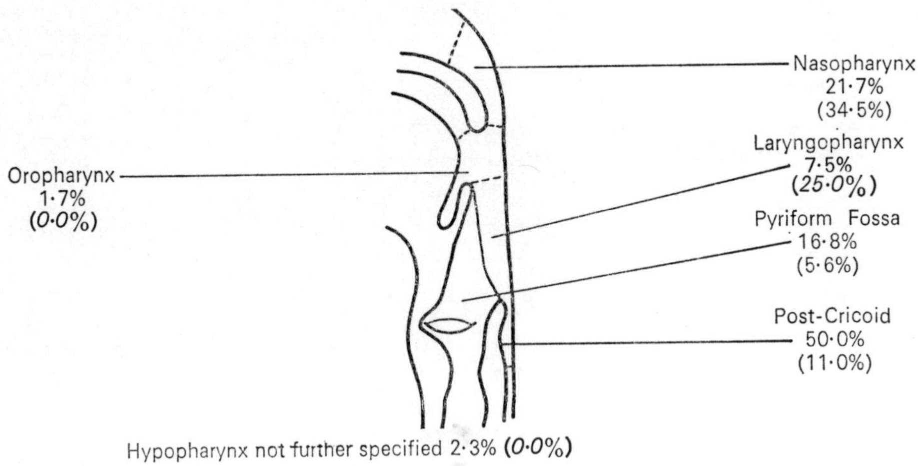

Females

BASES OF DISTRIBUTIONS

Anatomical only: 412 cases (Males); 346 cases (Females)
5 Year Survival Rates: 160 cases (Males); 134 cases (Females)

5 Year Survival Rates for cases without further specification of site detail:

Males (6 cases): *0·0%*
Females (0 cases): —

c

INCIDENCE RATE (per 100,000)

Male —— *Female* ----

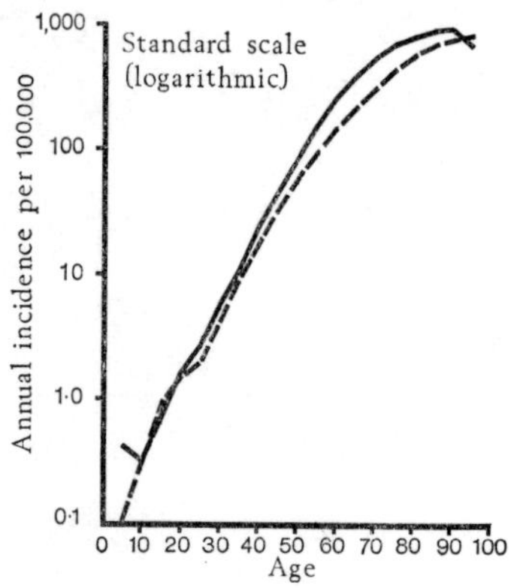

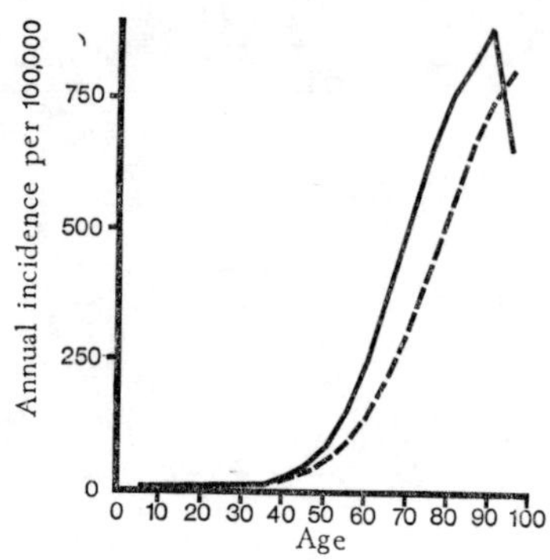

INCIDENCE RATES (per 100,000) by Age

Total cases 12414 *males*; 11072 *females* (of which age not stated for 8 *males* and 27 *females*)

Age	M	F	Age	M	F	Age	M	F
0–4	0·6	0·2	*35–39*	12·8	11·5	*70–74*	595·6	368·4
5–9	0·1	0·1	*40–44*	33·9	23·1	*75–79*	736·1	486·6
10–14	0·4	0·5	*45–49*	53·1	42·8	*80–84*	776·4	635·5
15–19	1·0	1·3	*50–54*	109·4	71·0	*85–89*	919·1	716·6
20–24	2·0	1·4	*55–59*	189·2	114·9	*90–94*	676·5	848·4
25–29	3·0	2·4	*60–64*	320·1	179·1	*95 +*	406·5	514·8
30–34	8·0	6·0	*65–69*	445·2	261·5	*All ages*	88·0	76·7

SEX AND AGE DISTRIBUTION

	Male	*Female*
Mean age (*years*)	65·3	68·6
95% between ages	40 & 86	41 & 89
Children under 15 (%)	0·1	0·1
Median age (*years*)	65·9	69·9
Proportion by sex (%)	52·9	47·1
Proportion of all cancers by sex (%)	28·8	27·3
Trend over 10 years	(–)	(+)

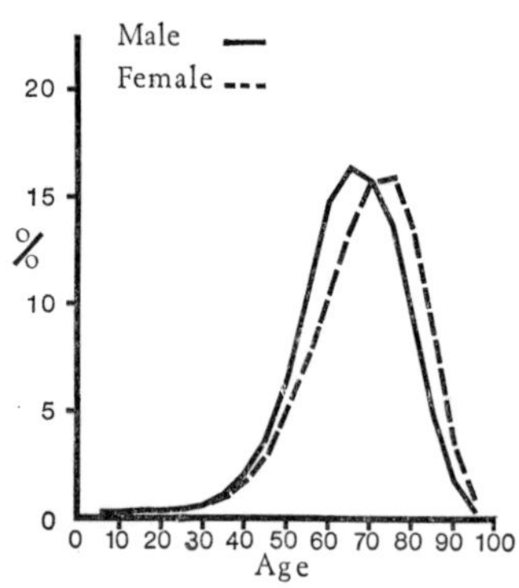

NOTES

Includes: Appendix (part of 153·0 in both 8th and 7th revisions), which is omitted from the separate site page-pairs.

Excludes: Peritoneum (158 in both 8th and 7th revisions), which is classified with BONE AND CONNECTIVE TISSUE; unspecified digestive organs (159 in both revisions) which are classified with UNKNOWN PRIMARY.

5-YEAR SURVIVAL RATES BY AGE

Crude —— *Corrected* ----

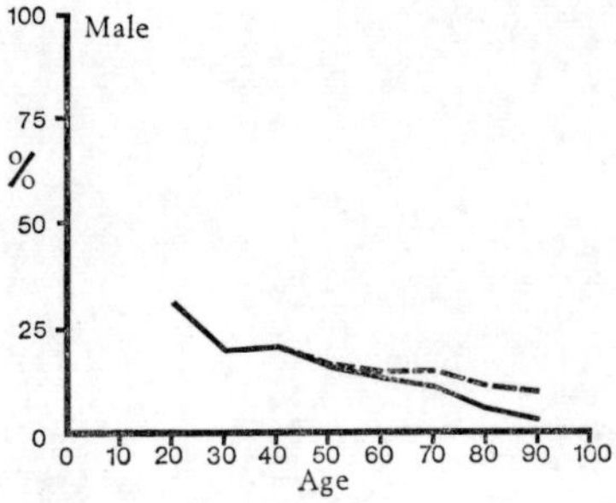

ALL CASES

Total 12351
Male 6618
Female 5733

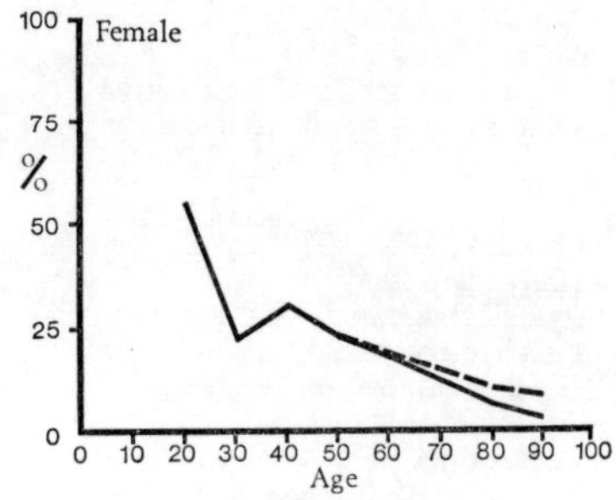

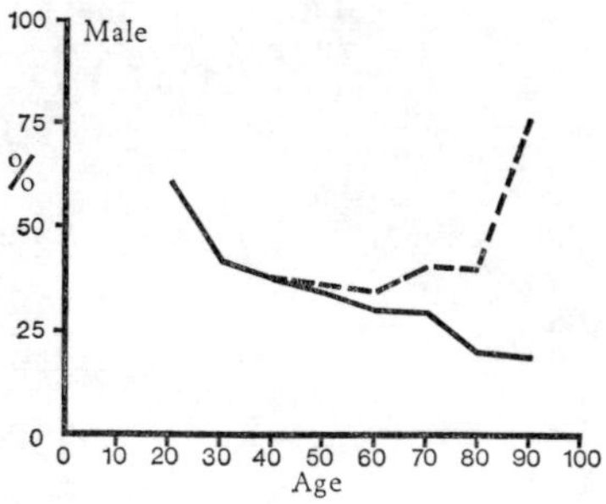

RADICAL TREATMENT

(34·0% of total)
34·1% *male*
33·9% *female*

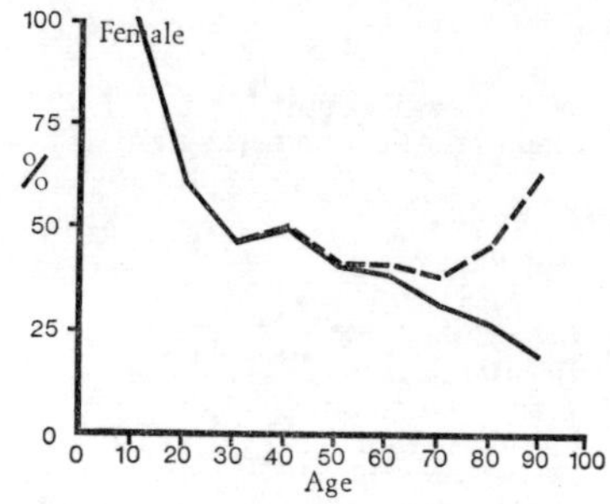

INDICES OF SURVIVAL

	All cases *Male*	All cases *Female*	Radical Treatment *Male*	Radical Treatment *Female*
FIVE YEAR SURVIVAL RATE (%)				
Crude	10·7	12·8	29·4	35·5
Corrected	*14·2*	*16·3*	*36·8*	*41·3*
Total cases†	6618	5733	2258	1944
TEN YEAR SURVIVAL RATE (%)				
Crude	8·0	9·9	19·8	24·6
Corrected	*14·3*	*15·2*	*31·9*	*34·1*
Total cases†	3838	3260	1467	1263
SURVIVAL TIME (*months*)				
First quartile (75% S.R.)	0·8	0·9	7·3	10·6
Median (50% S.R.)	**3·6**	**4·3**	**24·2**	**29·9**
Third quartile (25% S.R.)	16·0	18·4	>60	>60

†Number of cases on which survival rate is based

ANNUAL SURVIVAL RATES

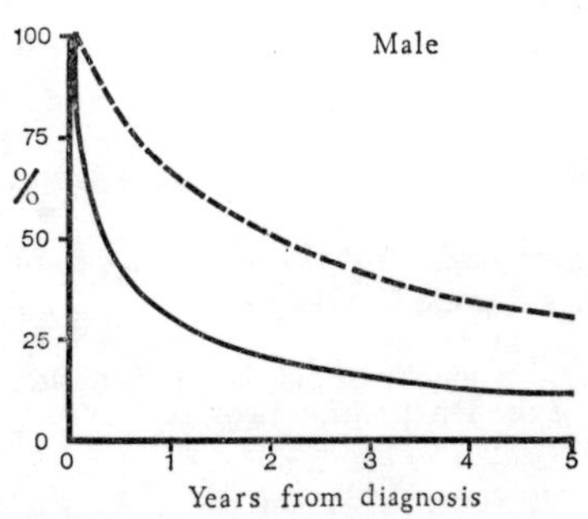

All cases ——
Radical treatment ----

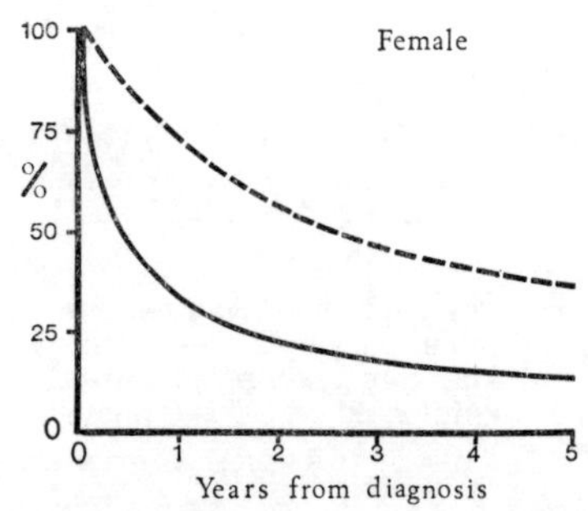

ALIMENTARY TRACT

	Distribution (%) of System		5-Year Survival Rate (%)	
	Male	*Female*	*Male*	*Female*
Oesophagus	**6·4**	**5·2**	**2·0**	**4·6**
Upper third	0·5	0·5	3·6	2·8
Middle third	1·7	1·5	0·0	6·3
Lower third	2·4	1·8	4·2	5·6
Gastro-oesophageal junction	0·2	0·1	8·3	*0·0*
Oesophagus, no further detail	1·6	1·3	0·0	1·8
Stomach	**37·0**	**29·8**	**3·9**	**3·3**
Cardia	2·1	0·9	3·6	2·0
Body	3·0	1·7	3·1	2·5
Pyloric antrum	7·5	5·7	7·7	6·3
Lesser curvature	3·4	2·1	6·7	11·4
Greater curvature	0·8	0·6	10·7	7·1
Anterior wall	0·1	0·1	26·7	*0·0*
Posterior wall	0·6	0·3	13·3	10·0
Stomach, no further detail	19·5	18·4	1·2	1·2
Small Intestine	**0·8**	**0·7**	**31·8**	**16·0**
Duodenum	0·2	0·2	*0·0*	20·0
Jejunum and ileum	0·5	0·4	45·2	18·5
Small intestine, no further detail	0·1	0·1	*0·0*	*0·0*
Large Intestine	**43·5**	**51·3**	**19·9**	**21·9**
Appendix	0·2	0·5	92·3	70·4
Caecum	3·1	5·1	17·1	24·2
Ascending colon	1·6	2·5	25·9	20·5
Hepatic flexure	0·8	1·0	34·0	12·7
Transverse colon	1·8	3·2	23·4	19·9
Splenic flexure	1·2	1·6	19·2	16·3
Descending colon	1·8	2·9	28·9	21·3
Pelvic colon	7·4	10·2	18·8	27·0
Rectosigmoid junction	2·1	2·5	14·7	24·8
Rectum	20·1	16·4	20·9	22·9
Anal canal	0·3	0·5	17·6	14·3
Colon, no further detail	3·1	4·9	4·3	7·2
Biliary System	**2·7**	**4·2**	**0·1**	**0·4**
Liver	1·0	0·5	0·0	0·0
Gallbladder	0·7	2·6	0·0	0·0
Bile ducts	1·0	1·1	1·6	1·5
Pancreas	**9·6**	**8·8**	**0·7**	**0·4**
Head of pancreas	4·8	4·4	0·0	0·0
Body of pancreas	0·7	0·6	0·0	0·0
Tail of pancreas	0·3	0·2	0·0	0·0
Ampulla of Vater	0·4	0·4	13·3	9·5
Pancreas, no further detail	3·4	3·2	0·0	0·0
Whole system	**100·0**	**100·0**	**10·7**	**12·8**
Total Cases	19,248	16,973	6,618	5,733

Rates printed in italics are based on less than ten cases

0·0* means (with*) that the number of cases is *not* actually zero, but only to the degree of accuracy quoted, i.e. it is less than 0·05.

0·0 means (without*) that there were in fact *no cases.*

— in the Survival Rate column means that no survival rate can be calculated because there were no cases in that category. This might not accord with the figure given in the Distribution column, which may indicate a non-zero number of cases; the reason for such apparent discrepancies is that the survival rates are based on a fewer number of years than that used as the base of the Distribution figures.

OESOPHAGUS

Distribution by detailed site of tumour
(5 Year Survival Rates in parenthesis)

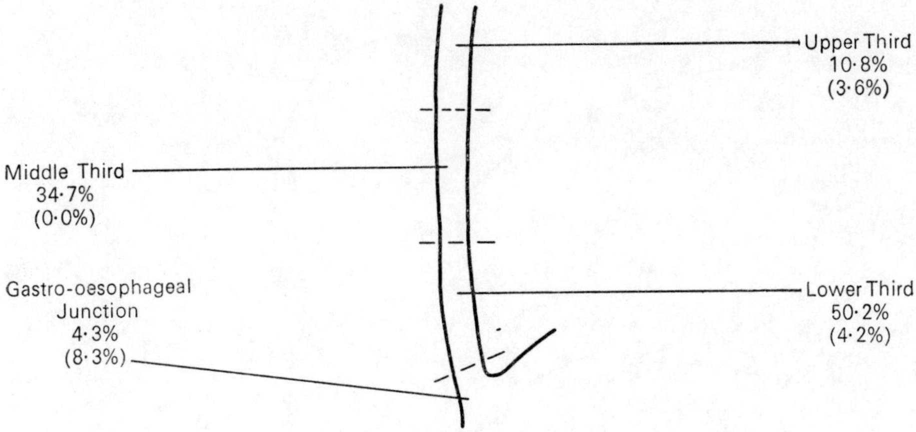

Males

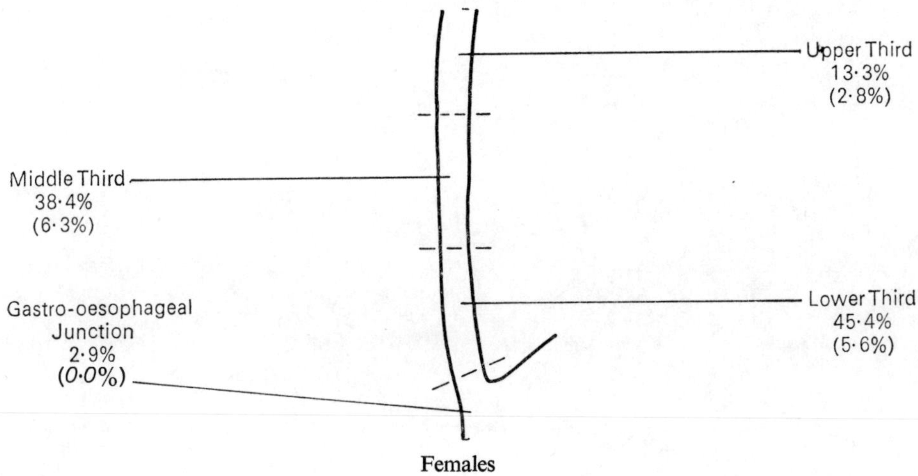

Females

BASES OF DISTRIBUTIONS

Anatomical only: 915 cases (Males); 667 cases (Females)
5 Year Survival Rates: 301 cases (Males); 227 cases (Females)

5 Year Survival Rates for cases without further specification of site detail:

Males (100 cases): 0·0%
Females (55 cases): 1·8%

Distributions by anatomical subdivisions are based only on those cases for which sufficient detail was available. Such cases form a selected subgroup which is not necessarily representative of the site as a whole (see discussion p. 8).

STOMACH

Distribution by detailed site of tumour
(5 Year Survival Rates in parenthesis)

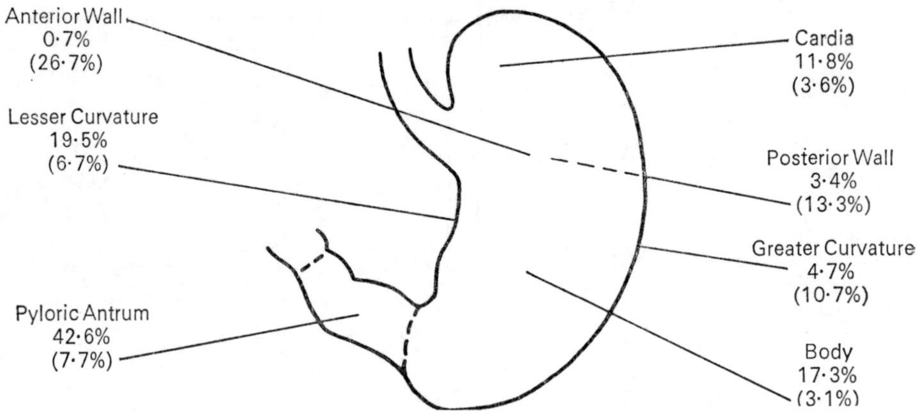

Males

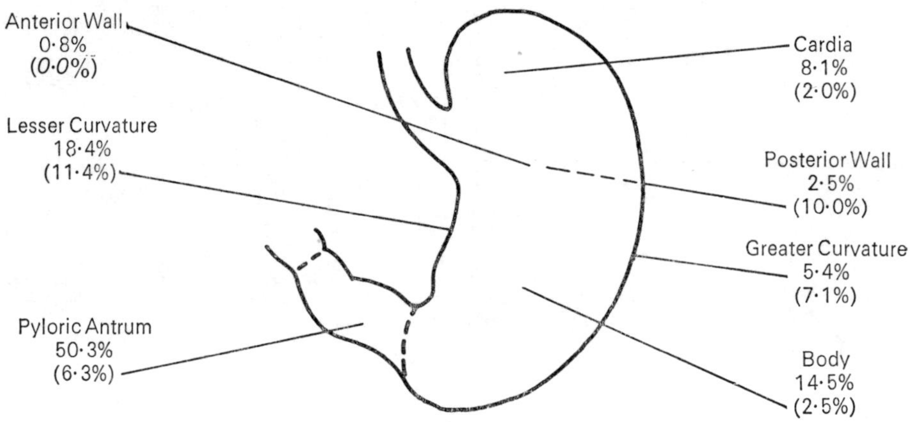

Females

BASES OF DISTRIBUTIONS

Anatomical only: 3371 cases (Males); 1939 cases (Females)
5 Year Survival Rates: 1204 cases (Males); 658 cases (Females)

5 Year Survival Rates for cases without further specification of site detail:

Males (1296 cases): 1·2%
Females (1022 cases): 1·2%

LARGE INTESTINE

Distribution by detailed site of tumour
(5 Year Survival Rates in parenthesis)

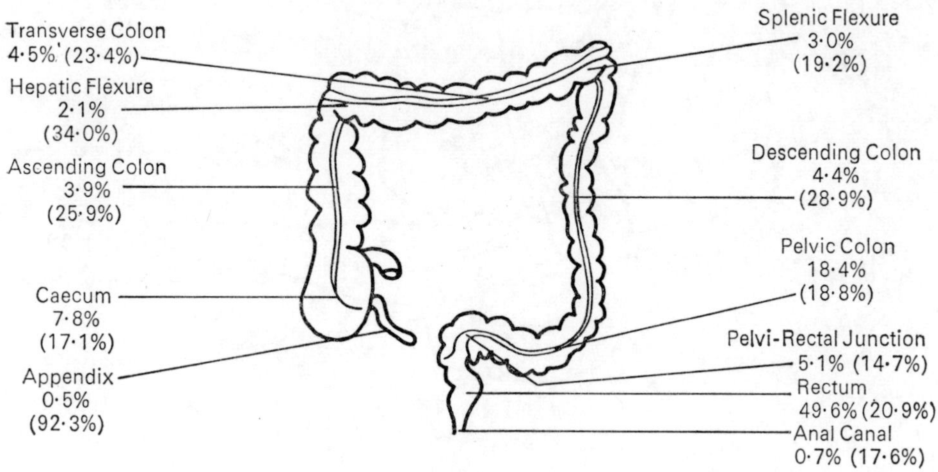

Males

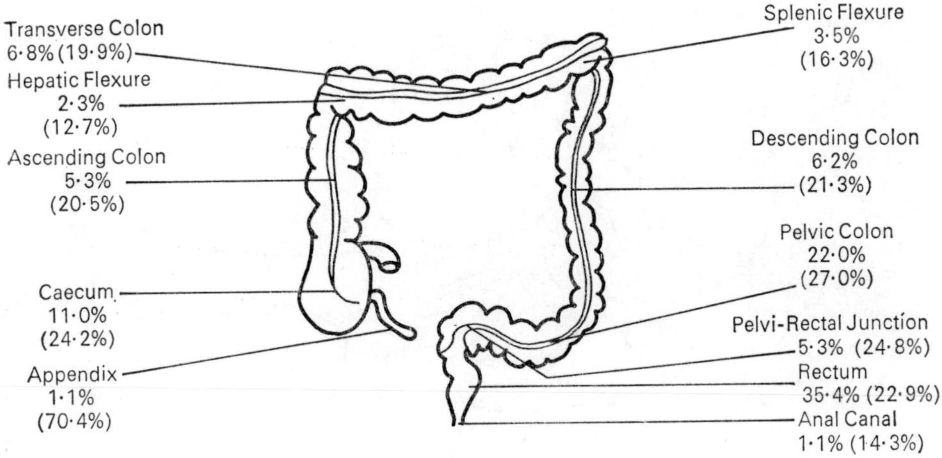

Females

BASES OF DISTRIBUTIONS

Anatomical only: 7791 cases (Males); 7859 cases (Females)
5 Year Survival Rates: 2750 cases (Males); 2713 cases (Females)

5 Year Survival Rates for cases without further specification of site detail:

Males (207 cases): 4·3%
Females (304 cases): 7·2%

BILIARY SYSTEM AND PANCREAS

Distribution by detailed site of tumour
(5 year Survival Rates in parentheses)

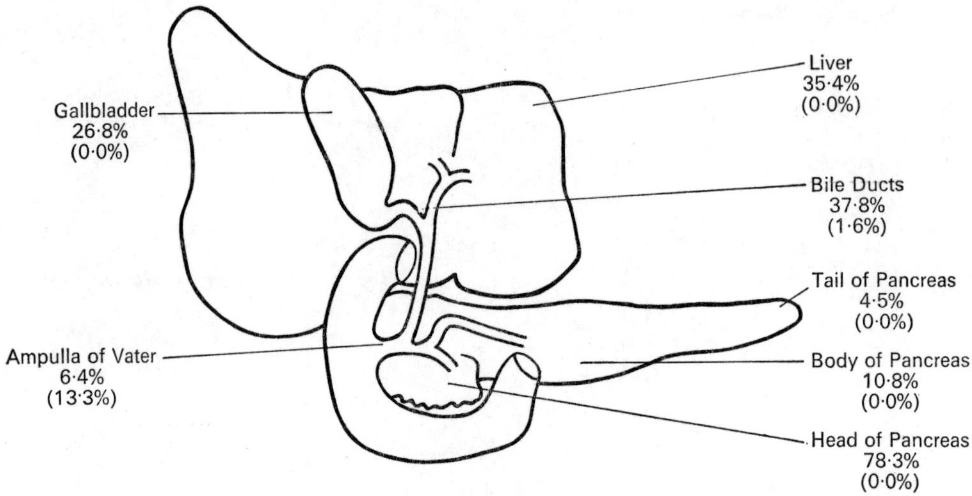

Males

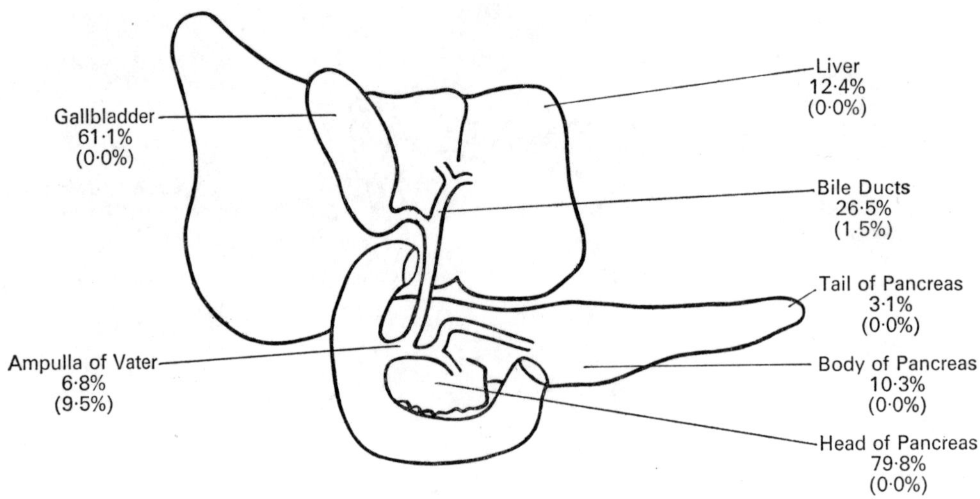

Females

BASES OF DISTRIBUTIONS

Biliary System Anatomical only: 519 cases (Males); 710 cases (Females)
5 Year Survival Rates: 161 cases (Males); 241 cases (Females)

No cases without specification of detail.

Pancreas Anatomical only: 1190 cases (Males); 935 cases (Females)
5 Year Survival Rates: 379 cases (Males); 283 cases (Females)

5 Year Survival Rates for cases without further specification of site detail:

Males (176 cases): 0·0%
Females (180 cases): 0·0%

INCIDENCE RATE (per 100,000)

Male ——— *Female* - - - -

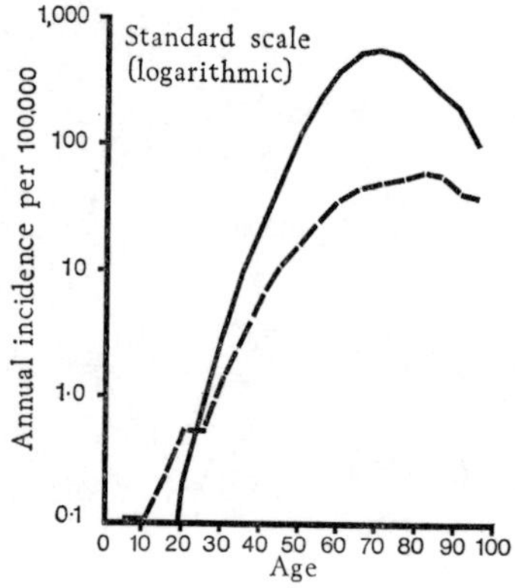

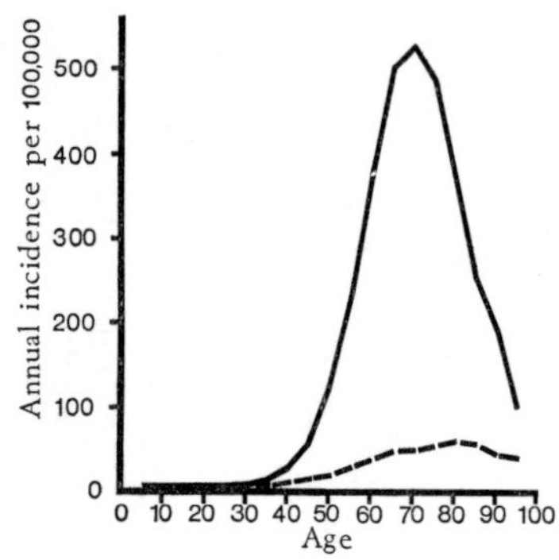

INCIDENCE RATES (per 100,000) by Age

Total cases 13610 *males*; 1929 *females* (of which age not stated for 11 *males* and 3 *females*)

Age	M	F	Age	M	F	Age	M	F
0–4	0·0	0·1	*35–39*	13·9	3·4	*70–74*	523·6	46·5
5–9	0·0	0·1	*40–44*	32·6	8·9	*75–79*	416·8	55·3
10–14	0·1	0·1	*45–49*	71·4	12·8	*80–84*	264·1	58·1
15–19	0·0	0·4	*50–54*	169·9	19·6	*85–89*	205·1	43·6
20–24	0·5	0·5	*55–59*	293·0	31·5	*90–94*	92·3	27·4
25–29	1·2	0·5	*60–64*	478·8	39·1	*95+*	135·5	96·5
30–34	4·7	2·1	*65–69*	524·5	49·3	*All ages*	96·5	13·4

SEX AND AGE DISTRIBUTION

	Male	*Female*
Mean age (*years*)	62·3	63·1
95% between ages	42 & 80	37 & 85
Children under 15 (%)	0·0	0·3
Median age (*years*)	62·4	63·7
Proportion by sex (%)	87·6	12·4
Proportion of all cancers by sex (%)	31·6	4·7
Trend over 10 years	+	+ +

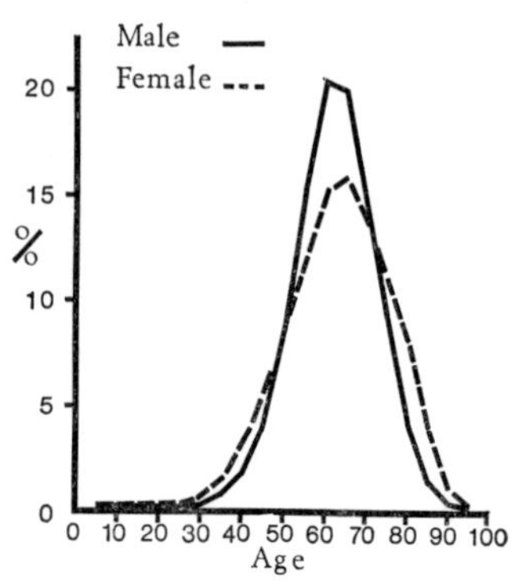

NOTES

Includes: Pleura (163.0 in 8th revision; 162.2 in 7th) and Mediastinum (163.1 in 8th revision; 164 in 7th), which are omitted from the separate site page-pairs.

Excludes: Eustachian tube and middle ear (160.1 in both 8th and 7th revisions) which are classified with NERVOUS SYSTEM, ETC.

5-YEAR SURVIVAL RATES BY AGE

Crude —— *Corrected* ----

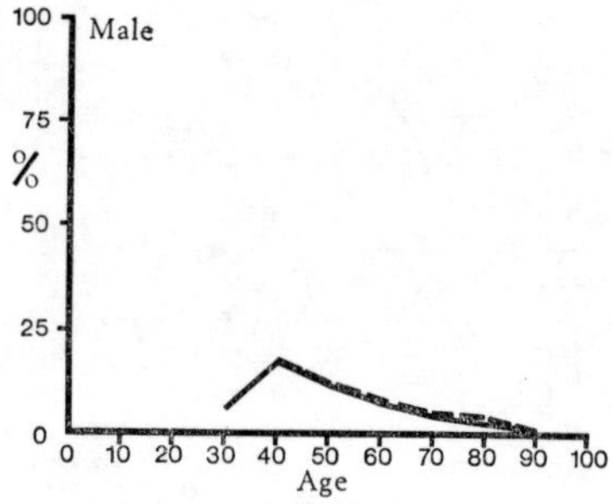

ALL CASES

Total 7550
Male 6691
Female 859

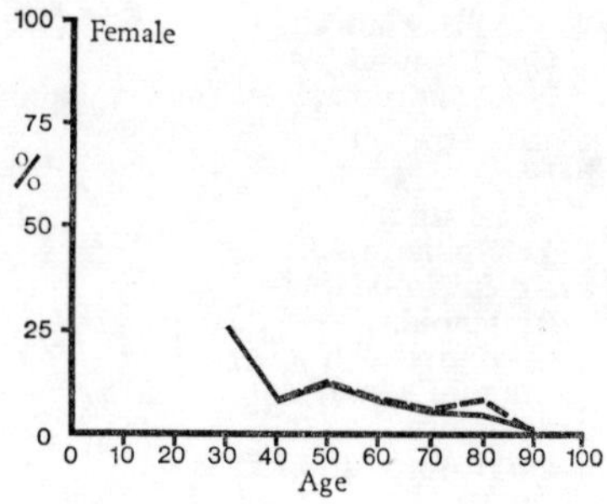

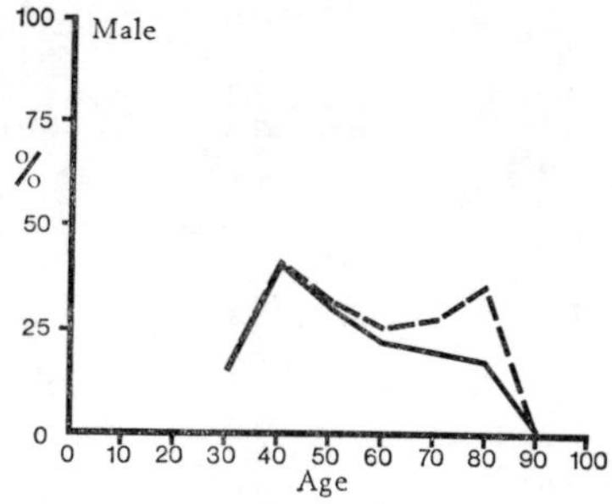

RADICAL TREATMENT

(25·0% of total)
25·2% *male*
23·2% *female*

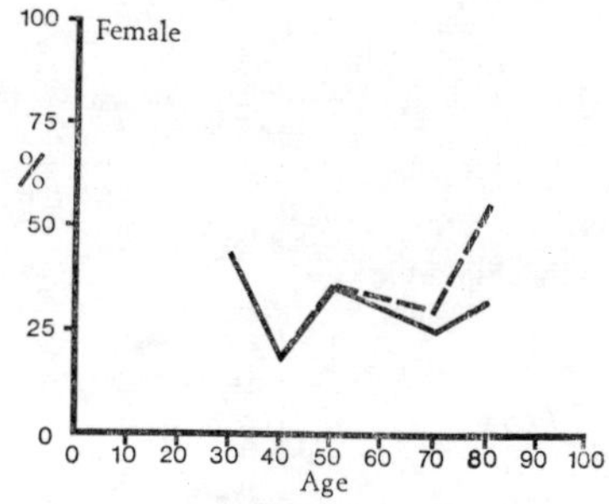

INDICES OF SURVIVAL

	All cases		Radical Treatment	
	Male	*Female*	*Male*	*Female*
FIVE YEAR SURVIVAL RATE (%)				
Crude	6·5	7·1	24·5	29·1
Corrected	*7·9*	*8·2*	*28·3*	*31·9*
Total cases†	6691	859	1688	199
TEN YEAR SURVIVAL RATE (%)				
Crude	5·3	5·8	18·5	21·6
Corrected	*7·6*	*7·8*	*25·4*	*27·8*
Total cases†	3782	497	1032	125

†Number of cases on which survival rate is based

SURVIVAL TIME (*months*)				
First quartile (75% S.R.)	1·1	1·0	4·9	5·5
Median (50% S.R.)	**3·6**	**3·1**	**13·1**	**16·5**
Third quartile (25% S.R.)	9·7	8·5	56.2	>60

ANNUAL SURVIVAL RATES

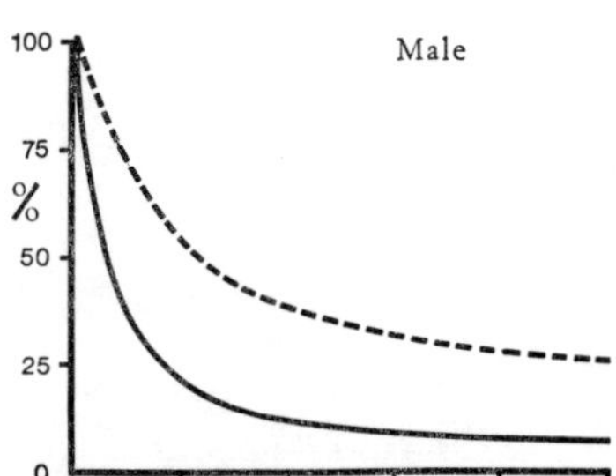

All cases ——
Radical treatment ----

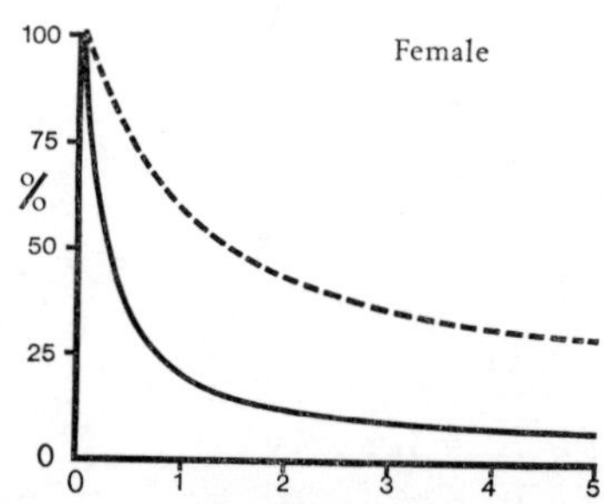

RESPIRATORY SYSTEM

	Distribution (%) of System		5-Year Survival Rate (%)	
	Male	*Female*	*Male*	*Female*
Nasal cavities and sinuses	**1·0**	**6·0**	**23·1**	**31·7**
Nasal cavity	0·2	1·5	25·0	50·0
Maxillary antrum	0·6	3·6	19·0	17·2
Other sinuses	0·2	0·9	36·4	30·8
Nose and sinuses, no further detail	0·0*	0·0*	—	*100·0*
Larynx	**5·0**	**4·6**	**33·2**	**39·5**
Vocal cords	2·7	1·7	50·5	64·3
Ventricular fold	0·0*	0·0*	*0·0*	—
Aryepiglottic fold	0·3	0·4	4·2	*33·3*
Arytenoid	0·1	0·2	18·2	0·0
Epiglottis	0·5	0·8	20·5	*33·3*
Anterior commissure	0·1	0·0*	*44·4*	—
Subglottic	0·1	0·2	25·0	50·0
Larynx, no further detail	1·2	1·3	10·8	16·7
Lung, etc.	**94·0**	**89·4**	**4·8**	**3·4**
Trachea	0·2	0·2	0·0	*0·0*
Main bronchus—right	4·0	4·0	2·6	5·3
—left	4·7	4·8	3·9	2·5
—unspecified	0·2	0·3	0·0	*0·0*
Upper lobe —right	15·9	11·9	6·3	3·0
—left	15·4	11·0	8·1	4·4
—unspecified	0·3	0·2	0·0	*0·0*
Middle lobe	2·2	2·1	6·1	0·0
Lower lobe —right	10·2	8·7	6·5	9·1
—left	9·0	8·1	7·0	6·8
—unspecified	0·2	0·2	*12·5*	*100·0*
Apex —right	0·4	0·2	0·0	*0·0*
—left	0·3	0·1	4·3	—
—unspecified	0·0*	0·0	*0·0*	—
Lung parenchyma	0·1	0·2	*0·0*	*0·0*
Pleura	0·2	0·5	*16·7*	—
Mediastinum	0·1	0·8	0·0	*0·0*
Lung, no further detail	30·6	36·1	1·1	1·0
Whole system	**100·0**	**100·0**	**6·5**	**7·1**
Total Cases	20,633	2,911	6,691	859

Rates printed in italics are based on less than ten cases

0·0* means (with*) that the number of cases is *not* actually zero, but only to the degree of accuracy quoted, i.e. it is less than 0·05.

0·0 means (without*) that there were in fact *no cases.*

— in the Survival Rate column means that no survival rate can be calculated because there were no cases in that category. This might not accord with the figure given in the Distribution column, which may indicate a non-zero number of cases; the reason for such apparent discrepancies is that the survival rates are based on a fewer number of years than that used as the base of the Distribution figures.

TRACHEA AND LUNGS

Distribution by detailed site of tumour
(5 Year Survival Rates in parenthesis)

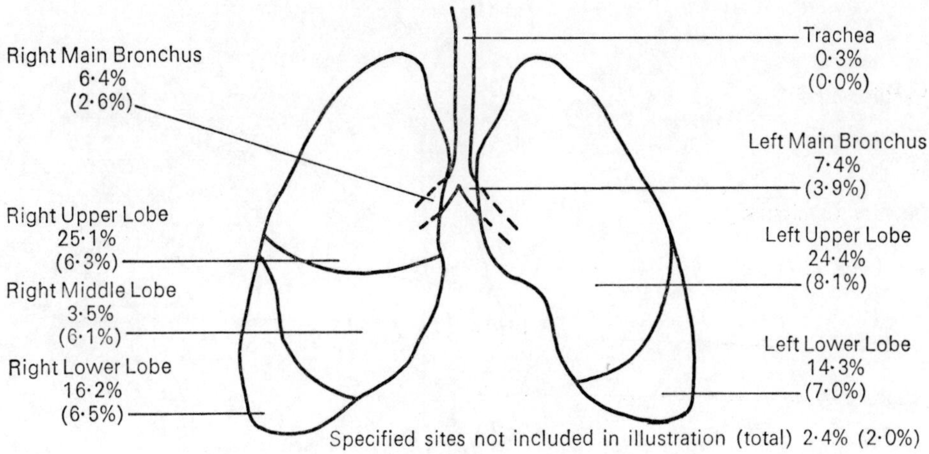

Males

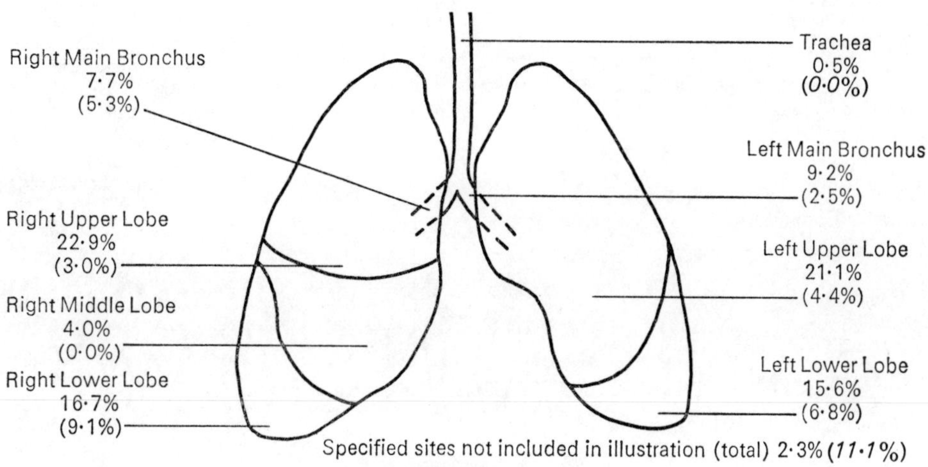

Females

BASES OF DISTRIBUTIONS

Anatomical only: 13026 cases (Males); 1513 cases (Females)
5 Year Survival Rates: 4399 cases (Males); 436 cases (Females)

5 Year Survival Rates for cases without further specification of site detail:

Males (1837 cases): 1·1%
Females (315 cases): 1·0%

LARYNX

Distribution by detailed site of tumour
(5 Year Survival Rates in parenthesis)

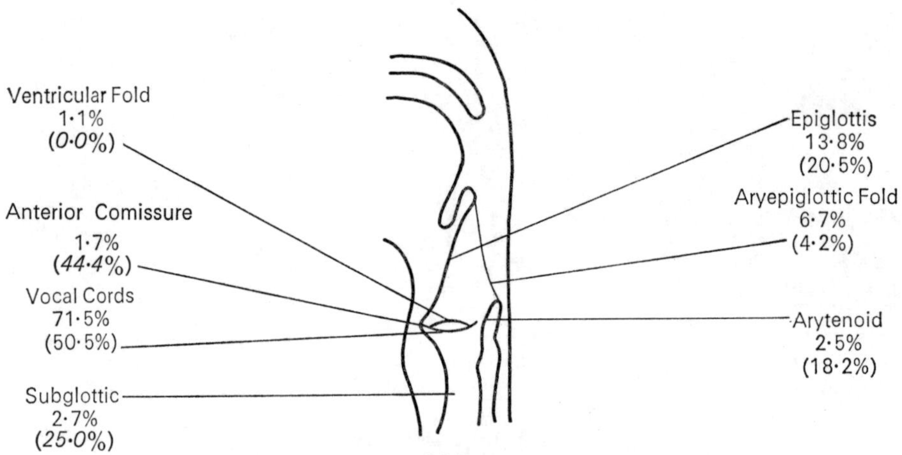

Males

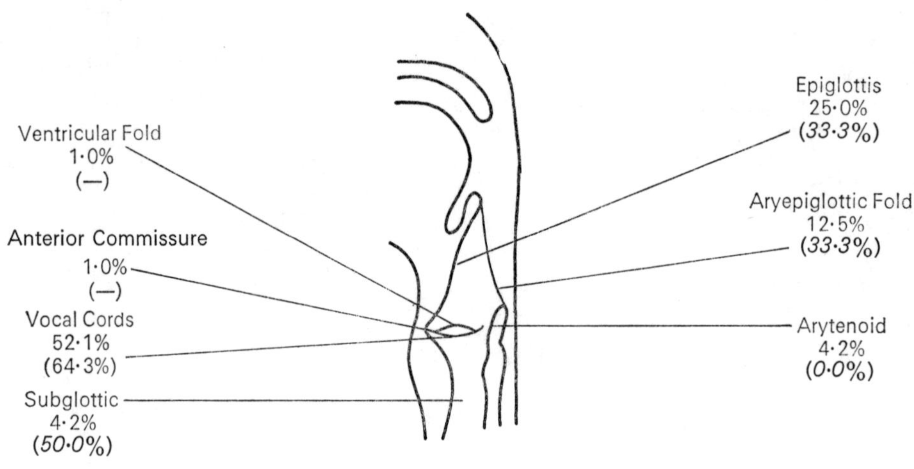

Females

Bases of Distributions

Anatomical only: 789 cases (Males); 96 cases (Females)
5 Year Survival Rates: 285 cases (Males); 26 cases (Females)

5 Year Survival Rates for cases without further specification of site detail:

Males (83 cases): 10·8%
Females (12 cases): 16·7%

BONE AND CONNECTIVE TISSUE ICD (8th) **158, 170, 171**

INCIDENCE RATE (per 100,000)

Male —— *Female* ----

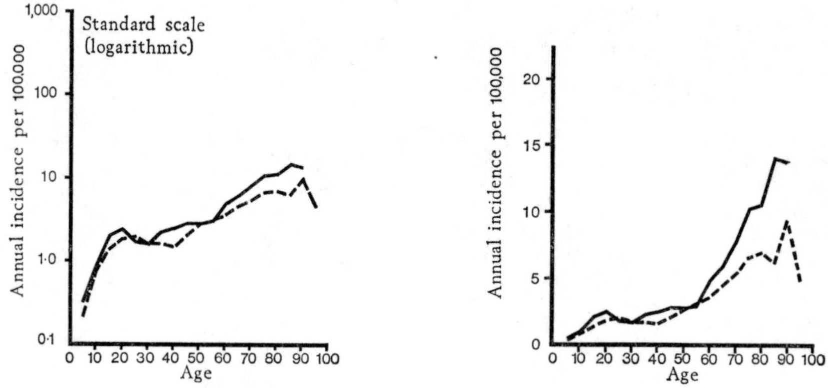

INCIDENCE RATES (per 100,000) by Age

Total cases 365 *males*; 314 *females* (of which age not stated for 0 *males* and 0 *females*)

Age	M	F	Age	M	F	Age	M	F
0–4	0·4	0·3	*35–39*	2·4	1·4	*70–74*	10·7	5·1
5–9	0·2	0·2	*40–44*	2·1	1·3	*75–79*	9·0	8·1
10–14	1·4	1·1	*45–49*	3·1	2·4	*80–84*	13·1	4·5
15–19	2·5	1·4	*50–54*	2·0	2·5	*85–89*	16·0	10·0
20–24	2·0	2·0	*55–59*	3·7	3·2	*90–94*	0·0	5·5
25–29	1·3	1·6	*60–64*	6·2	3·7	*95 +*	0·0	0·0
30–34	1·8	1·5	*65–69*	5·4	5·2	*All ages*	2·6	2·2

SEX AND AGE DISTRIBUTION

	Male	*Female*
Mean age (*years*)	48·9	51·7
95% between ages	11 & 84	11 & 86
Children under 15 (%)	2·0	0·9
Median age (*years*)	50·7	55·4
Proportion by sex (%)	53·8	46·2
Proportion of all cancers by sex (%)	0·85	0·77
Trend over 10 years	(-)	(-)

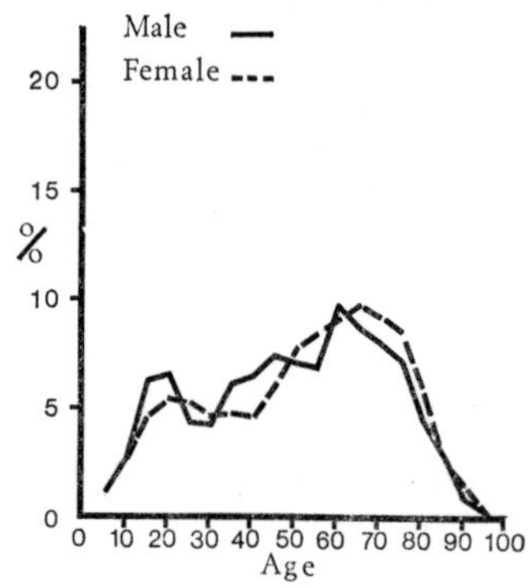

NOTES

Includes: Peritoneum and retroperitoneal tissue (158 in both 8th and 7th revisions), which are omitted from the separate site page-pairs.

5-YEAR SURVIVAL RATES BY AGE

Crude —— *Corrected* ----

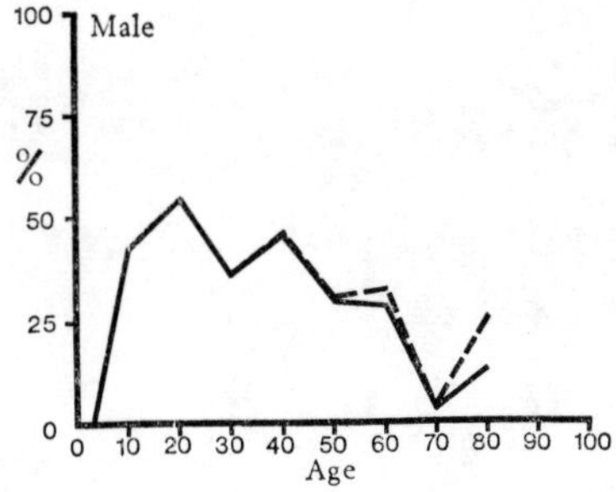

ALL CASES

Total 404
Male 205
Female 199

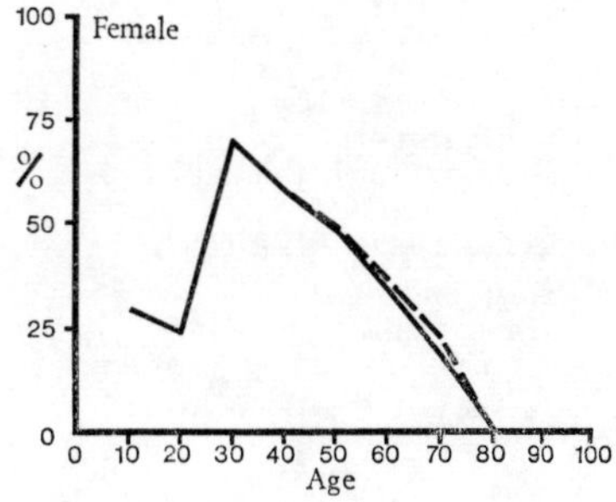

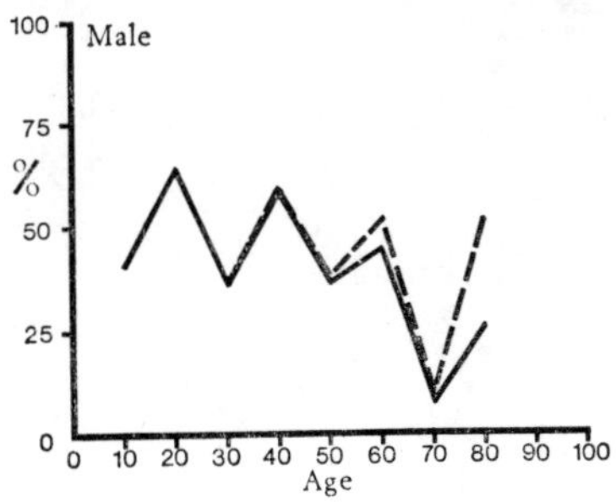

RADICAL TREATMENT

(63·9% of total)
61·0% *male*
66·8% *female*

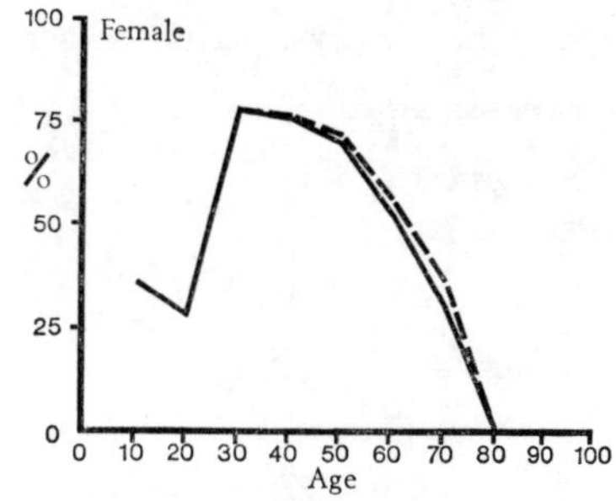

INDICES OF SURVIVAL

	All cases *Male*	All cases *Female*	Radical Treatment *Male*	Radical Treatment *Female*
FIVE YEAR SURVIVAL RATE (%)				
Crude	25·9	32·7	37·6	47·4
Corrected	*30·0*	*36·4*	*41·9*	*51·6*
Total cases†	205	199	125	133
TEN YEAR SURVIVAL RATE (%)				
Crude	19·4	29·7	32·7	43·0
Corrected	*25·3*	*37·5*	*40·5*	*51·5*
Total cases†	165	148	98	93
†Number of cases on which survival rate is based				
SURVIVAL TIME (*months*)				
First quartile (75% S.R.)	3·1	4·5	9·5	15·0
Median (50% S.R.)	**13·5**	**18·8**	**32·8**	**54·5**
Third quartile (25% S.R.)	>60	>60	>60	>60

ANNUAL SURVIVAL RATES

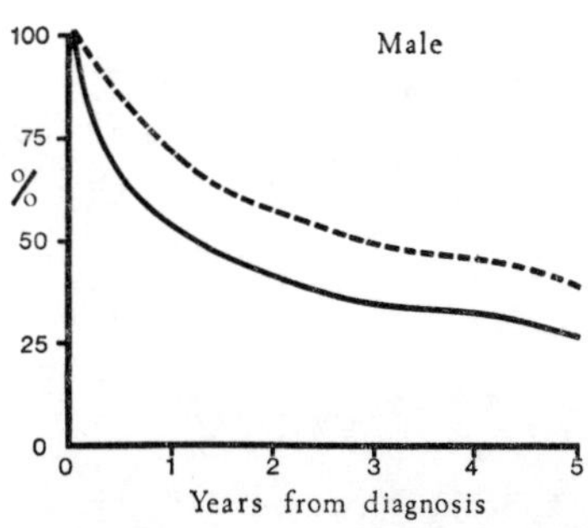

All cases ——————
Radical treatment - - - -

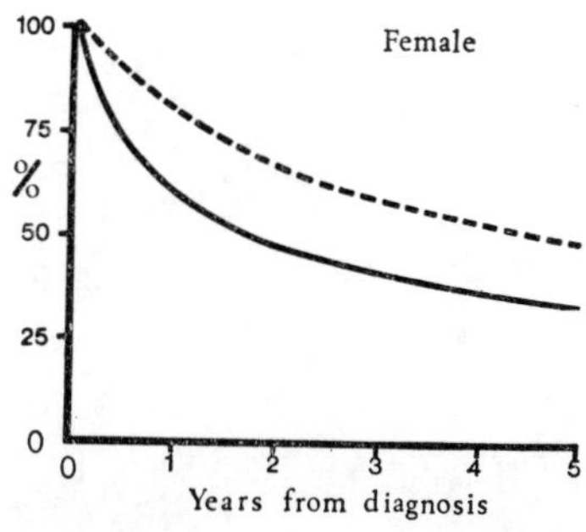

BONE, CONNECTIVE TISSUE AND MUSCULAR SYSTEM

	Distribution (%) of System		5-Year Survival Rate (%)	
	Male	*Female*	*Male*	*Female*
Bones	**39·1**	**34·1**	**18·1**	**23·1**
Skull and face	3·9	5·6	*20·0*	40·0
Limbs—right	10·8	9·5	18·2	39·1
—left	10·2	9·9	39·1	6·7
—unspecified	1·6	0·2	*0·0*	*33·3*
Other specified	12·2	8·9	0·0	10·0
Bone, no further detail	0·4	0·0	0·0	—
Connective Tissue, Muscle etc.	**60·4**	**65·1**	**30·8**	**38·1**
Head and Neck	3·2	2·9	*50·0*	*66·7*
Upper limb—right	4·4	6·2	*62·5*	*50·0*
—left	3·2	3·9	*50·0*	*66·7*
—unspecified	0·0	0·2	*100·0*	*0·0*
Lower limb—right	8·1	7·7	27·8	50·0
—left	9·5	12·8	25·0	42·9
—unspecified	0·9	0·8	*33·3*	*50·0*
Trunk	31·1	29·8	24·2	26·7
Connective tissue, no further detail	0·0	0·8	—	*0·0*
Peritoneum, mesentery	**0·5**	**0·8**	***50·0***	***66·7***
Whole system	**100·0**	**100·0**	**25·9**	**32·7**
Total Cases	566	516	205	199

Tumours of retroperitoneal tissue, other than reticuloses, are classified with connective tissue.

Rates printed in italics are based on less than ten cases.

0·0* means (with*) that the number of cases is *not* actually zero, but only to the degree of accuracy quoted, i.e. it is less than 0·05.

0·0 means (without*) that there were in fact *no cases.*

— in the Survival Rate column means that no survival rate can be calculated because there were no cases in that category. This might not accord with the figure given in the Distribution column, which may indicate a non-zero number of cases; the reason for such apparent discrepancies is that the survival rates are based on a fewer number of years than that used as the base of the Distribution figures.

SKIN (All histological types) ICD (8th) **172, 173**

INCIDENCE RATE (per 100,000)

Male —— *Female* - - - -

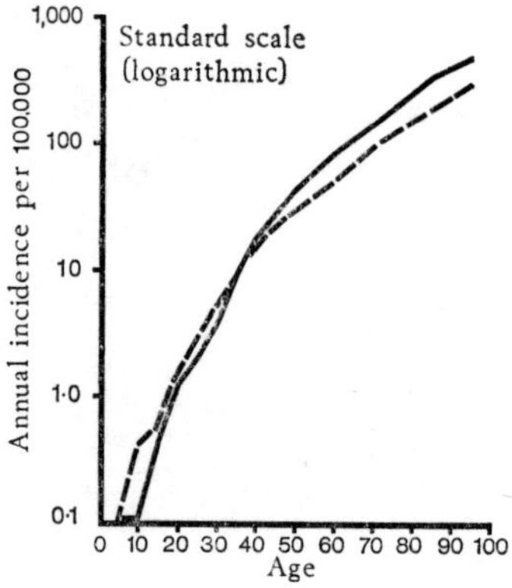

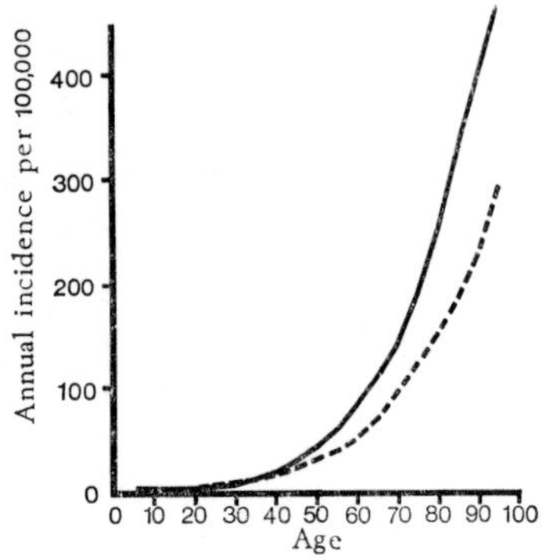

INCIDENCE RATES (per 100,000) by Age

Total cases 4544 *males*; 3925 *females* (of which age not stated for 37 *males* and 28 *females*)

Age	M	F	Age	M	F	Age	M	F
0–4	0·1	0·0	*35–39*	12·2	11·0	*70–74*	168·8	109·1
5–9	0·1	0·2	*40–44*	22·8	19·3	*75–79*	221·2	138·3
10–14	0·1	0·5	*45–49*	32·2	25·5	*80–84*	308·1	169·3
15–19	0·7	0·7	*50–54*	51·6	32·3	*85–89*	397·0	216·8
20–24	1·7	2·5	*55–59*	67·0	42·1	*90–94*	399·8	262·7
25–29	2·2	3·3	*60–64*	102·4	57·3	*95+*	1084·0	450·7
30–34	5·1	7·2	*65–69*	117·1	82·2	*All ages*	32·2	27·2

SEX AND AGE DISTRIBUTION

	Male	*Female*
Mean age (*years*)	62·9	64·6
95% between ages	35 & 87	32 & 89
Children under 15 (%)	0·0	0·1
Median age (*years*)	63·1	66·5
Proportion by sex (%)	53·7	46·3
Proportion of all cancers by sex (%)	10·5	9·7
Trend over 10 years	(+)	(+)

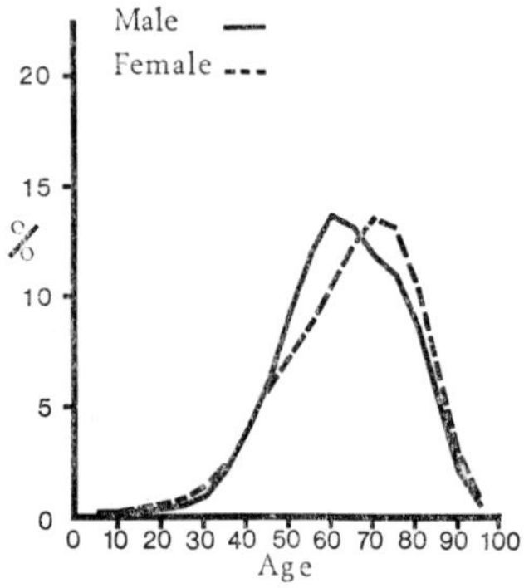

NOTES

Excludes: Scrotum (172.5, 173.5 in 8th revision; 179.1 in 7th), which is classified with GENITAL SYSTEM (Male) (p. 58), and separately as a page-pair on p. 162-3.

Important. Only cases of melanoma or of squamous-cell carcinoma are followed up routinely. The remainder, chiefly basal-cell carcinoma (rodent ulcers), are not followed up. For this reason Fate pages are available only for cases of melanoma, and for cases of squamous-cell carcinoma of skin.

ICD (7th) 190, 191 (part) **SKIN (Squamous and melanoma only)**

5-YEAR SURVIVAL RATES BY AGE

Crude —— *Corrected* ----

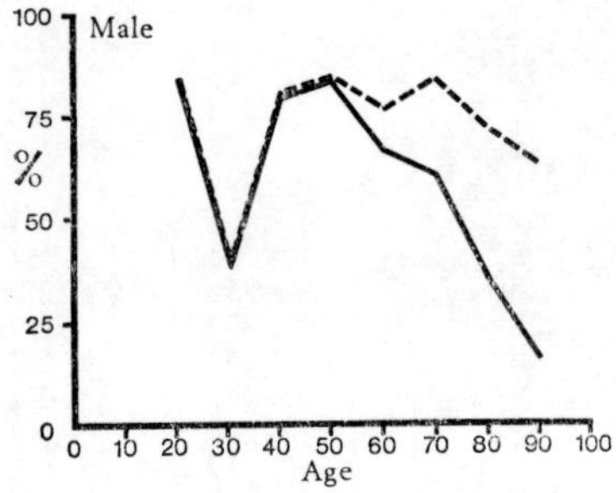

ALL CASES

Total 1237
Male 733
Female 504

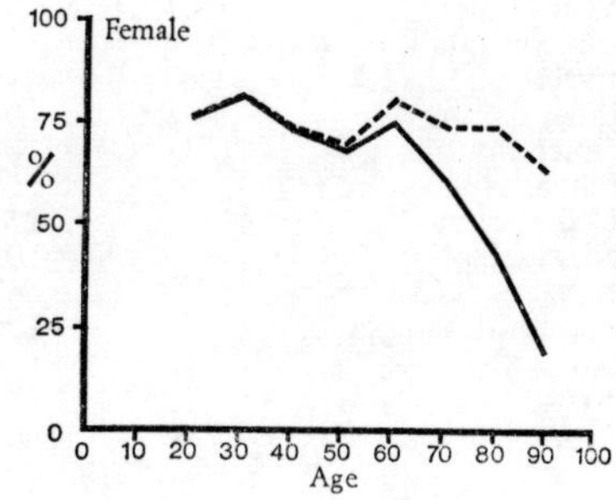

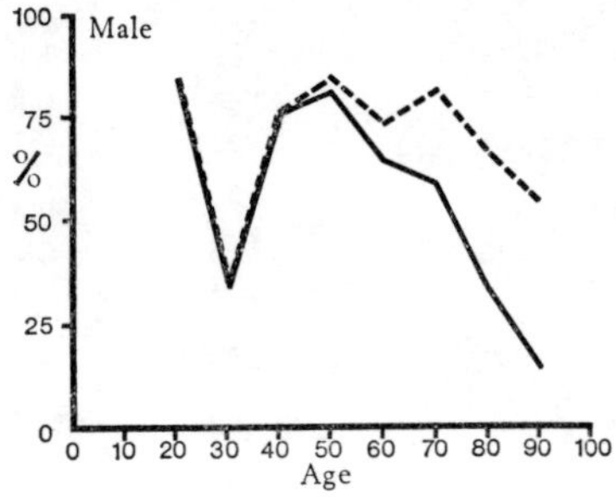

RADICAL TREATMENT

(92·2% of total)
93·2% *male*
90·9% *female*

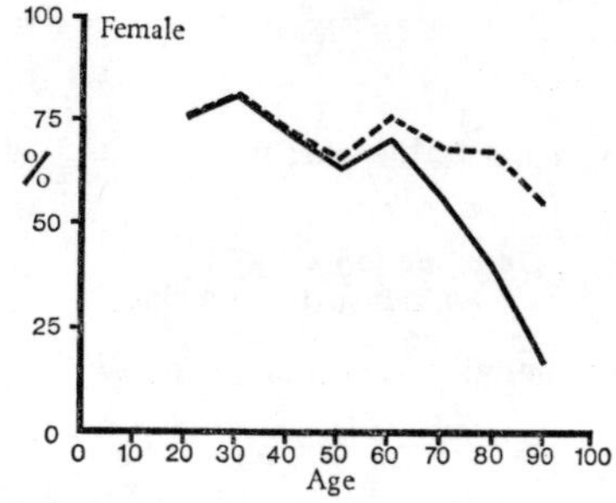

INDICES OF SURVIVAL

	All cases *Male*	All cases *Female*	Radical Treatment *Male*	Radical Treatment *Female*
FIVE YEAR SURVIVAL RATE (%)				
Crude	54·8	56·2	57·7	60·0
Corrected	*75·9*	*70·5*	*79·1*	*74·3*
Total cases†	733	504	683	458
TEN YEAR SURVIVAL RATE (%)				
Crude	35·0	44·6	36·7	47·5
Corrected	*67·0*	*72·5*	*68·8*	*75·9*
Total cases†	569	390	537	362

†Number of cases on which survival rate is based

SURVIVAL TIME (*months*)				
First quartile (75% S.R.)	22·8	21·9	26·6	29·3
Median (50% S.R.)	**>60**	**>60**	**>60**	**>60**
Third quartile (25% S.R.)	>60	>60	>60	>60

ANNUAL SURVIVAL RATES

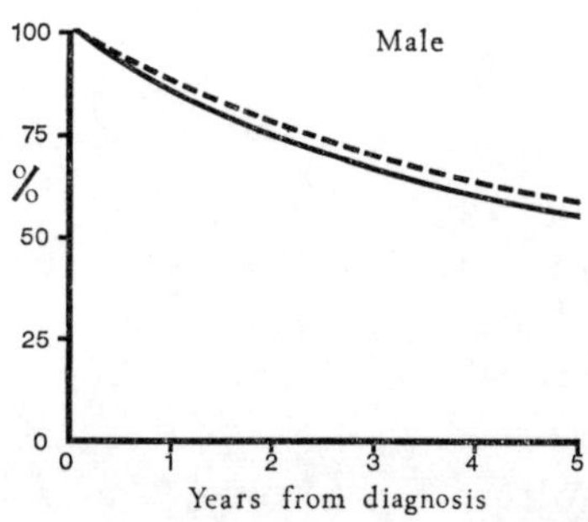

All cases ————
Radical treatment ----

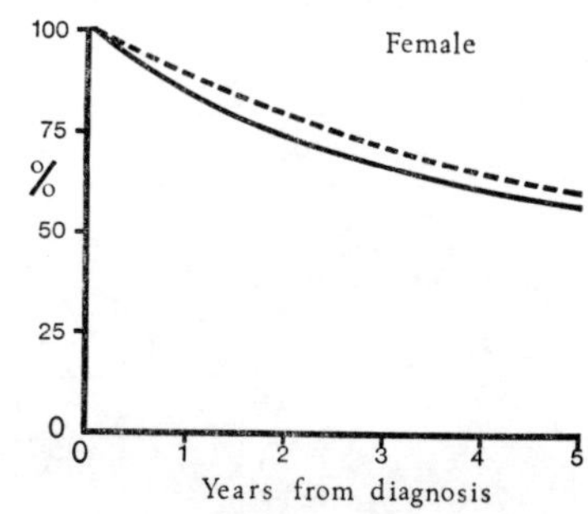

SKIN

Distribution by site and type of growth

MALE

	TYPE OF GROWTH				TOTAL	
	Melanoma	Squamous	Basal	Other	No.	(%)
Skin of lip	0	60	45	4	109	1·5
Lip, vermilion or unspecified	2	**	72	9	83	1·1
Eyelid	1	64	471	552	16	7·6
Inner canthus	0	14	413	6	433	6·0
Outer canthus	0	8	68	2	78	1·1
Pinna, post-auricular	5	446	317	31	799	11·0
Cheek, chin	25	191	1,211	39	1,466	20·1
Naso-labial	0	10	71	2	83	1·1
Nose	3	98	811	26	938	12·9
Forehead, temple	12	94	809	22	937	12·9
Scalp	7	34	106	10	157	2·2
Neck	9	46	114	8	177	2·4
Trunk	49	49	117	33	248	3·4
Groin	3	6	5	3	17	0·2
Anus, perineum	1	27	7	7	42	0·6
Hand	18	316	23	37	394	5·4
Forearm	18	57	33	6	114	1·6
Upper arm	15	13	16	12	56	0·8
Arm, not further specified	0	10	1	2	13	0·2
Foot	39	19	0	2	60	0·8
Leg, excluding foot	42	72	34	20	168	2·3
Lower limb, not further specified	2	3	1	1	7	0·1
Site unspecified or multiple sites	3	41	287	12	343	4·7
TOTAL	254	1,678	5,032	310	7,274	100·0

NOTES

Tumour sites in the table above are arranged in the order of the ICD 8th revision, which is also the same order as that of the 7th revision, except for the inclusion in the former list of *Scrotum.*

Scrotum: Tumours of the scrotum are not included here, but are classified separately (see p. 60), and also in GENITAL SYSTEM (male).

** Tumours of Lip: *Skin of lip* includes lip tumours specified as not of the vermilion. In the remaining group are classified together tumours specified as of the vermilion and those where no more detail than "lip" is given. In this latter group, however, when the histology is squamous they are classified with *Lip vermilion* in the system BUCCAL CAVITY AND PHARYNX.

Multiple coincidental tumours, if limited to a single site description as given in the above list, are included as a single entry for each patient. When more than one site description is involved, they appear within the last category (*Site unspecified, or multiple*), again as one entry per patient.

The division into right or left side is not given for the sites in these tables. When it was examined, only two sites showed a statistically significant excess on either side. They were *Pinna, post auricular*, basal cell carcinoma, which showed an excess on the left side in the male, and on the right side in the female; and *Lower limb, not further specified*, which in the male, for all histological groups together, showed an excess on the left side.

SKIN

Distribution by site and type of growth

FEMALE

	TYPE OF GROWTH				TOTAL	
	Melanoma	Squamous	Basal	Other	No.	(%)
Skin of lip	1	14	86	1	102	1·6
Lip, vermilion or unspecified	1	**	86	5	92	1·4
Eyelid	2	40	397	17	456	7·2
Inner canthus	0	16	344	3	363	5·7
Outer canthus	2	4	64	2	72	1·1
Pinna, post-auricular	8	51	107	5	171	2·7
Cheek, chin	43	144	970	51	1,208	19·0
Naso-labial	0	6	58	0	64	1·0
Nose	3	74	793	25	895	14·0
Forehead, temple	13	57	913	30	1,013	15·9
Scalp	1	40	105	20	166	2·6
Neck	13	34	144	13	204	3·2
Trunk	70	70	156	70	366	5·7
Groin	5	7	13	7	32	0·5
Anus, perineum	5	38	8	7	58	0·9
Hand	13	78	10	17	118	1·9
Forearm	26	31	20	10	87	1·4
Upper arm	16	13	26	9	64	1·0
Arm, not further specified	4	4	1	2	11	0·2
Foot	78	10	1	3	92	1·4
Leg, excluding foot	196	142	41	62	441	6·9
Lower limb, not further specified	4	11	1	5	21	0·3
Site unspecifiea or multiple sites	3	24	234	19	280	4·4
TOTAL	507	908	4,578	383	6,376	100·0

NOTES

Tumour sites in the table above are arranged in the order of the ICD 8th revision, which is also the same order as that of the 7th revision.

**Tumours of Lip: *Skin of lip* includes lip tumours specified as not of the vermilion. In the remaining group are classified together tumours specified as of the vermilion and those where no more detail than "lip" is given. In this latter group, however, when the histology is squamous they are classified with *Lip vermilion* in the system BUCCAL CAVITY AND PHARYNX.

Multiple coincidental tumours, if limited to a single site description as given in the above list, are included as a single entry for each patient. When more than one site description is involved, they appear within the last category (*Site unspecified, or multiple*), again as one entry per patient.

The division into right or left side is not given for the sites in these tables. When it was examined, only two sites showed a statistically significant excess on either side. They were *Pinna, post auricular*, basal cell carcinoma, which showed an excess on the left side in the male, and on the right side in the female; and *Lower limb, not further specified*, which in the male, for all histological groups together, showed an excess on the left side.

SKIN

5-Year Survival rate by site and type of growth

	Melanoma		Squamous	
	Male	*Female*	*Male*	*Female*
Skin of lip	—	*100·0*	82·1	*71·4*
Lip, vermilion or unspecified	*0·0*	—	**	**
Eyelid	—	*100·0*	75·0	73·3
Inner canthus	—	—	63·6	*80·0*
Outer canthus	—	—	—	*0·0*
Pinna, post-auricular	*0·0*	—	58·1	76·2
Cheek, chin	*28·6*	35·7	59·0	60·9
Naso-labial	—	—	*66·7*	*100·0*
Nose	*0·0*	*0·0*	43·2	74·1
Forehead, temple	*50·0*	*50·0*	55·6	81·0
Scalp	*100·0*	—	58·3	36·4
Neck	*25·0*	*60·0*	60·0	50·0
Trunk	*25·0*	42·4	47·6	42·1
Groin	*0·0*	*33·3*	*50·0*	*0·0*
Anus, perineum	*0·0*	*0·0*	36·4	40·0
Hand	*40·0*	*50·0*	62·4	75·9
Forearm	*100·0*	58·3	76·0	50·0
Upper arm	*33·3*	*25·0*	*75·0*	*0·0*
Arm, not further specified	—	—	*80·0*	*0·0*
Foot	21·4	44·0	40·0	*66·7*
Leg, excluding foot	30·8	57·8	34·8	52·9
Lower limb, not further specified	*0·0*	*50·0*	*50·0*	*71·4*
Site unspecified or multiple sites	*0·0*	*0·0*	*30·8*	*50·0*
TOTAL	32·1	50·0	57·6	59·4
TOTAL CASES	78	174	655	330

NOTES

Tumour sites in the table above are arranged in the order of the ICD 8th revision, which is also the same order as that of the 7th revision, except for the inclusion in the former list of *Scrotum.*

Scrotum: Tumours of the scrotum are not included here, but are classified separately (see p. 60), and also in GENITAL SYSTEM (male).

**Tumours of Lip: *Skin of lip* includes lip tumours specified as not of the vermilion. In the remaining group are classified together tumours specified as of the vermilion and those where no more detail than "lip" is given. In this latter group, however, when the histology is squamous they are classified with *Lip vermilion* in the system BUCCAL CAVITY AND PHARYNX.

Multiple coincidental tumours, if limited to a single site description as given in the above list, are included as a single entry for each patient. When more than one site description is involved, they appear within the last category (*Site unspecified, or multiple*), again as one entry per patient.

The division into right or left side is not given for the sites in these tables. When it was examined, only two sites showed a statistically significant excess on either side. They were *Pinna, post auricular*, basal cell carcinoma, which showed an excess on the left side in the male, and on the right side in the female: and *Lower limb, not further specified*, which in the male, for all histological groups together, showed an excess on the left side.

Survival rates are given only for those cases where the histology is *melanoma* or *squamous cell carcinoma.* It is common practice not to follow up cases of basal cell carcinoma, and in consequence survival data are not available. The fourth histological group (*Other histological types*) is too heterogeneous to warrant the quotation of separate survival rates.

Rates printed in italics are based on less than ten cases.

0·0* means (with*) that the number of cases is *not* actually zero, but only to the degree of accuracy quoted, i.e. it is less than 0·05.

0·0 means (without*) that there were in fact *no cases.*

— in the Survival Rate column means that no survival rate can be calculated because there were no cases in that category. This might not accord with the figure given in the Distribution column, which may indicate a non-zero number of cases; the reason for such apparent discrepancies is that the survival rates are based on a fewer number of years than that used as the base of the Distribution figures.

SKIN (Melanoma) ICD (8th) **172**

INCIDENCE RATE (per 100,000)

Male ——— *Female* - - - -

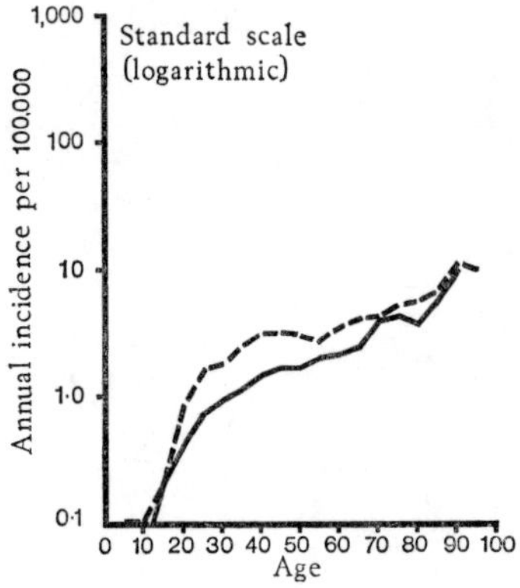

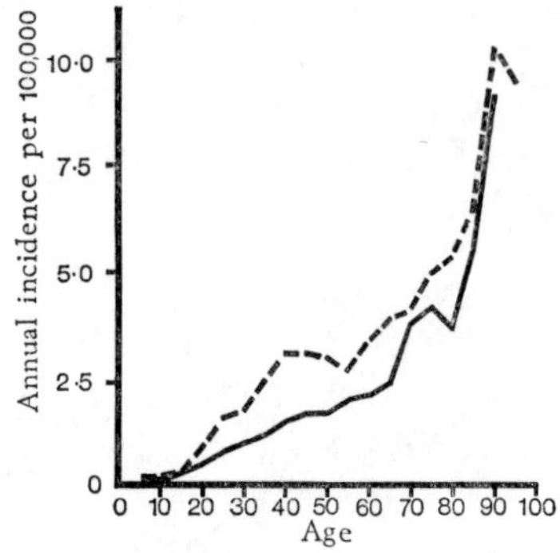

INCIDENCE RATES (per 100,000) by Age

Total cases 162 *males*; 304 *females* (of which age not stated for 0 *males* and 1 *female*)

Age	M	F	Age	M	F	Age	M	F
0–4	0·1	0·0	*35–39*	1·1	3·0	*70–74*	4·4	4·5
5–9	0·0	0·2	*40–44*	1·6	3·0	*75–79*	3·5	5·5
10–14	0·1	0·1	*45–49*	1·6	3·1	*80–84*	3·7	5·0
15–19	0·4	0·4	*50–54*	1·7	2·6	*85–89*	10·7	10·0
20–24	0·5	1·3	*55–59*	2·3	2·7	*90–94*	0·0	10·9
25–29	0·8	1·7	*60–64*	1·7	4·0	*95+*	0·0	0·0
30–34	1·0	1·8	*65–69*	3·1	3·5	*All ages*	1·1	2·1

SEX AND AGE DISTRIBUTION

	Male	*Female*
Mean age (*years*)	52·1	52·7
95% between ages	18 & 85	20 & 87
Children under 15 (%)	1·2	1·0
Median age (*years*)	52·5	51·9
Proportion by sex (%)	34·8	65·2
Proportion of all cancers by sex (%)	0·4	0·8
Trend over 10 years	(+)	(−)

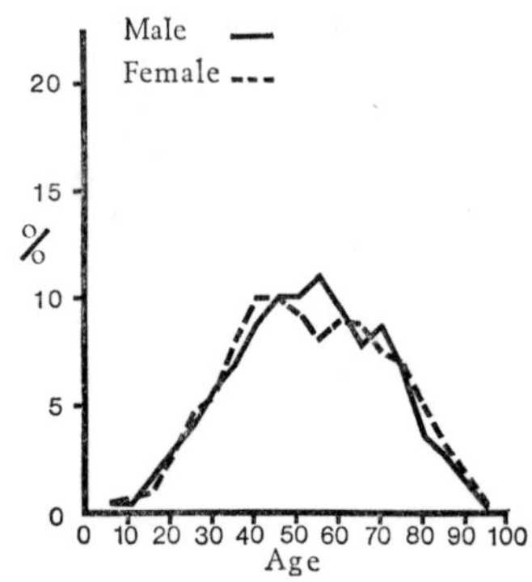

5-YEAR SURVIVAL RATES BY AGE

Crude —— *Corrected* ----

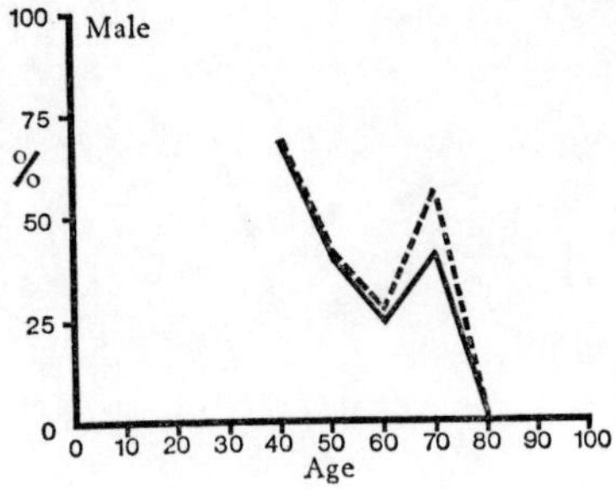

ALL CASES

Total 252
Male 78
Female 174

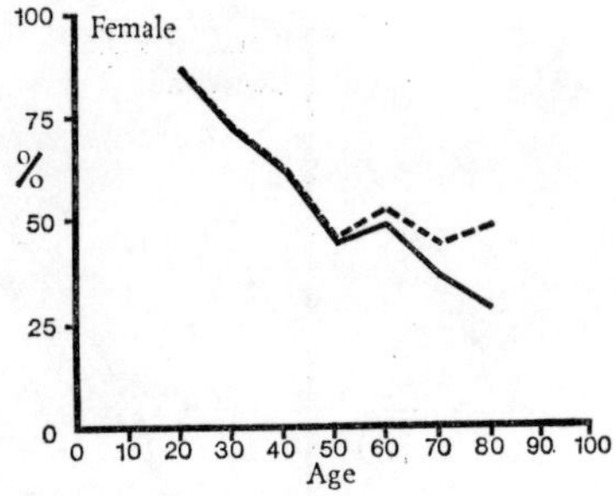

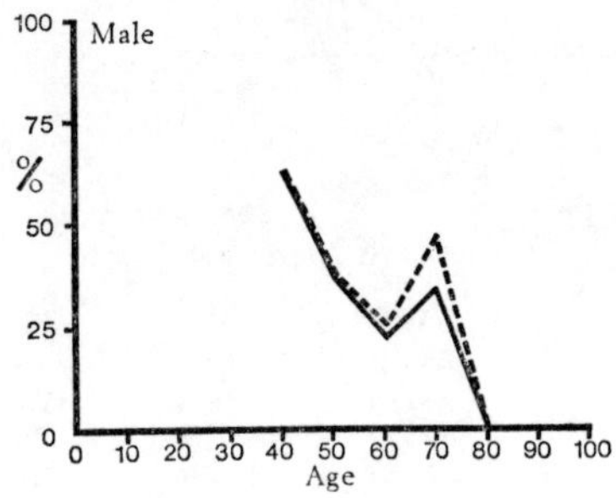

RADICAL TREATMENT

(90·5% of total)
87·2% *male*
92·0% *female*

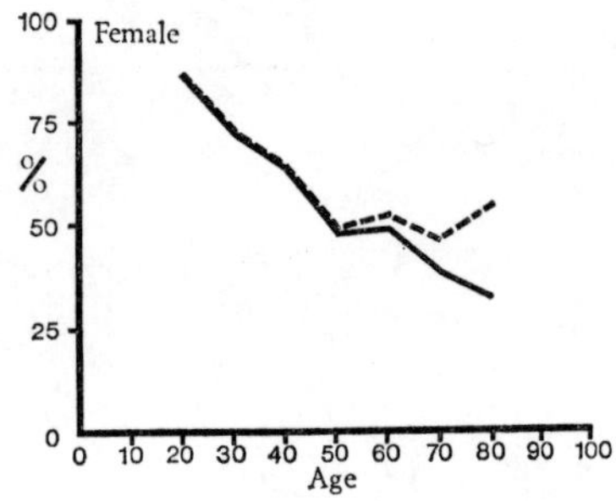

INDICES OF SURVIVAL

	All cases		Radical Treatment	
	Male	*Female*	*Male*	*Female*
FIVE YEAR SURVIVAL RATE (%)				
Crude	32·1	50·0	36·8	52·5
Corrected	*38·5*	*55·2*	*43·4*	*57·4*
Total cases†	78	174	68	160
TEN YEAR SURVIVAL RATE (%)				
Crude	14·8	34·9	17·4	37·7
Corrected	*22·1*	*44·3*	*24·5*	*47·1*
Total cases†	54	83	46	77
†Number of cases on which survival rate is based				
SURVIVAL TIME (*months*)				
First quartile (75% S.R.)	9·1	18·4	16·1	22·6
Median (50% S.R.)	**29·7**	**60·0**	**29·0**	**>60**
Third quartile (25% S.R.)	>60	>60	>60	>60

ANNUAL SURVIVAL RATES

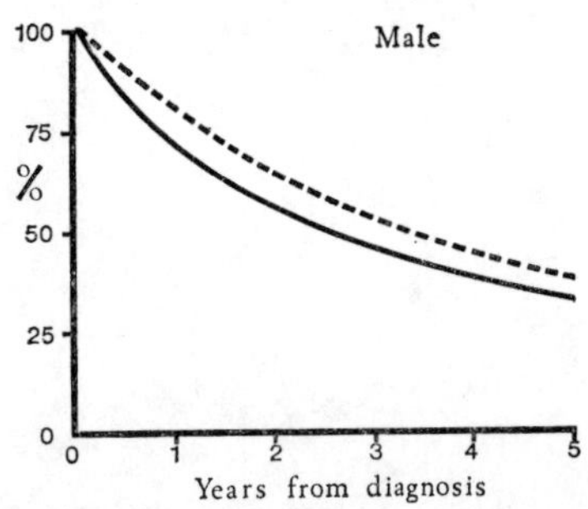

All cases ——
Radical treatment ----

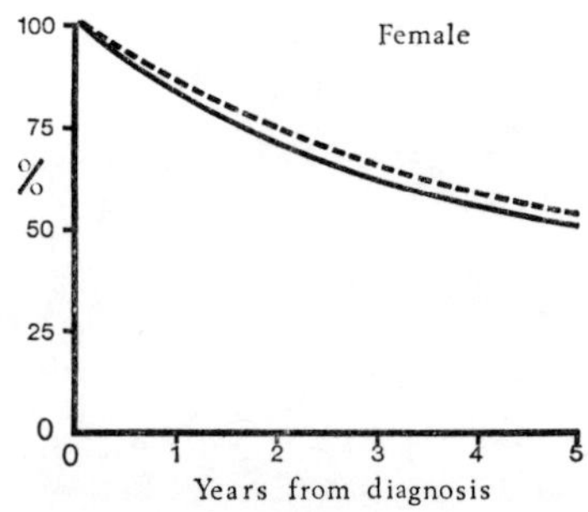

SKIN (Squamous cell carcinoma) ICD (8th) **173 (part)**

INCIDENCE RATE (per 100,000)

Male —— *Female* ----

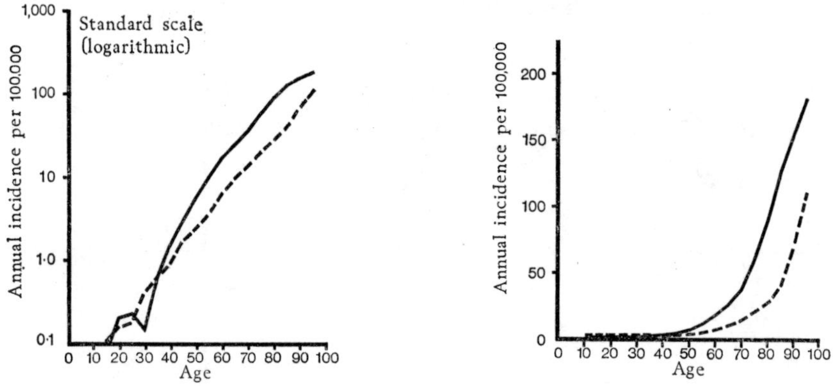

INCIDENCE RATES (per 100,000) by Age

Total cases 1017 *males*; 545 *females* (of which age not stated for 3 *males* and 2 *females*)

Age	M	F	Age	M	F	Age	M	
0–4	0·0	0·0	*35–39*	0·9	0·7	*70–74*	48·1	16·1
5–9	0·0	0·0	*40–44*	2·0	1·2	*75–79*	73·6	24·2
10–14	0·0	0·2	*45–49*	3·9	2·1	*80–84*	116·1	30·3
15–19	0·0	0·0	*50–54*	7·7	2·6	*85–89*	149·2	61·1
20–24	0·4	0·1	*55–59*	12·6	4·7	*90–94*	169·1	98·5
25–29	0·0	0·2	*60–64*	22·7	8·0	*95+*	271·0	160·9
30–34	0·3	0·5	*65–69*	27·1	11·4	*All ages*	7·2	3·8

SEX AND AGE DISTRIBUTION

	Male	*Female*
Mean age (*years*)	68·3	69·9
95% between ages	42 & 89	38 & 93
Children under 15 (%)	0·0	0·4
Median age (*years*)	69·4	71·5
Proportion by sex (%)	65·1	34·9
Proportion of all cancers by sex (%)	2·3	1.3
Trend over 10 years	(–)	(–)

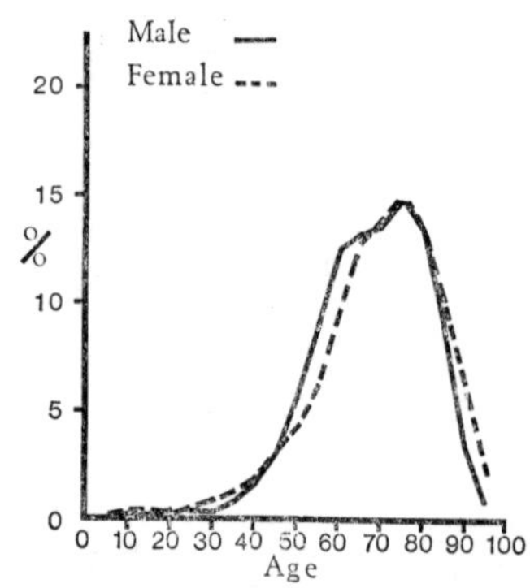

5-YEAR SURVIVAL RATES BY AGE

Crude —— *Corrected* ----

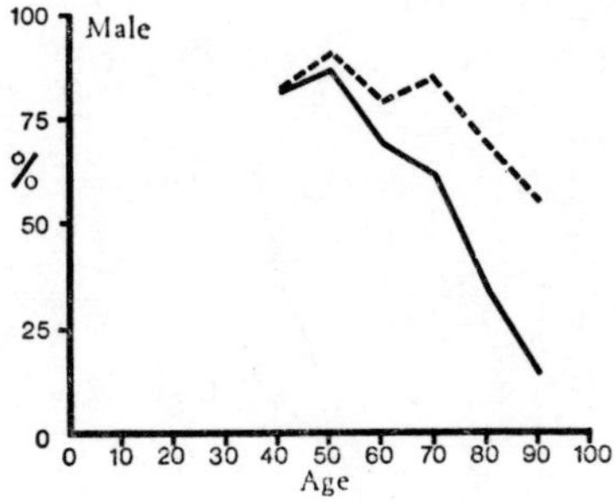

ALL CASES

Total 985
Male 655
Female 330

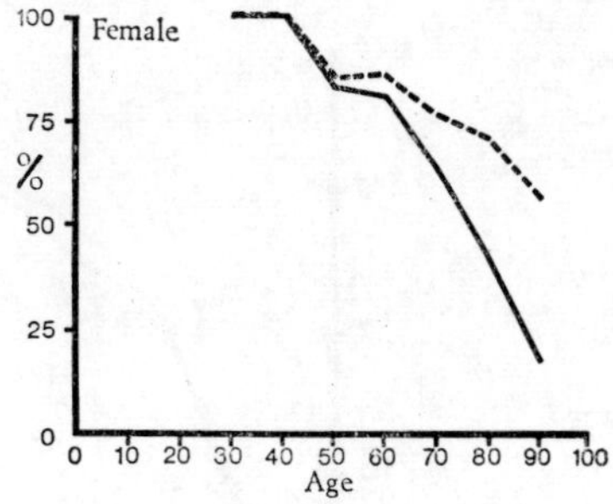

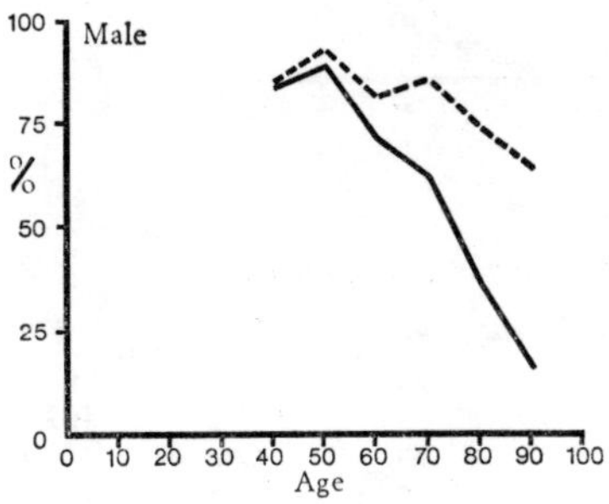

RADICAL TREATMENT

(92·7% of total)
93·9% *male*
90·3% *female*

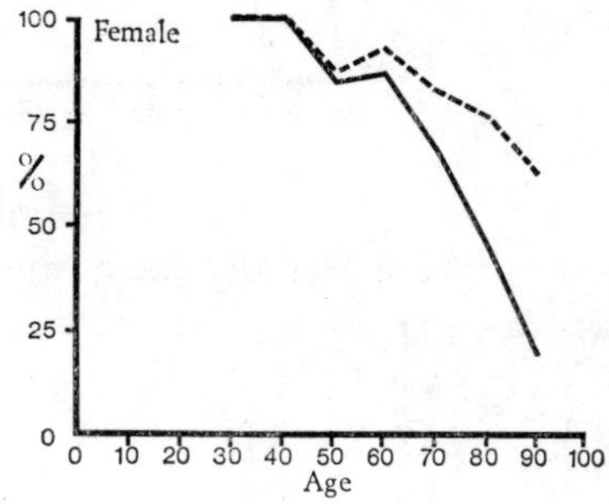

INDICES OF SURVIVAL

	All cases *Male*	All cases *Female*	Radical Treatment *Male*	Radical Treatment *Female*
FIVE YEAR SURVIVAL RATE (%)				
Crude	57·6	59·4	60·0	64·1
Corrected	*81·3*	*80·3*	*83·7*	*85·4*
Total cases†	655	330	615	298
TEN YEAR SURVIVAL RATE (%)				
Crude	46·8	47·2	48·7	50·5
Corrected	*92·3*	*82·8*	*94·2*	*87·0*
Total cases†	515	307	491	285
SURVIVAL TIME (*months*)				
First quartile (75% S.R.)	25·7	25·7	30·1	37·5
Median (50% S.R.)	**>60**	**>60**	**>60**	**>60**
Third quartile (25% S.R.)	>60	>60	>60	>60

†Number of cases on which survival rate is based

ANNUAL SURVIVAL RATES

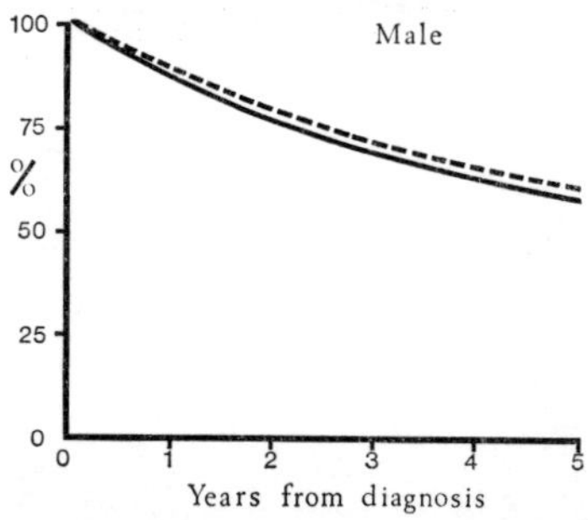

All cases ——
Radical treatment ----

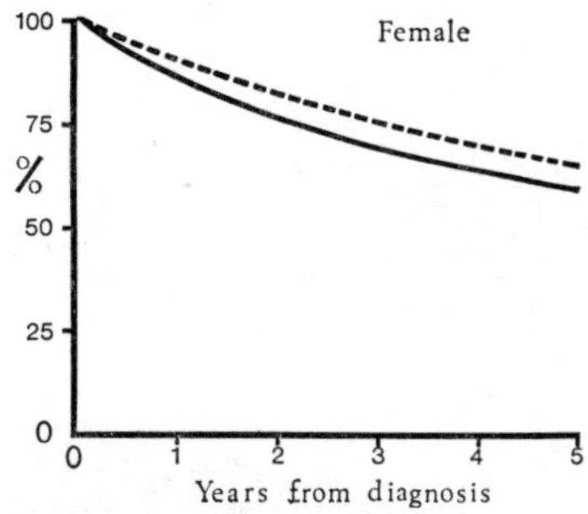

SKIN (Basal cell carcinoma) ICD (8th) **173 (part)**

INCIDENCE RATE (per 100,000)

Male —— *Female* ----

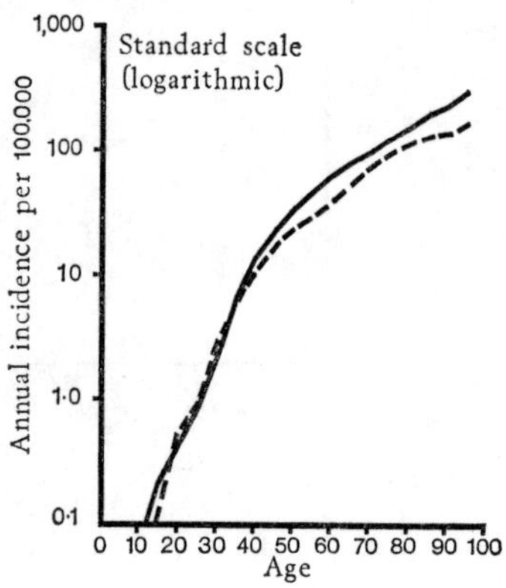

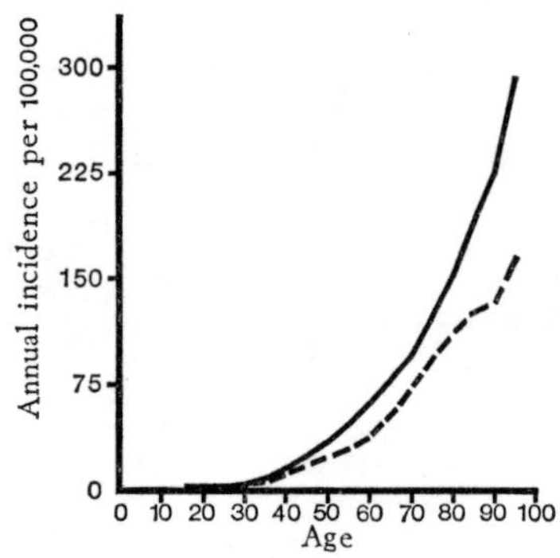

INCIDENCE RATES (per 100,000) by Age

Total cases 3200 *males*; 2849 *females* (of which age not stated for 33 *males* and 23 *females*)

Age	M	F	Age	M	F	Age	M	F
0–4	0·0	0·0	*35–39*	9·1	6·9	*70–74*	111·0	83·6
5–9	0·0	0·0	*40–44*	18·4	13·9	*75–79*	136·1	102·0
10–14	0·0	0·2	*45–49*	25·8	19·2	*80–84*	179·8	123·1
15–19	0·4	0·1	*50–54*	40·4	25·4	*85–89*	223·8	128·4
20–24	0·5	0·9	*55–59*	49·9	31·5	*90–94*	230·6	147·8
25–29	1·1	0·9	*60–64*	75·0	42·4	*95+*	813·0	257·4
30–34	3·4	4·5	*65–69*	82·0	61·3	*All ages*	22·7	19·7

SEX AND AGE DISTRIBUTION

	Male	*Female*
Mean age (*years*)	61·9	64·9
95% between ages	36 & 87	36 & 88
Children under 15 (%)	0·0	0·1
Median age (*years*)	61·9	66·5
Proportion by sex (%)	52·9	47·1
Proportion of all cancers by sex (%)	7·4	7·0
Trend over 10 years	(+)	(+)

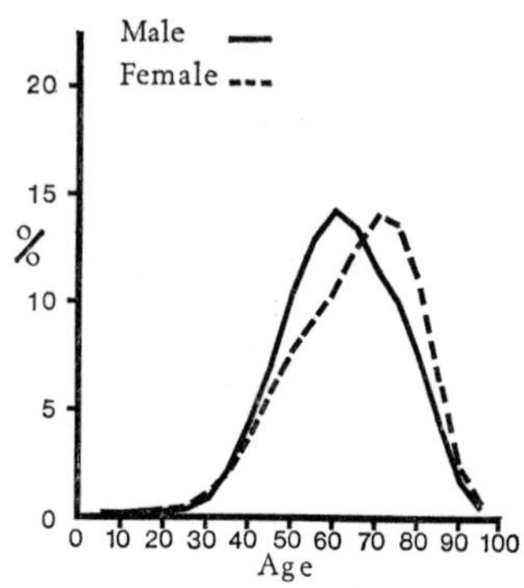

No survival rates are available. See note p. 46.

SKIN (Other histological types) ICD (8th) **173 (part)**

INCIDENCE RATE (per 100,000)

Male —— *Female* ----

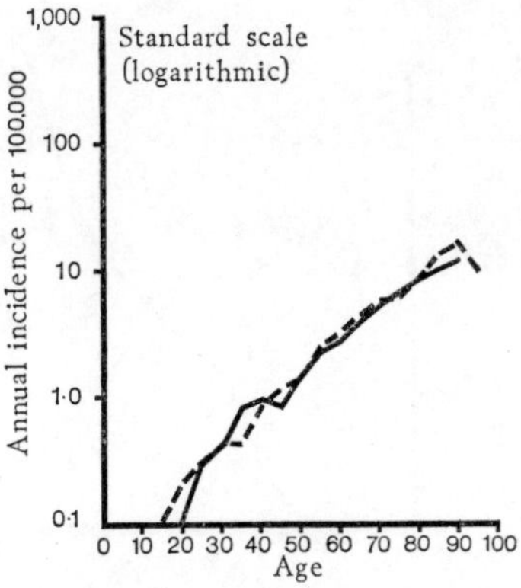

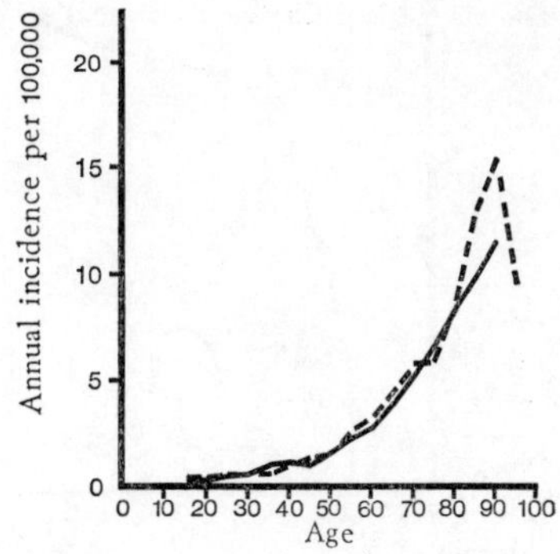

INCIDENCE RATES (per 100,000) by Age

Total cases 165 *males*; 227 *females* (of which age not stated for 1 *male* and 2 *females*)

Age	M	F	Age	M	F	Age	M	F
0–4	0·0	0·0	*35–39*	1·0	0·4	*70–74*	5·4	4·9
5–9	0·1	0·0	*40–44*	0·8	1·2	*75–79*	8·0	6·6
10–14	0·0	0·1	*45–49*	0·9	1·0	*80–84*	8·4	10·9
15–19	0·0	0·2	*50–54*	2·0	1·7	*85–89*	13·3	17·4
20–24	0·2	0·2	*55–59*	2·3	3·1	*90–94*	0·0	5·5
25–29	0·3	0·5	*60–64*	3·0	2·9	*95+*	0·0	32·2
30–34	0·5	0·3	*65–69*	4·7	6·0	*All ages*	1·2	1·6

SEX AND AGE DISTRIBUTION

	Male	*Female*
Mean age (*years*)	59·9	64·2
95% between ages	27 & 86	26 & 89
Children under 15 (%)	0·6	0·4
Median age (*years*)	61·3	66·3
Proportion by sex (%)	42·1	57·9
Proportion of all cancers by sex (%)	0·4	0·6
Trend over 10 years	(−)	(+)

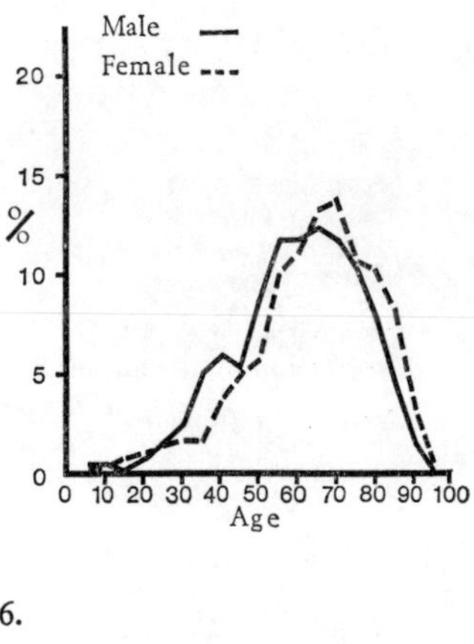

No survival rates are available. See note p. 46.

BREAST ICD (8th) **174**

INCIDENCE RATE (per 100,000)

Male —— *Female* ----

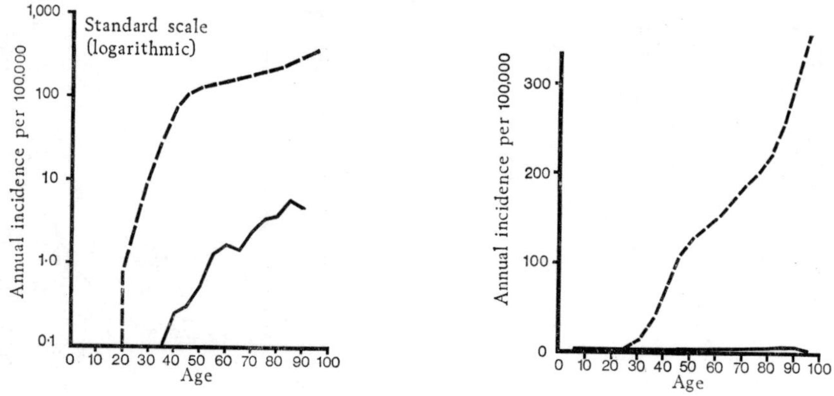

INCIDENCE RATES (per 100,000) by Age

Total cases 70 *males*; 9976 *females* (of which age not stated for 0 *males* and 10 *females*)

Age	M	F	Age	M	F	Age	M	F
0–4	0·0	0·0	*35–39*	0·2	43·1	*70–74*	3·8	191·9
5–9	0·0	0·0	*40–44*	0·3	89·4	*75–79*	2·5	208·3
10–14	0·0	0·0	*45–49*	0·3	120·2	*80–84*	5·6	236·3
15–19	0·0	0·1	*50–54*	0·7	128·9	*85–89*	5·3	295·3
20–24	0·0	1·4	*55–59*	1·8	144·8	*90–94*	0·0	339·4
25–29	0·0	5·2	*60–64*	1·4	154·8	*95+*	0·0	450·5
30–34	0·0	18·0	*65–69*	1·3	179·5	*All ages*	0·5	69·1

SEX AND AGE DISTRIBUTION

	Male	*Female*
Mean age (*years*)	63·9	59·6
95% between ages	39 & 86	35 & 86
Children under 15 (%)	0·0	0·0
Median age (*years*)	62·8	59·0
Proportion by sex (%)	0·7	99·3
Proportion of all cancers by sex (%)	0·2	24·6
Trend over 10 years	(−)	(−)

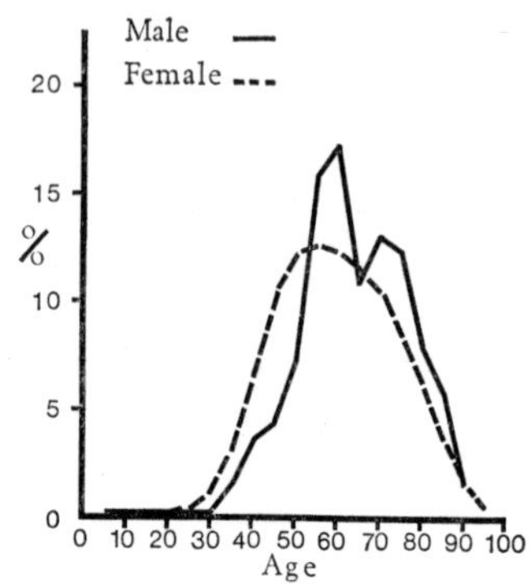

NOTES

Includes: All malignant tumours of breast. No attempt has been made to include subdivisions by any system of clinical staging (e.g. TNM).

5-YEAR SURVIVAL RATES BY AGE

Crude —— *Corrected* ----

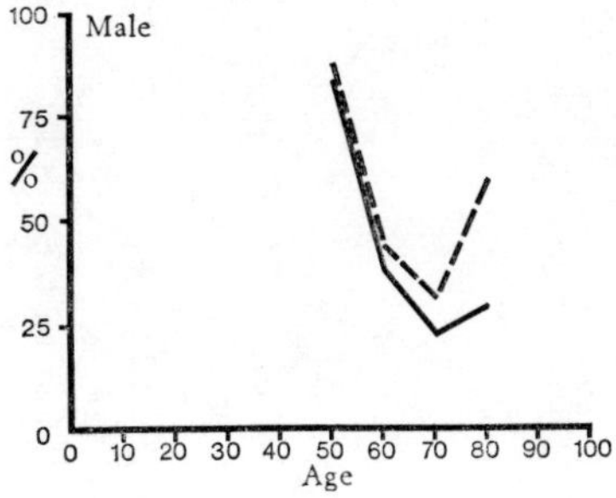

ALL CASES

Total 5805
Male 49
Female 5756

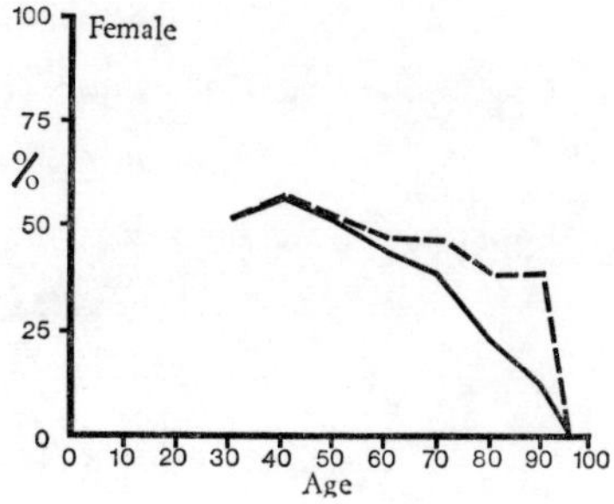

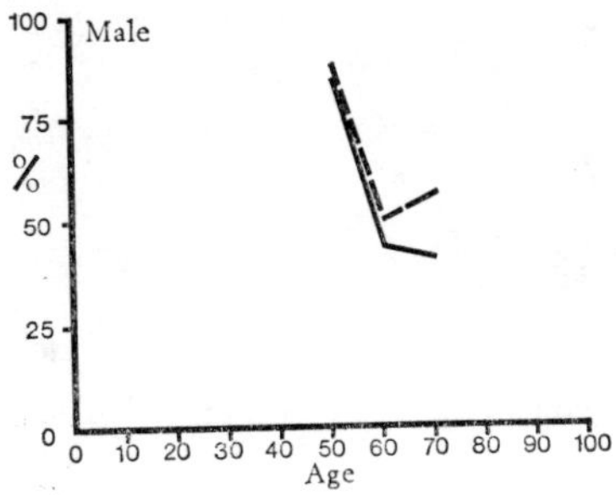

RADICAL TREATMENT

(78·9% of total)
75·5% *male*
78·9% *female*

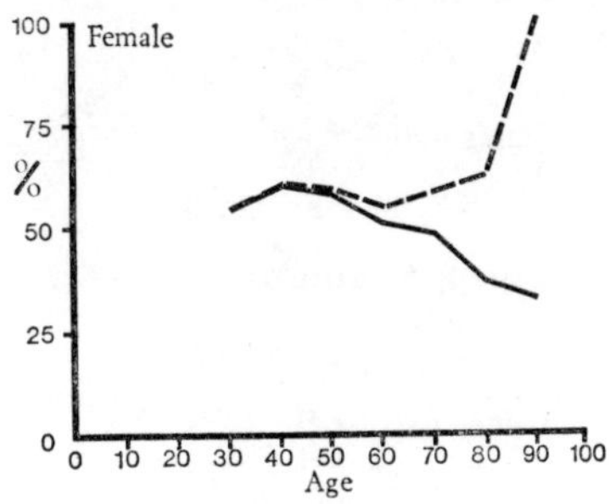

INDICES OF SURVIVAL

	All cases		Radical Treatment	
	Male	*Female*	*Male*	*Female*
FIVE YEAR SURVIVAL RATE (%)				
Crude	44·9	42·6	59·5	52·2
Corrected	*58·2*	*49·0*	*71·2*	*57·8*
Total cases†	49	5756	37	4544
TEN YEAR SURVIVAL RATE (%)				
Crude	21·9	28·8	26·5	34·5
Corrected	*31·6*	*38·2*	*42·1*	*43·6*
Total cases†	41	4283	34	3495

†Number of cases on which survival rate is based

SURVIVAL TIME (*months*)				
First quartile (75% S.R.)	16·3	15·7	41·0	25·9
Median (50% S.R.)	**45·5**	**44·7**	**>60**	**>60**
Third quartile (25% S.R.)	>60	>60	>60	>60

ANNUAL SURVIVAL RATES

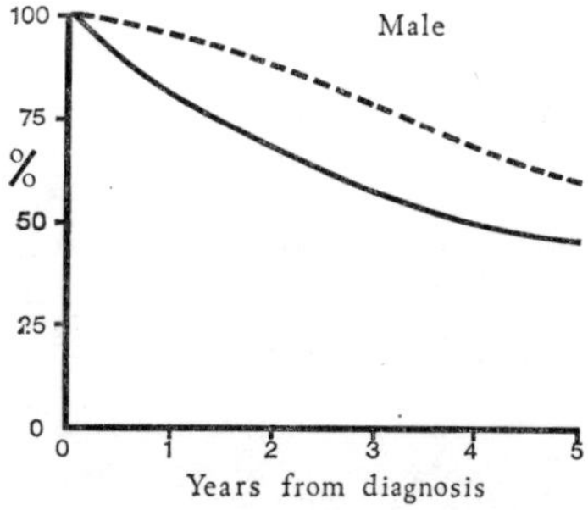

All cases ——
Radical treatment ----

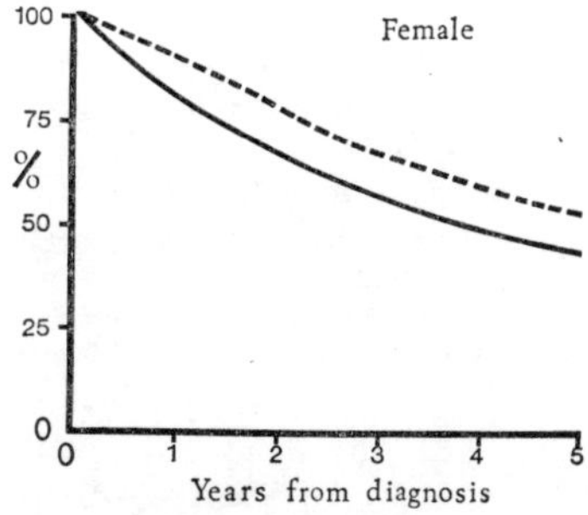

BREAST

	Distribution (%) of organ		5-Year Survival Rate (%)	
	Male	*Female*	*Male*	*Female*
Upper inner quadrant—right	1·7	4·3	—	55·3
—left	1·7	5·0	*100·0*	56·8
—unspecified	0·0	0·0	—	*0·0*
Upper outer quadrant—right	1·7	11·8	0·0	51·2
—left	0·9	12·7	—	47·1
—unspecified	0·0	0·0*	—	*100·0*
Lower inner quadrant—right	0·9	1·5	—	50·6
—left	0·0	1·9	*0·0*	55·1
—unspecified	0·0	0·0*	—	*0·0*
Lower outer quadrant—right	2·6	2·5	*0·0*	45·0
—left	0·0	2·9	—	50·6
—unspecified	0·0	0·0	—	—
Central—right	22·6	5·2	57·1	43·0
—left	27·8	6·2	57·1	42·7
—unspecified	0·0	0·1	—	*0·0*
Outer half—right	1·7	2·2	*0·0*	40·0
—left	0·9	2·0	*100·0*	52·0
—unspecified	0·0	0·0*	—	*100·0*
Inner half—right	0·0	0·8	—	59·5
—left	0·0	1·2	—	47·2
—unspecified	0·0	0·0*	—	*0·0*
Upper half—right	1·7	3·0	*100·0*	48·0
—left	0·0	3·6	—	54·3
—unspecified	0·0	0·0*	—	*0·0*
Lower half—right	0·9	1·4	—	54·8
—left	0·9	1·4	—	35·8
—unspecified	0·0	0·0	—	*0·0*
Axillary tail—right	0·9	1·3	*100·0*	51·3
—left	0·0	1·5	—	47·4
—unspecified	0·0	0·0*	—	*0·0*
Breast, no further detail—right	18·3	12·2	*0·0*	27·5
—left	14·8	13·6	*40·0*	26·6
—unspecified	0·0	1·7	—	11·3
Breast, all sites—right	53·0	46·1	37·0	43·9
—left	47·0	52·0	54·5	43·5
—unspecified	0·0	1·9	—	12·2
Breast	**100·0**	**100·0**	**44·9**	**42·6**
Total cases	115	16,003	49	5,756

Rates printed in italics are based on less than ten cases

0·0* means (with*) that the number of cases is *not* actually zero, but only to the degree of accuracy quoted, i.e. it is less than 0·05.

0·0 means (without*) that there were in fact *no cases.*

— in the Survival Rate column means that no survival rate can be calculated because there were no cases in that category. This might not accord with the figure given in the Distribution column, which may indicate a non-zero number of cases; the reason for such apparent discrepancies is that the survival rates are based on a fewer number of years than that used as the base of the Distribution figures.

GENTIAL SYSTEM

ICD (8th) **172.5, 173.5, 180–187**

INCIDENCE RATE (per 100,000)

Male —— *Female* ----

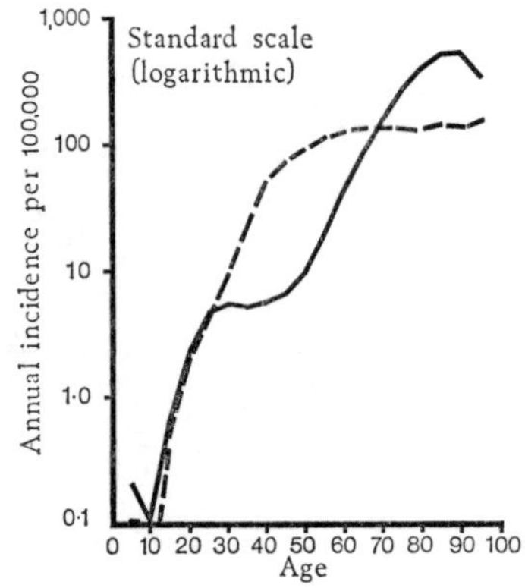

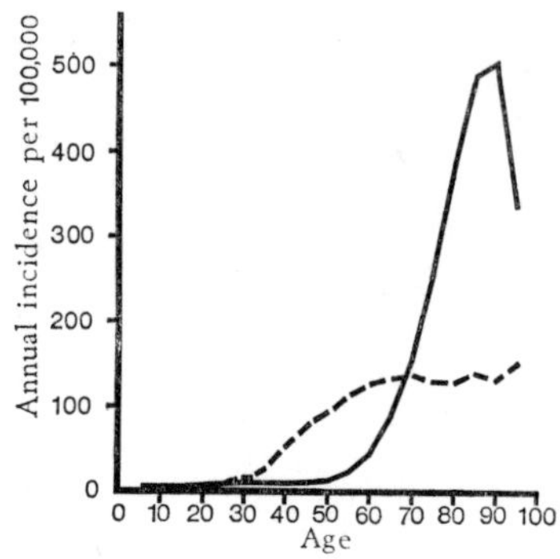

INCIDENCE RATES per (100,000) by Age

Total cases 3611 *males*; 7243 *females* (of which age not stated for 10 *males* and 10 *females*)

Age	M	F	Age	M	F	Age	M	F
0–4	0·4	0·1	*35–39*	5·3	33·4	*70–74*	206·1	132·0
5–9	0·0	0·1	*40–44*	5·6	66·1	*75–79*	333·3	119·9
10–14	0·2	0·0	*45–49*	6·9	76·7	*80–84*	474·9	136·5
15–19	1·2	1·1	*50–54*	11·1	102·6	*85–89*	527·5	130·9
20–24	3·5	2·9	*55–59*	27·0	118·8	*90–94*	353·6	131·4
25–29	5·5	5·4	*60–64*	60·1	126·7	*95+*	135·5	225·2
30–34	4·7	12·9	*65–69*	113·1	133·4	*All ages*	25·6	50·2

SEX AND AGE DISTRIBUTION

	Male	*Female*
Mean age (*years*)	69·0	58·5
95% between ages	29 & 88	34 & 84
Children under 15 (%)	0·1	0·0
Median age (*years*)	71·9	58·3
Proportion by sex (%)	33·0	67·0
Proportion of all cancers by sex (%)	8·4	17·8
Trend over 10 years	(–)	(–)

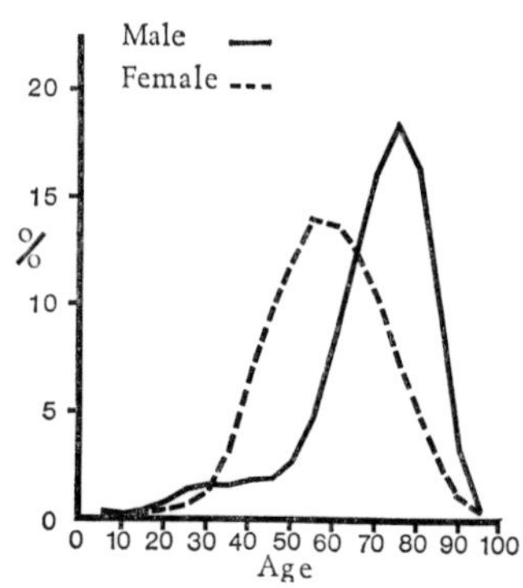

NOTES

Includes: All sites of male or female genital systems. Tumours of the scrotum, which are classified in the 8th revision among skin tumours, are included here.

Excludes: BREAST.

5-YEAR SURVIVAL RATES BY AGE

Crude —— *Corrected* ----

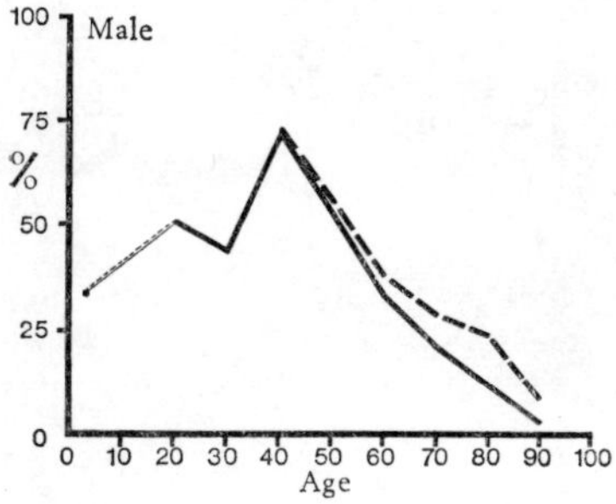

ALL CASES

Total 6092
Male 2036
Female 4056

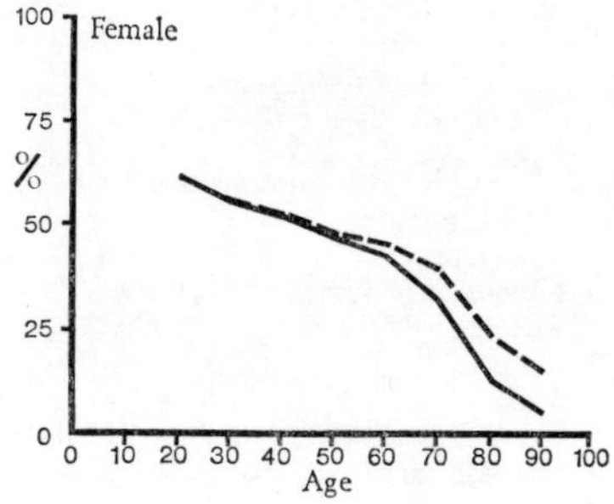

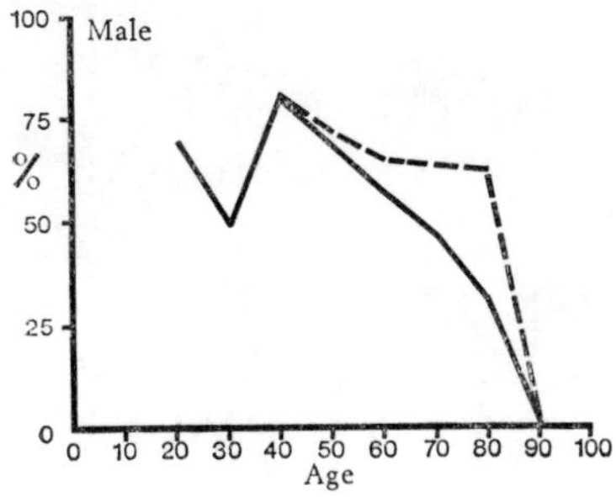

RADICAL TREATMENT

(53·9% of total)
14·2% *male*
73·9% *female*

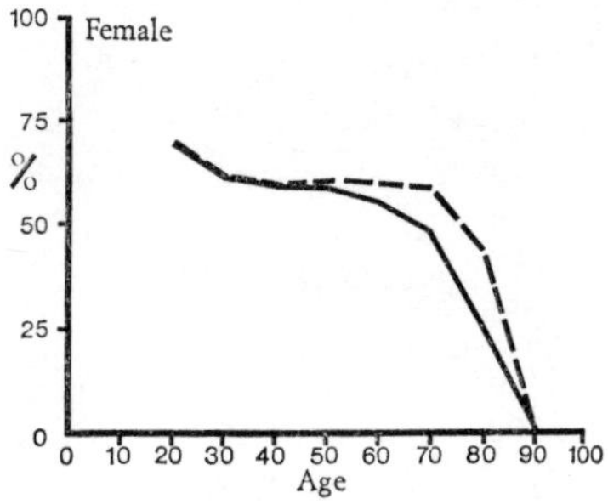

INDICES OF SURVIVAL

	All cases *Male*	All cases *Female*	Radical Treatment *Male*	Radical Treatment *Female*
FIVE YEAR SURVIVAL RATE (%)				
Crude	22·2	39·7	56·4	53·1
Corrected	*33·3*	*44·4*	*64·5*	*58·1*
Total cases†	2036	4056	289	2996
TEN YEAR SURVIVAL RATE (%)				
Crude	16·3	33·2	43·9	42·4
Corrected	*35·4*	*42·3*	*65·2*	*52·8*
Total cases†	1232	3199	305	2453
SURVIVAL TIME (*months*)				
First quartile (75% S.R.)	2·9	5·9	16·0	16·0
Median (50% S.R.)	**19·6**	**26·3**	**>60**	**>60**
Third quartile (25% S.R.)	52·5	>60	>60	>60

†Number of cases on which survival rate is based

ANNUAL SURVIVAL RATES

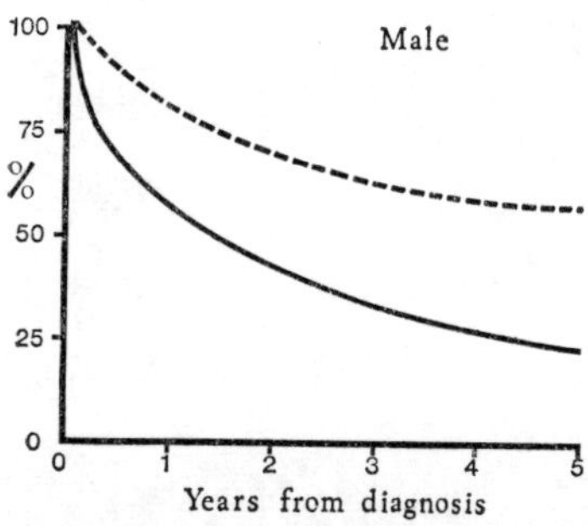

All cases ——
Radical treatment ----

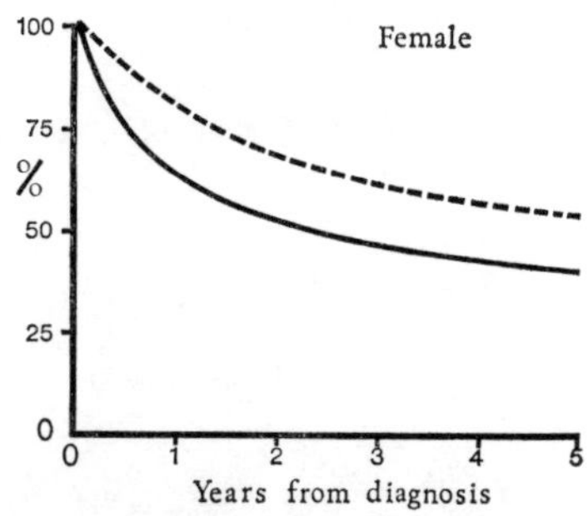

GENITAL SYSTEM

	Distribution (%) of system *Male*	Distribution (%) of system *Female*	5-Year Survival Rate (%) *Male*	5-Year Survival Rate (%) *Female*
Female Genital System				
Ovary—right		7·4		32·4
—left		7·1		29·6
—both		5·7		18·9
—unspecified		8·3		12·4
Fallopian tube—right		0·1		*100·0*
—left		0·1		*40·0*
—unspecified		0·1		*33·3*
Endometrium		24·8		62·2
Endocervix		3·3		43·9
Cervix, not further specified		31·6		39·1
Uterus, other and unspecified		3·6		27·0
Vagina		1·6		16·1
Vulva		5·7		40·6
Female genitalia, other and multiple sites		0·5		35·3
Female genitalia, no further detail		0·1		*0·0*
Whole system		**100·0**		**39·7**
Total cases		11,430		4,056
Male Genital System				
Prostate	84·1		17·0	
Testis—right	4·4		55·7	
—left	3·9		45·8	
—unspecified	0·5		*44·4*	
Epididymis	0·0*		*0·0*	
Spermatic cord	0·0*		*100·0*	
Seminal vesicle	0·0*		*0·0*	
Penis	4·6		48·1	
Scrotum	2·5**		50·0	
Male genitalia, no further detail	0·0*		—	
Whole system	**100·0**		**22·2**	
Total cases	5,678		2,036	

In the subdivisions of the female genital system which are included in the section by site sequence, certain minor variations from ICD definitions may be noted. They include for example the placing of tumours of the broad ligament (an extremely rare location) with "Other Female Genitalia" rather than with "Ovary", and the use of the term "Endometrium" as the description for 182·0 (8th) or 172 (7th), so that for this reason cases of sarcoma of the corpus uteri are included in "Other Uterus". In each case the numbers involved are small, and moreover the magnitude of the difference has been given, either in the Table above, or in the Notes on one of the page-pairs.

**The incidence of epitheliomatous tumours of the scrotum (see p. 162) is approximately four times greater than it is in the rest of Britain. The region from which these figures come includes the greater part of the light engineering manufactories of the country, and men in such work who also come into close contact with mineral oils show an increased incidence of scrotal epitheliomata.

Rates printed in italics are based on less than ten cases

0·0* means (with*) that the number of cases is *not* actually zero, but only to the degree of accuracy quoted, i.e. it is less than 0·05.

0·0 means (without*) that there were in fact *no cases.*

— in the Survival Rate column means that no survival rate can be calculated because there were no cases in that category. This might not accord with the figure given in the Distribution column, which may indicate a non-zero number of cases; the reason for such apparent discrepancies is that the survival rates are based on a fewer number of years than that used as the base of the Distribution figures.

FEMALE GENITAL SYSTEM

Distribution by detailed site of tumour
(5 Year Survival Rates in parenthesis)

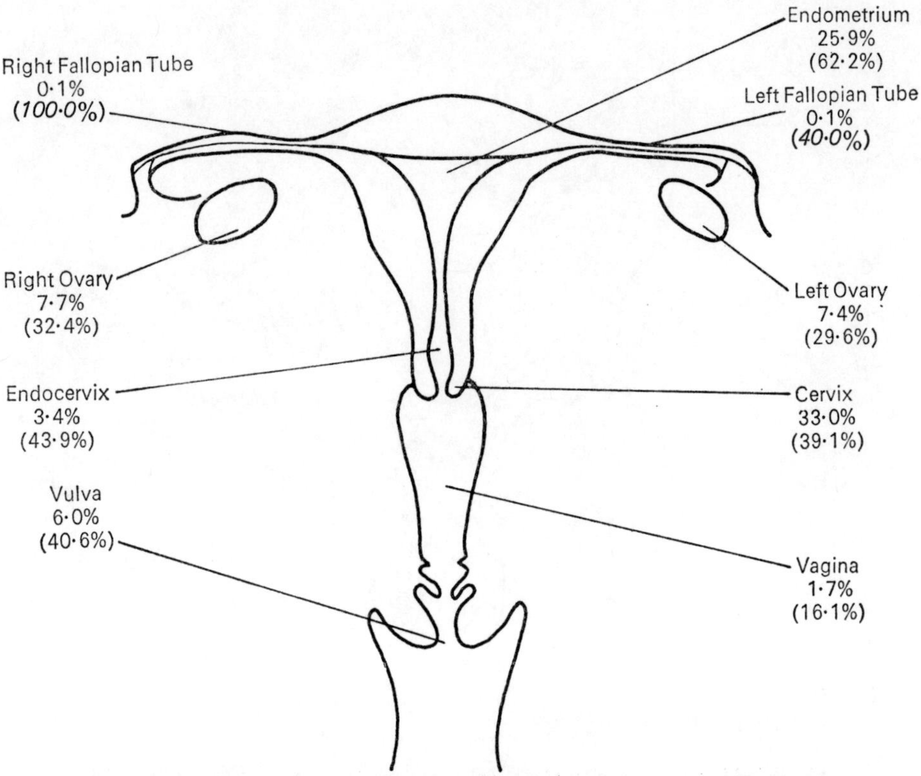

Not included in the illustration above are cases specified as Ovary or Fallopian Tube but where the tumours were bilateral or the side was not known: 14·7% (15·4%)

BASES OF DISTRIBUTIONS

Anatomical only: 10948 cases
5 Year Survival Rates: 3884 cases

5 Year Survival Rates for cases without further specification of site detail:
(172 cases): 27·3%

MALE GENITAL SYSTEM

Distribution by detailed site of tumour
(5 Year Survival Rates in parenthesis)

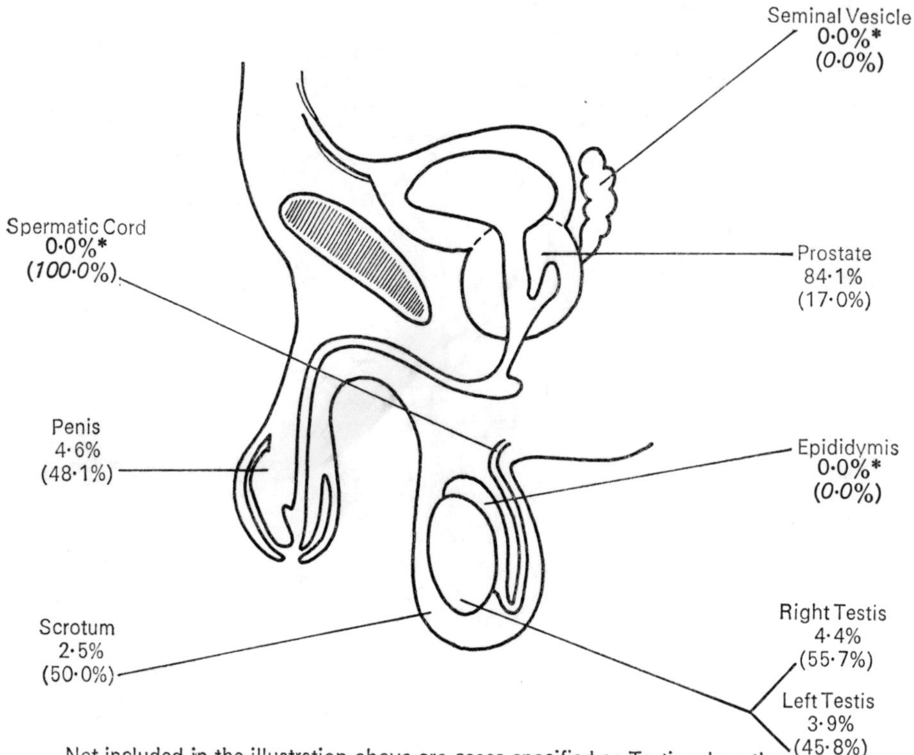

Not included in the illustration above are cases specified as Testis when the side was not known: 0·5% *(44·4%)*

BASES OF DISTRIBUTIONS

Anatomical only: 5677 cases
5 Year Survival Rates: 2036 cases

There were no cases lacking site detail.

INCIDENCE RATE (per 100,000)

Male ——— *Female* - - - -

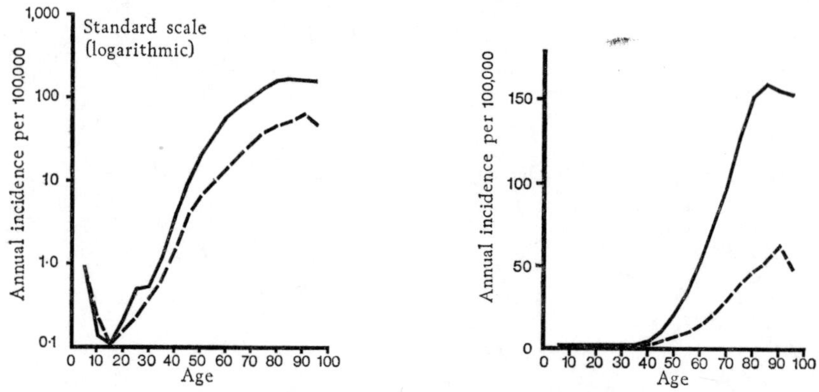

INCIDENCE RATES (per 100,000) by Age

Total cases 2527 *males*; 1011 *females* (of which age not stated for 2 *males* and 0 *females*)

Age	M	F	Age	M	F	Age	M	F
0–4	1·6	1·3	*35–39*	1·9	0·8	*70–74*	114·8	33·2
5–9	0·2	0·5	*40–44*	5·3	1·9	*75–79*	146·6	45·2
10–14	0·1	0·0	*45–49*	12·8	5·2	*80–84*	159·2	47·2
15–19	0·1	0·2	*50–54*	25·8	7·3	*85–89*	154·5	63·6
20–24	0·3	0·1	*55–59*	40·6	11·0	*90–94*	153·8	49·3
25–29	0·6	0·3	*60–64*	67·9	16·2	*95+*	135·5	32·2
30–34	0·4	0·4	*65–69*	82·9	22·7	*All ages*	17·9	7·0

SEX AND AGE DISTRIBUTION

	Male	*Female*
Mean age (*years*)	64·7	66·6
95% between ages	41 & 86	30 & 89
Children under 15 (%)	0·9	1·9
Median age (*years*)	65·0	68·9
Proportion by sex (%)	71·4	28·6
Proportion of all cancers by sex (%)	5·86	2·49
Trend over 10 years	(+)	(+)

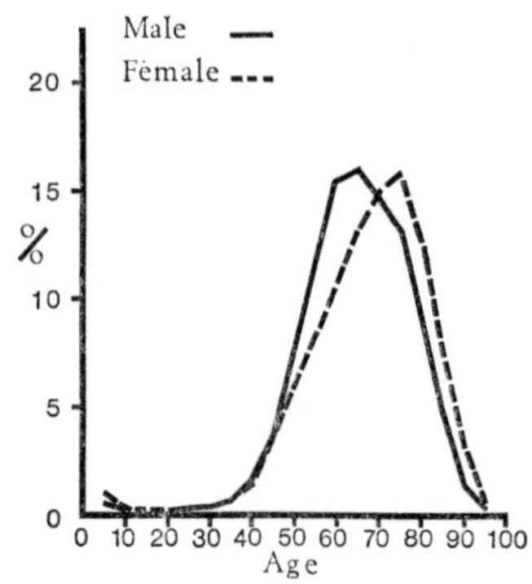

NOTES

Excludes: Urachus (189.9 in 8th revision; 181.7 in 7th), which is classified among extra-gonadal developmental tumours with ENDOCRINE, ETC.

5-YEAR SURVIVAL RATES BY AGE

Crude —— *Corrected* ----

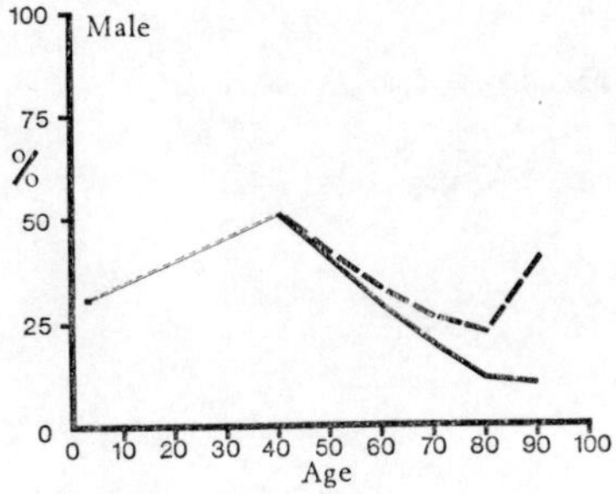

ALL CASES

Total 1791
Male 1280
Female 511

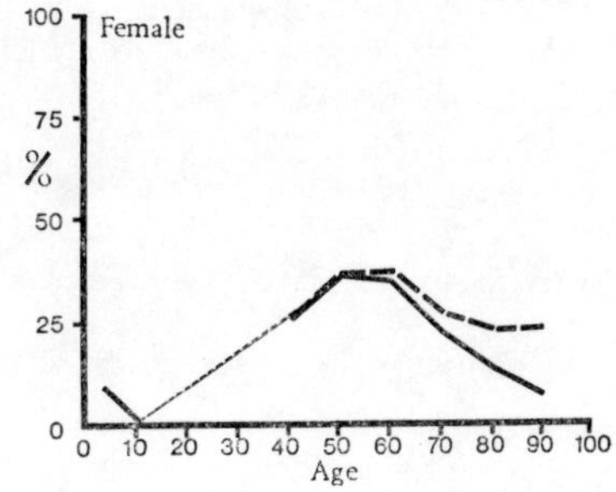

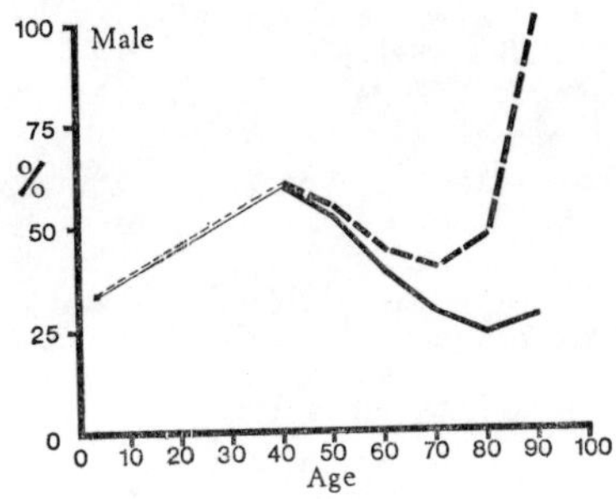

RADICAL TREATMENT

(62·5% of total)
64·0% *male*
58·7% *female*

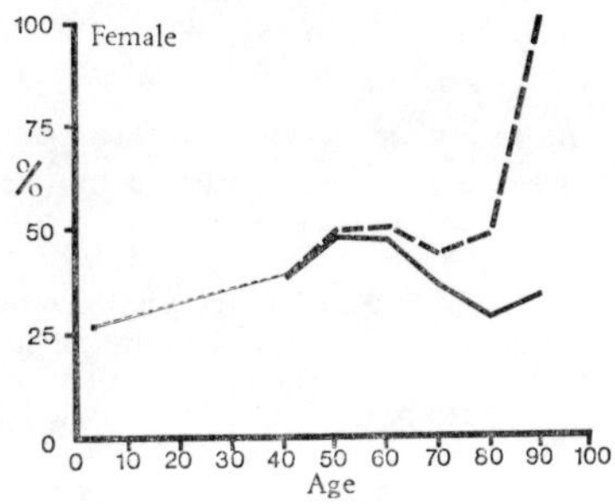

INDICES OF SURVIVAL

	All cases		Radical Treatment	
	Male	*Female*	*Male*	*Female*
FIVE YEAR SURVIVAL RATE (%)				
Crude	24·4	23·3	37·0	38·3
Corrected	*32·2*	*29·1*	*46·3*	*45·3*
Total cases†	1280	511	819	300
TEN YEAR SURVIVAL RATE (%)				
Crude	17·3	16·0	25·4	27·2
Corrected	*31·0*	*24·8*	*41·2*	*38·9*
Total cases†	984	401	619	228
†Number of cases on which survival rate is based				
SURVIVAL TIME (*months*)				
First quartile (75% S.R.)	2·9	2·1	8·9	12·4
Median (50% S.R.)	**12·3**	**12·6**	**31·8**	**36·0**
Third quartile (25% S.R.)	56·1	54·3	>60	>60

ANNUAL SURVIVAL RATES

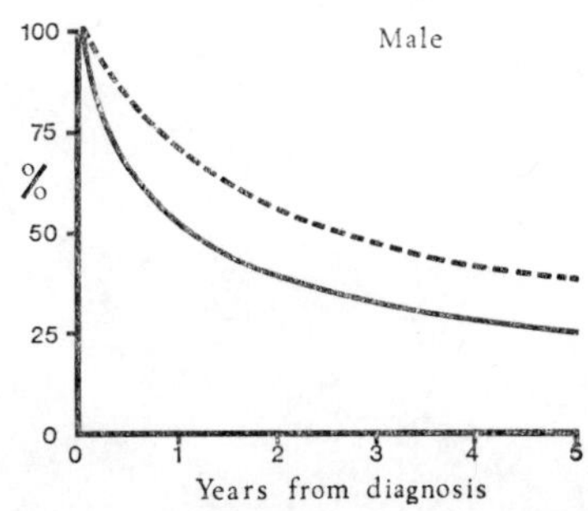

All cases ——
Radical treatment ----

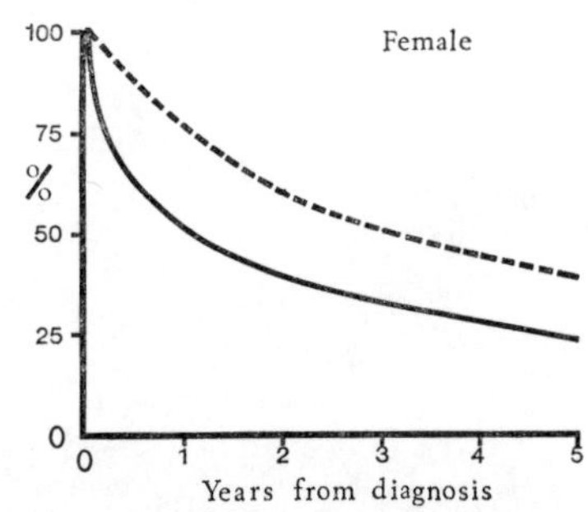

URINARY SYSTEM

	Distribution (%) of System		5-Year Survival Rate (%)	
	Male	*Female*	*Male*	*Female*
Kidney pelvis—right	1·2	1·8	38·5	10·0
—left	1·4	1·3	12·5	*0·0*
—unspecified	0·2	0·2	*33·3*	—
Kidney other and unspecified—right	9·0	14·9	24·2	16·7
—left	9·3	13·5	32·2	25·0
—unspecified	2·3	2·3	0·0	9·1
Ureter—right	0·4	0·8	*0·0*	*50·0*
—left	0·4	0·4	*83·3*	*0·0*
—unspecified	0·1	0·1	*100·0*	*0·0*
Bladder	75·0	62·7	23·8	25·0
Urethra	0·6	2·0	14·3	35·7
Urinary system, no further detail	0·1	0·0	—	—
Whole system	**100·0**	**100·0**	**24·4**	**23·3**
Total Cases	3,932	1,582	1,280	511

Rates printed in italics are based on less than ten cases

0·0* means (with*) that the number of cases is *not* actually zero, but only to the degree of accuracy quoted, i.e. it is less than 0·05.

0·0 means (without*) that there were in fact *no cases.*

— in the Survival Rate column means that no survival rate can be calculated because there were no cases in that category. This might not accord with the figure given in the Distribution column, which may indicate a non-zero number of cases; the reason for such apparent discrepancies is that the survival rates are based on a fewer number of years than that used as the base of the Distribution figures.

URINARY

Distribution by detailed site of tumour
(5 Year Survival Rates in parenthesis)

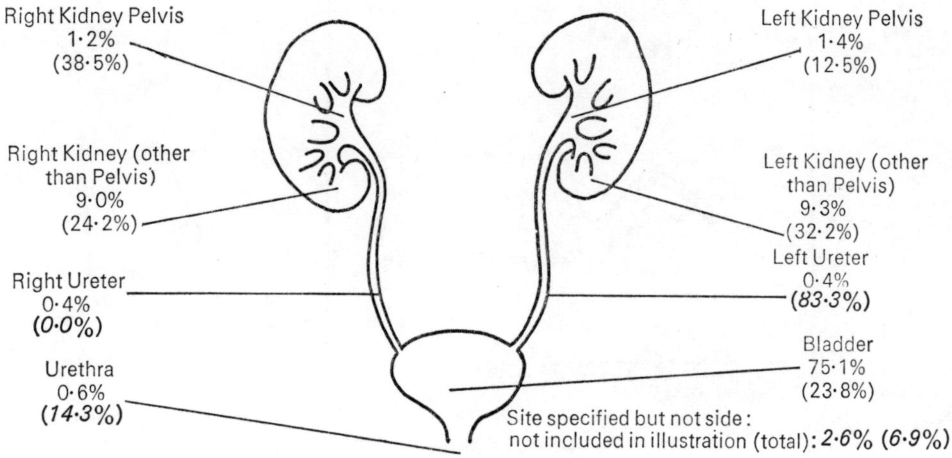

Males

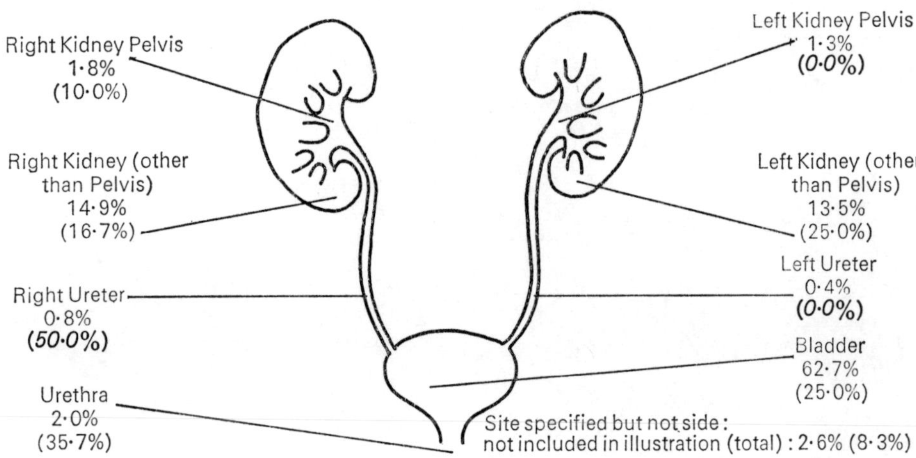

Females

Bases of Distributions

Anatomical only: 3929 cases (Males); 1582 cases (Females)
5 Year Survival Rates: 1280 cases (Males); 511 cases (Females)

There were no cases lacking site detail.

NERVOUS SYSTEM,
EYE AND EAR

ICD (8th) **190–192, 160.1, 225.0, .2, .3, .4, .9, 238.1, .3, .4, .5, .9**

INCIDENCE RATE (per 100,000)

Male ——— *Female* - - - -

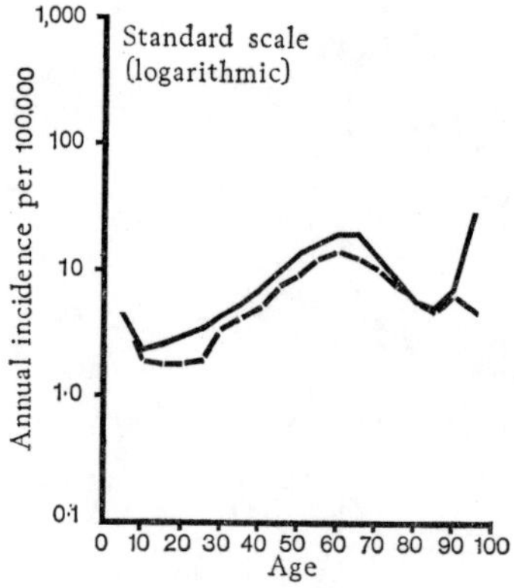

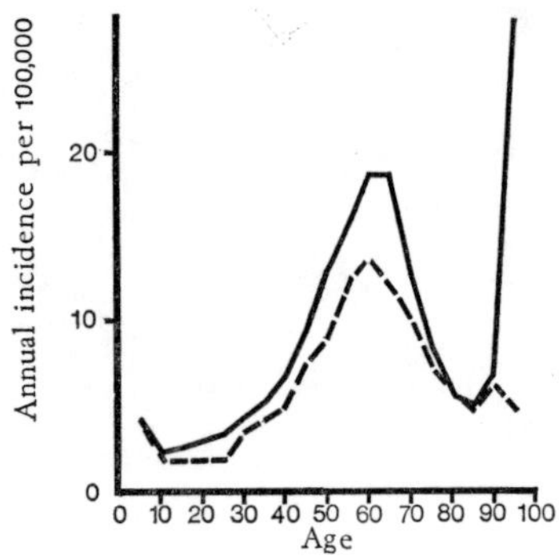

INCIDENCE RATES (per 100,000) by Age

Total cases 1033 *males*; 845 *females* (of which age not stated for 2 *males* and 1 *female*)

Age	M	F	Age	M	F	Age	M	F
0–4	5·6	6·2	*35–39*	5·4	3·5	*70–74*	10·1	7·8
5–9	2·4	2·0	*40–44*	7·8	6·3	*75–79*	5·5	6·3
10–14	2·0	1·7	*45–49*	10·7	8·4	*80–84*	5·6	4·0
15–19	2·9	1·7	*50–54*	15·0	9·4	*85–89*	2·7	6·2
20–24	2·7	1·7	*55–59*	16·0	14·8	*90–94*	30·8	5·5
25–29	3·8	1·9	*60-64*	21·5	12·1	*95+*	0·0	0·0
30–34	4·7	4·9	*65–69*	14·1	11·7	*All ages*	7·3	5·9

SEX AND AGE DISTRIBUTION

	Male	*Female*
Mean age (*years*)	45·6	46·9
95% between ages	2 & 74	2 & 78
Children under 15 (%)	6·9	7·7
Median age (*years*)	50·5	51·9
Proportion by sex (%)	55·0	45·0
Proportion of all cancers by sex (%)	2·4	2·1
Trend over 10 years	(+)	(+)

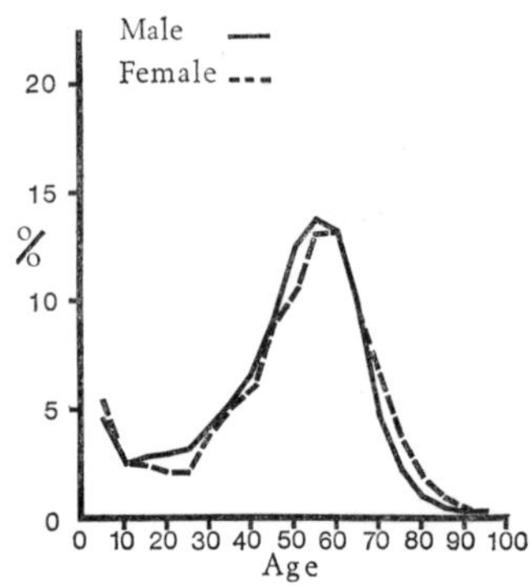

NOTES

Includes: Benign and unspecified tumours of the central nervous system (225 and 238 in 8th revision; 223 and 237 in 7th; but excluding peripheral nervous system).
Ear (other than skin of ear), which is omitted from the separate site page-pairs.

ICD (7th) **192, 193, 160.1, 223 (part), 237 (part)**

NERVOUS SYSTEM

5-YEAR SURVIVAL RATES BY AGE

Crude —— *Corrected* ----

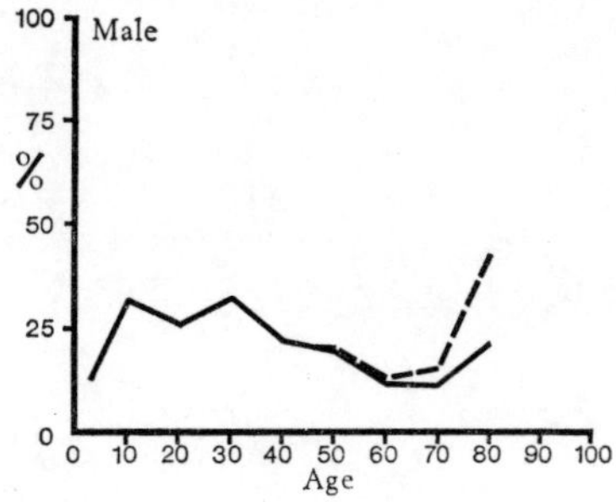

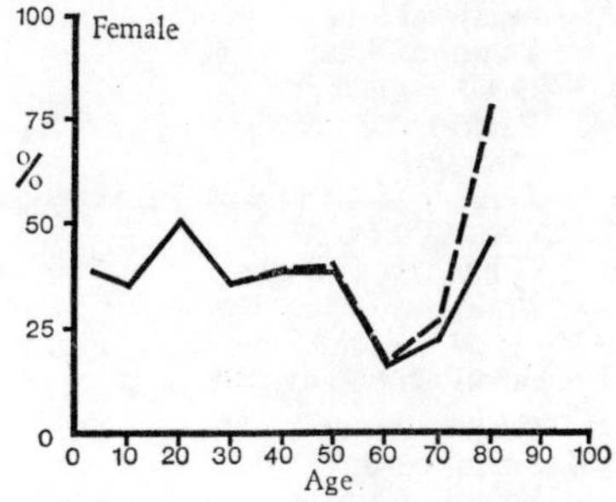

ALL CASES

Total 958
Male 504
Female 454

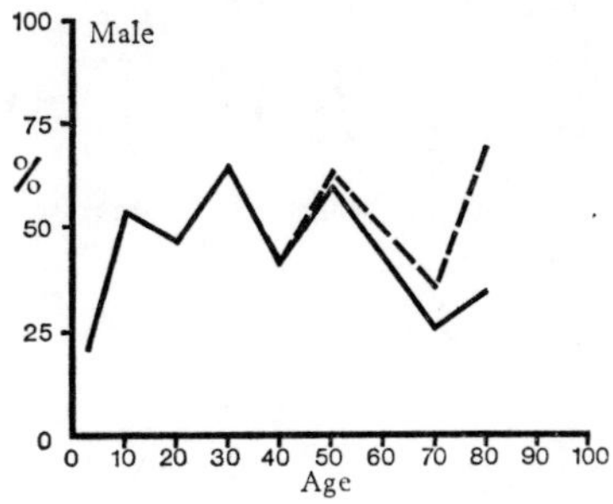

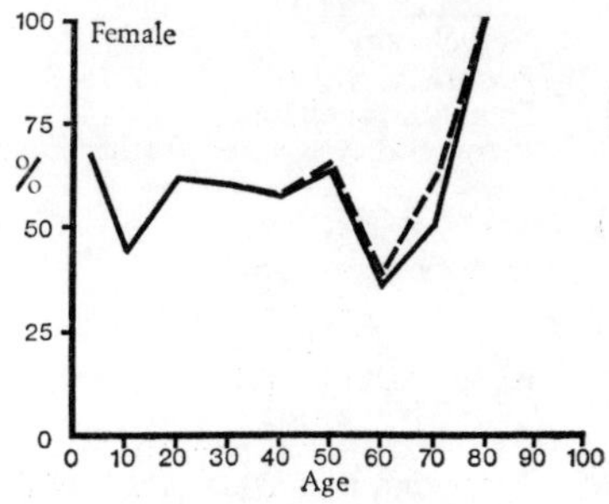

RADICAL TREATMENT

(36·6% of total)
31·2% *male*
42·7% *female*

INDICES OF SURVIVAL

	All cases		Radical Treatment	
	Male	*Female*	*Male*	*Female*
FIVE YEAR SURVIVAL RATE (%)				
Crude	17·5	30·6	43·9	54·6
Corrected	*19·1*	*32·4*	*48·0*	*57·8*
Total cases†	504	454	157	194
TEN YEAR SURVIVAL RATE (%)				
Crude	18·1	24·3	45·4	56·6
Corrected	*21·0*	*27·1*	*52·3*	*63·5*
Total cases†	404	411	141	158
SURVIVAL TIME (*months*)				
First quartile (75% S.R.)	0·8	0·9	10·0	13·1
Median (50% S.R.)	**3·5**	**8·4**	**37·5**	**>60**
Third quartile (25% S.R.)	26·3	>60	>60	>60

†Number of cases on which survival rate is based

ANNUAL SURVIVAL RATES

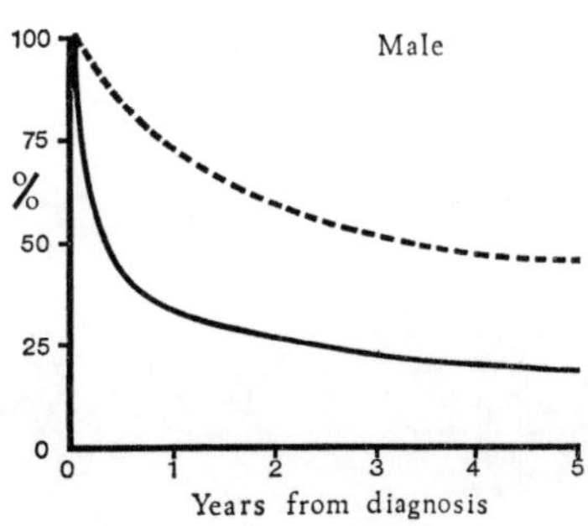

All cases ——
Radical treatment ----

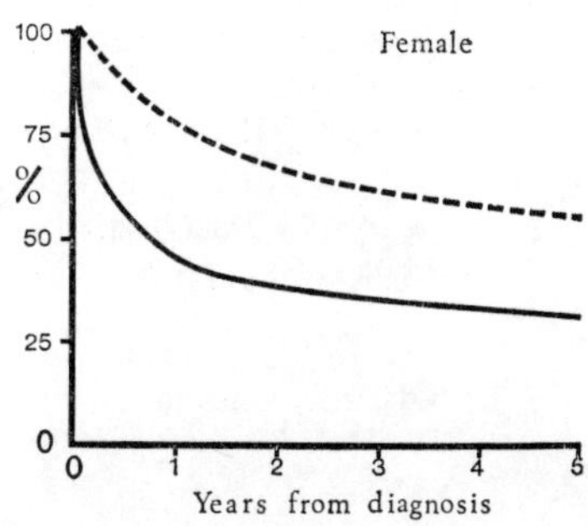

CENTRAL AND PERIPHERAL NERVOUS SYSTEM, EYE AND EAR

	Distribution (%) of System		5-Year Survival Rate (%)	
	Male	*Female*	*Male*	*Female*
Central nervous system	**80·8**	**74·9**	**11·5**	**24·3**
Frontal lobe	15·2	14·8	12·5	20·5
Parietal lobe	12·9	10·7	11·1	27·5
Occipital lobe	3·1	3·8	23·5	38·9
Temporal lobe	15·9	10·6	3·0	22·2
Basal ganglia	0·5	0·5	—	*0·0*
Lateral and third ventricles	2·5	2·8	38·5	7·7
Mid brain	1·0	1·3	*20·0*	*37·5*
Pons, medulla and fourth ventricle	4·3	3·5	14·3	43·8
Cerebellum	4·9	5·3	31·8	47·8
Other specified site	9·2	8·3	6·6	16·7
Brain, no further detail	11·3	13·3	6·0	18·5
Peripheral nervous system	**8·4**	**11·5**	**35·4**	**47·6**
Cranial nerves	0·8	2·8	*60·0*	53·8
Spinal cord	2·6	3·2	60·0	*66·7*
Spinal meninges	0·3	0·6	*50·0*	*66·7*
Cauda equina	0·3	0·1	*0·0*	—
Nerve roots	0·3	0·5	*100·0*	*50·0*
Peripheral nerves	1·1	0·9	*0·0*	*60·0*
Sympathetic chain	2·9	2·9	11·8	23·1
Peripheral system, no further detail	0·1	0·5	—	—
Eye and orbit	**8·2**	**11·6**	**57·5**	**58·0**
Intra-ocular—right	3·0	5·4	62·5	76·9
—left	3·4	4·7	66·7	40·0
—unspecified	0·4	0·1	—	—
Extra-ocular—right	0·4	0·4	*75·0*	*100·0*
—left	0·3	0·4	*33·3*	*66·7*
—unspecified	0·1	0·0	—	—
Eye, orbit, no further detail—right	0·1	0·3	—	*0·0*
—left	0·4	0·2	*0·0*	—
—unspecified	0·1	0·1	—	—
Ear	**2·6**	**2·0**	**11·8**	**41·7**
External meatus—right	0·7	0·1	*100·0*	*100·0*
—left	0·4	0·5	*33·3*	*50·0*
—unspecified	0·0	0·0	—	—
Middle ear—right	0·6	0·5	*0·0*	*50·0*
—left	0·7	0·8	*0·0*	*33·3*
—unspecified	0·1	0·0	—	—
Inner ear	0·0	0·0	—	—
Ear, no further detail—right	0·0	0·0	*0·0*	—
—left	0·0	0·1	—	—
—unspecified	0·1	0·0	—	—
Whole system	**100·0**	**100·0**	**17·5**	**30·6**
Total cases	1,568	1,331	504	454

Benign and unspecified tumours of the central nervous system (225 and 238 in 8th revision; 223 and 237 in 7th; but excluding peripheral nervous system) are included in the table above.

No separate diagram is included for the peripheral nervous system.

No separate diagram is included for the eye.

No separate diagram is included for the ear.

Rates printed in italics are based on less than ten cases

0·0* means (with*) that the number of cases is *not* actually zero, but only to the degree of accuracy quoted, i.e. it is less than 0·05.

0·0 means (without*) that there were in fact *no cases.*

— in the Survival Rate column means that no survival rate can be calculated because there were no cases in that category. This might not accord with the figure given in the Distribution column, which may indicate a non-zero number of cases; the reason for such apparent discrepancies is that the survival rates are based on a fewer number of years than that used as the base of the Distribution figures.

BRAIN

Distribution by detailed site of tumour
(5 Year Survival Rates in parenthesis)

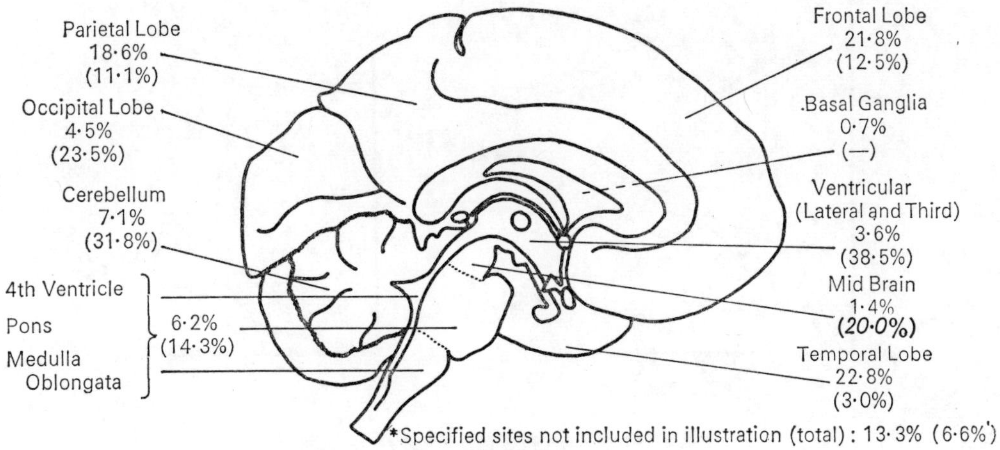

Males

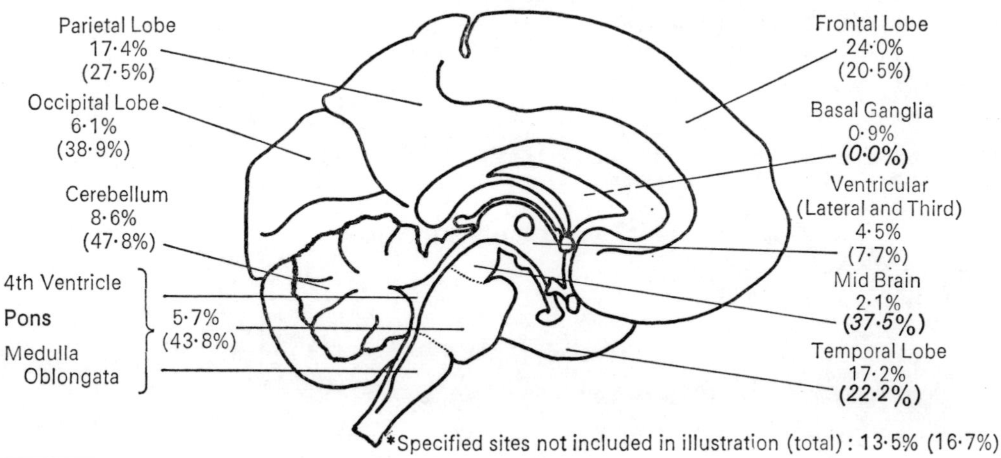

Females

Bases of Distributions

Anatomical only: 1091 cases (Males); 821 cases (Females)
5 Year Survival Rates: 349 cases (Males); 296 cases (Females)

5 Year Survival Rates for cases without further specification of site detail:

Males	(50 cases):	6·0%
Females	(54 cases):	18·5%

* Refers chiefly to cases which do not fall clearly into one of the listed categories, i.e. to ill-defined cases, but also includes some cases which were grouped together in the form of anatomical coding used.

ENDOCRINE GLANDS, ETC. ICD (8th) **193, 194**

INCIDENCE RATE (per 100,000)

Male —— *Female* ----

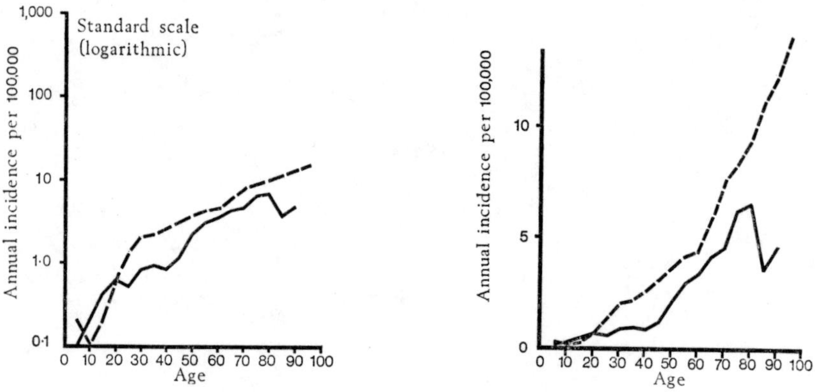

INCIDENCE RATES (per 100,000) by Age

Total cases 198 *males*; 391 *females* (of which age not stated for 1 *male* and 1 *female*)

Age	M	F	Age	M	F	Age	M	F
0–4	0·2	0·4	*35–39*	0·7	1·9	*70–74*	4·7	8·2
5–9	0·1	0·0	*40–44*	0·9	3·1	*75–79*	8·5	8·4
10–14	0·2	0·3	*45–49*	1·4	2·9	*80–84*	2·8	10·9
15–19	0·6	0·1	*50–54*	2·9	4·3	*85–89*	5·3	11·2
20–24	0·5	1·1	*55–59*	2·9	3·9	*90–94*	0·0	16·4
25–29	0·5	1·6	*60–64*	3·9	4·7	*95+*	0·0	0·0
30–34	1·0	2·3	*65–69*	4·3	6·9	*All ages*	1·4	2·7

SEX AND AGE DISTRIBUTION

	Male	*Female*
Mean age (*years*)	53·9	56·6
95% between ages	13 & 80	21 & 86
Children under 15 (%)	3·0	1·8
Median age (*years*)	56·4	58·1
Proportion by sex (%)	33·6	66·4
Proportion of all cancers by sex (%)	0·46	0·96
Trend over 10 years	(−)	(+)

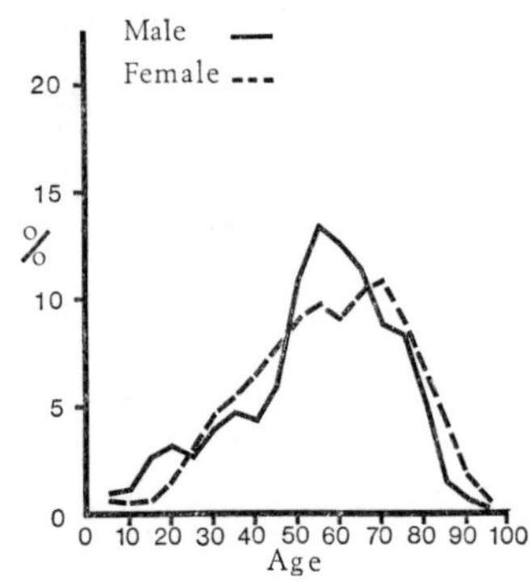

NOTES

Includes: Extra-gonadal developmental tumours, which are omitted from the separate site page-pairs. These comprise chiefly craniopharyngioma (21 cases) and chordoma (16 cases), the remainder being made up of teratoma, urachus, branchial cleft, etc.

5-YEAR SURVIVAL RATES BY AGE

Crude —— *Corrected* ----

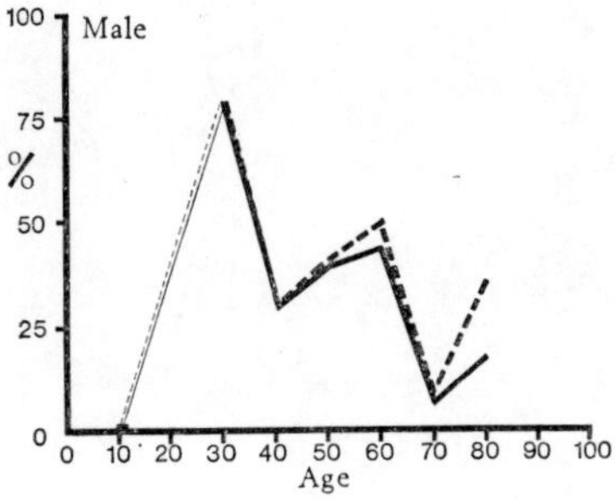

ALL CASES

Total 286
Male 113
Female 173

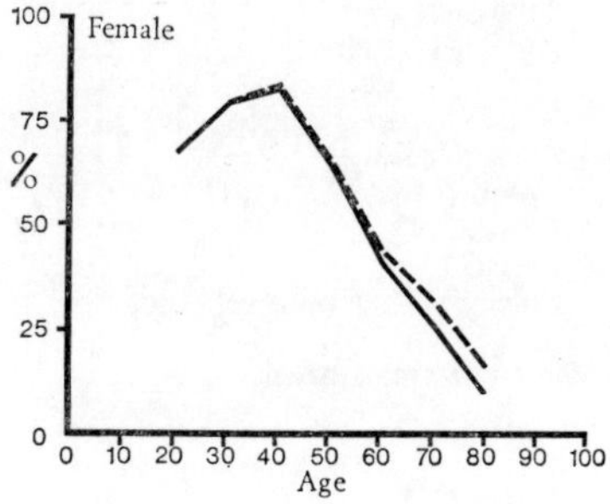

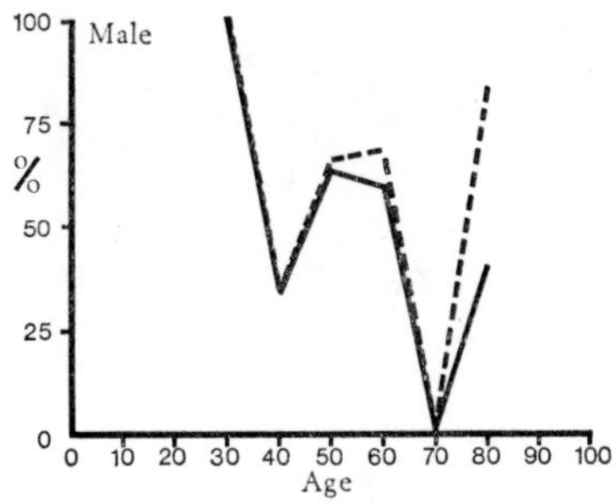

RADICAL TREATMENT

(60·8% of total)
52·2% *male*
66·5% *female*

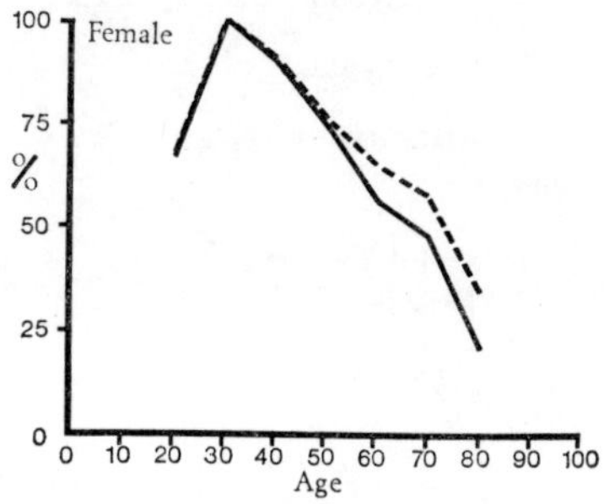

INDICES OF SURVIVAL

	All cases *Male*	All cases *Female*	Radical Treatment *Male*	Radical Treatment *Female*
FIVE YEAR SURVIVAL RATE (%)				
Crude	31·9	47·4	52·5	68·7
Corrected	*37·7*	*53·6*	*60·0*	*74·0*
Total cases†	113	173	59	115
TEN YEAR SURVIVAL RATE (%)				
Crude	29·5	37·0	48·9	57·3
Corrected	*38·3*	*47·6*	*59·8*	*67·9*
Total cases†	88	138	47	82

†Number of cases on which survival rate is based

SURVIVAL TIME (*months*)				
First quartile (75% S.R.)	1·0	2·4	15·5	33·5
Median (50% S.R.)	**17·3**	**47·5**	**>60**	**>60**
Third quartile (25% S.R.)	>60	>60	>60	>60

ANNUAL SURVIVAL RATES

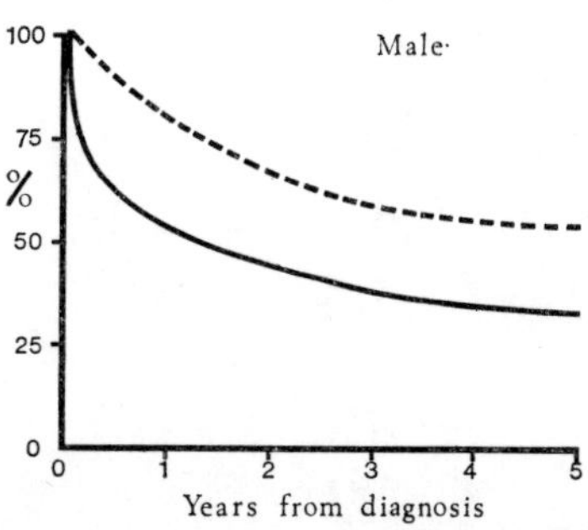

All cases ——
Radical treatment - - - -

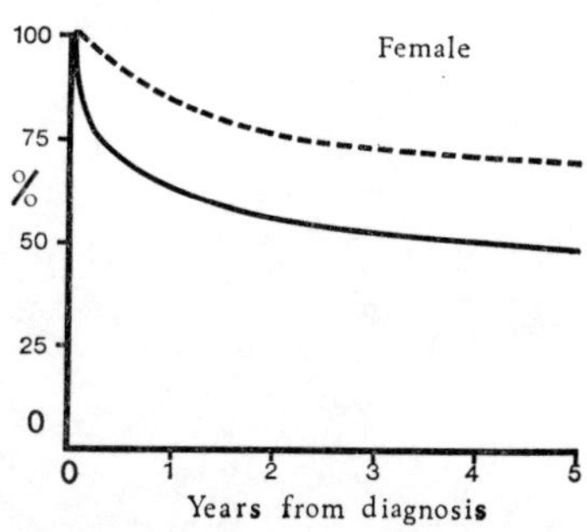

ENDOCRINE GLANDS, CHEMORECEPTOR AND DEVELOPMENTAL TUMOURS

	Distribution (%) of System		5-Year Survival Rate (%)	
	Male	*Female*	*Male*	*Female*
Endocrine Glands				
(excluding pancreas and gonads)				
Thyroid	51·8	80·7	23·9	48·9
Adrenal—right	3·6	1·5	*0·0*	*0·0*
—left	2·1	2·5	*25·0*	*50·0*
—unspecified	4·3	0·7	*0·0*	*0·0*
Parathyroid	0·7	0·2	0·0	—
Thymus	5·0	2·3	25·0	50·0
Pituitary	29·6	11·5	53·3	38·9
Pineal	2·9	0·6	0·0	—
Spleen (other than reticulosis)	0·0	0·0	—	—
Whole endocrine system	**100·0**	**100·0**	**32·3**	**48·5**
Total cases	280	529	99	167
Chemoreceptor				
Chemodectoma—carotid body	41·7	36·8	50·0	66·7
—other sites	8·3	5·3	—	—
Glomus jugulare	50·0	57·9	100·0	100·0
Whole chemoreceptor system	**100·0**	**100·0**	**66·7**	**85·7**
Total cases	12	19	3	7
Developmental Tumours (Extra-gonadal)**	**100·0**	**100·0**	**28·6**	**16·7**
Total cases	30	26	14	6

No separate diagram is included for these tumours.

**Extra-gonadal developmental tumours comprise chiefly craniopharyngioma (21 cases) and chordoma (16 cases), the remainder being made up of teratoma, urachus, branchial cleft, etc.

Rates printed in italics are based on less than ten cases

0·0* means (with*) that the number of cases is *not* actually zero, but only to the degree of accuracy quoted, i.e. it is less than 0·05.

0·0 means (without*) that there were in fact *no cases.*

— in the Survival Rate column means that no survival rate can be calculated because there were no cases in that category. This might not accord with the figure given in the Distribution column, which may indicate a non-zero number of cases; the reason for such apparent discrepancies is that the survival rates are based on a fewer number of years than that used as the base of the Distribution figures.

MALIGNANT LYMPHOMAS **ICD (8th) 200–203**

INCIDENCE RATE (per 100,000)

Male —— *Female* - - - -

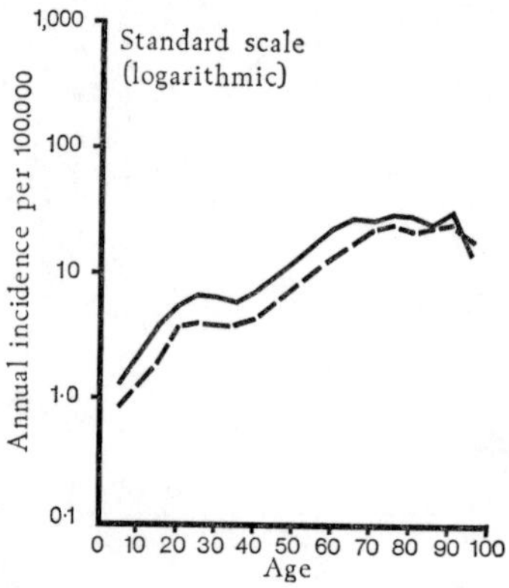

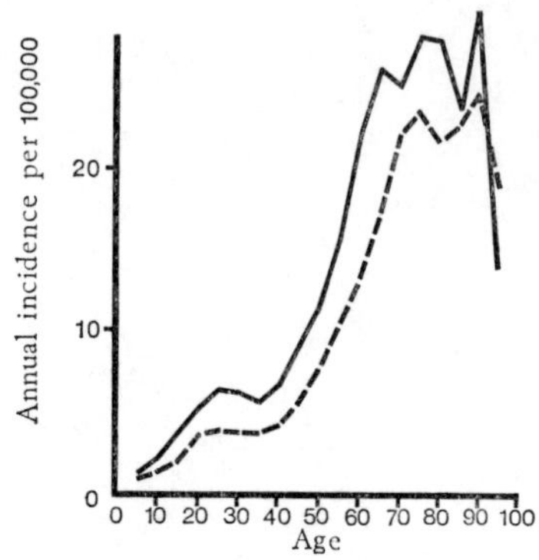

INCIDENCE RATES (per 100,000) by Age

Total cases 1262 *males*; 985 *females* (of which age not stated for 0 *males* and 1 *female*)

Age	M	F	Age	M	F	Age	M	F
0–4	1·1	0·4	*35–39*	5·2	3·5	*70–74*	25·6	24·5
5–9	1·4	1·3	*40–44*	8·0	4·8	*75–79*	31·5	21·6
10–14	2·7	1·0	*45–49*	9·9	6·0	*80–84*	20·6	21·3
15–19	4·5	2·7	*50–54*	13·0	9·0	*85–89*	32·0	24·9
20–24	6·1	3·9	*55–59*	18·3	11·4	*90–94*	15·4	21·9
25–29	6·6	3·4	*60–64*	27·0	14·9	*95+*	0·0	0·0
30–34	5·7	3·8	*65–69*	24·4	19·6	*All ages*	8·9	6·8

SEX AND AGE DISTRIBUTION

	Male	*Female*
Mean age (*years*)	50·5	56·3
95% between ages	11 & 81	11 & 88
Children under 15 (%)	4·8	3·0
Median age (*years*)	54·3	60·2
Proportion by sex (%)	56·2	43·8
Proportion of all cancers by sex (%)	2·9	2·4
Trend over 10 years	(+)	(+)

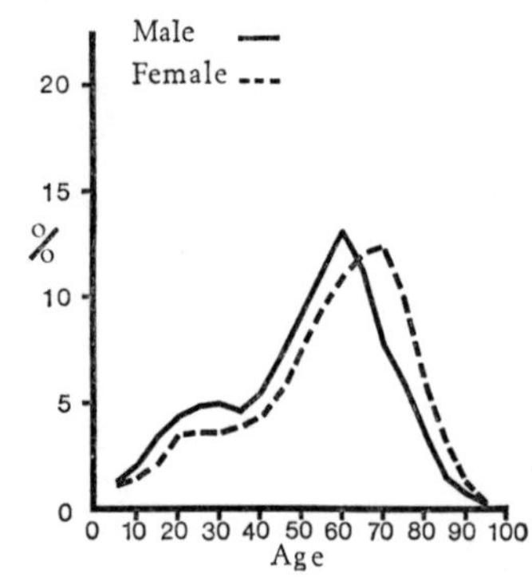

NOTES

Includes: Unifocal tumours of the lymphoid system.

5-YEAR SURVIVAL RATES BY AGE

Crude —— *Corrected* ----

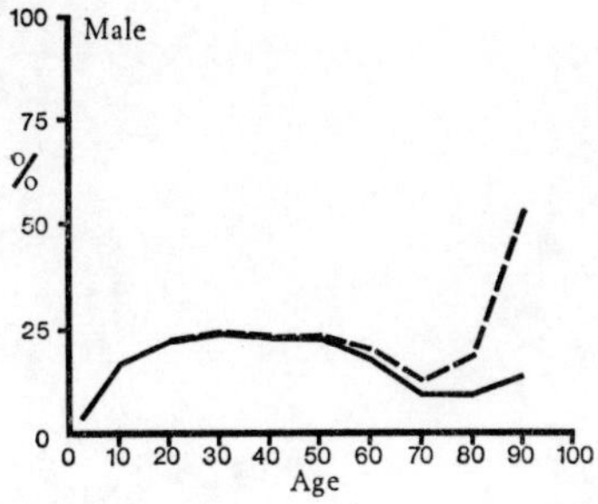

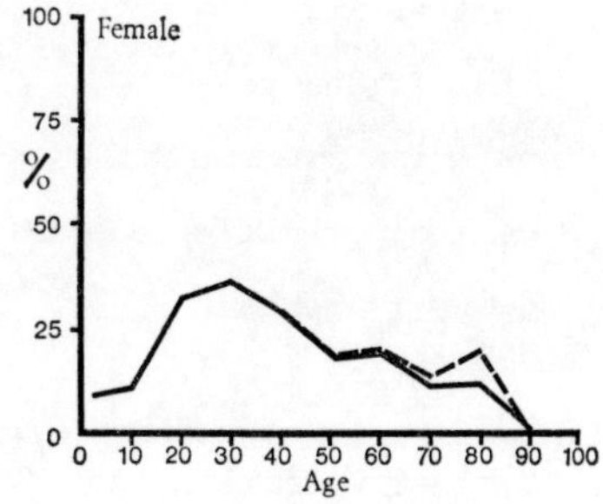

ALL CASES

Total 1213
Male 685
Female 528

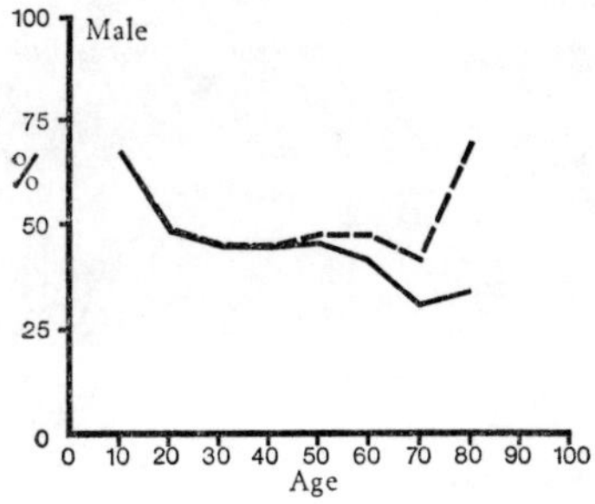

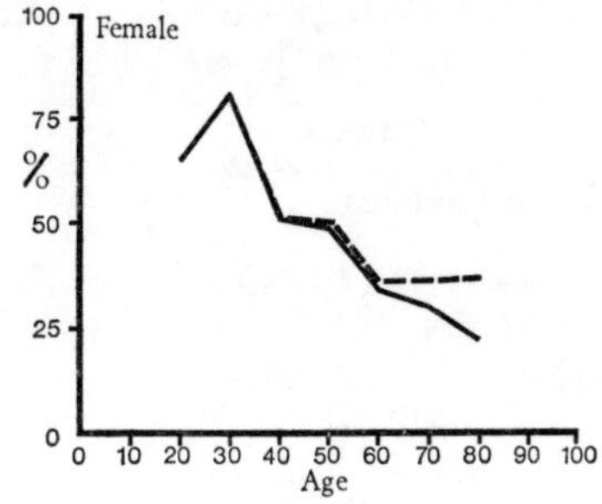

RADICAL TREATMENT

(27·4% of total)
28·2% *male*
26·3% *female*

INDICES OF SURVIVAL

	All cases		Radical Treatment	
	Male	*Female*	*Male*	*Female*
FIVE YEAR SURVIVAL RATE (%)				
Crude	20·2	22·7	42·5	46·0
Corrected	*22·8*	*25·9*	*46·4*	*50·7*
Total cases†	685	528	193	139
TEN YEAR SURVIVAL RATE (%)				
Crude	15·7	16·4	36·4	32·8
Corrected	*20·4*	*20·9*	*44·4*	*40·4*
Total cases†	407	336	121	116
SURVIVAL TIME (*months*)				
First quartile (75% S.R.)	2·0	2·8	9·0	14·4
Median (50% S.R.)	**8·8**	**11·9**	**41·6**	**53·4**
Third quartile (25% S.R.)	43·0	52·1	>60	>60

†Number of cases on which survival rate is based

ANNUAL SURVIVAL RATES

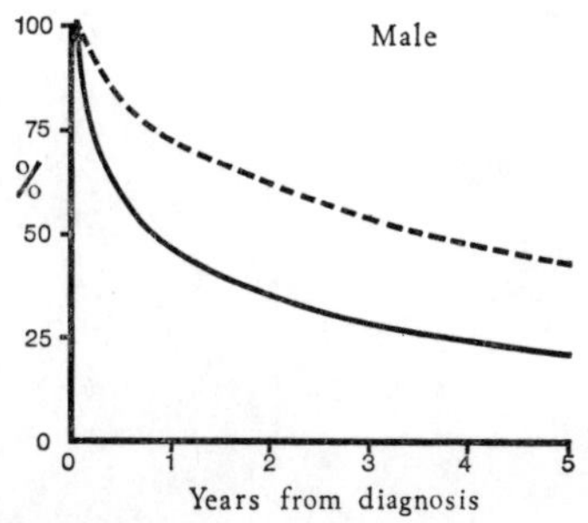

All cases ——
Radical treatment ----

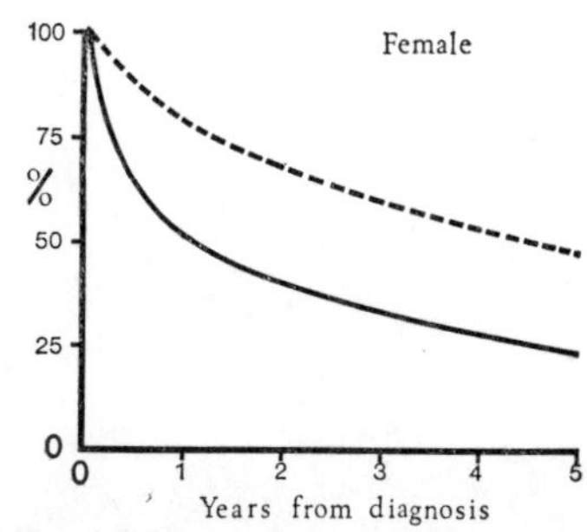

LYMPHOID AND HAEMOPOIETIC SYSTEMS

	Distribution (%) of System		5-Year Survival Rate (%)	
	Male	*Female*	*Male*	*Female*
Malignant lymphomas				
Giant follicular lymphoma	3·2	3·8	50·0	57·9
Lymphosarcoma	20·2	18·5	17·8	20·0
Reticulosarcoma	21·3	22·9	18·1	22·6
Hodgkin's disease	30·6	25·1	20·8	23·6
Mycosis fungoides	1·2	1·2	50·0	*50·0*
Other specified reticulosis	2·2	2·3	57·9	61·1
Myelomatosis	15·2	19·2	6·7	5·6
Malignant reticulosis, no further detail	6·1	7·0	22·2	27·6
All malignant lymphomas	**100·0**	**100·0**	**20·2**	**22·7**
Total Cases	2,028	1,531	685	528
Leukaemias and myeloproliferative diseases				
Leukaemia—acute	45·6	49·5	0·5	1·2
—chronic myelocytic	15·8	20·6	5·8	9·4
—chronic lymphocytic	23·7	18·5	17·2	14·6
—chronic monocytic	0·7	0·4	*0·0*	*66·7*
—other and unspecified	5·8	5·3	0·0	8·0
Polycythaemia	8·0	5·1	63·9	80·0
Thrombocythaemia	0·4	0·5	*50·0*	*50·0*
Myelofibrosis	0·0	0·1	—	*0·0*
All leukaemias, etc.	**100·0**	**100·0**	**10·8**	**10·3**
Total Cases	1,364	1,184	453	407

Rates printed in italics are based on less than ten cases

0·0* means (with*) that the number of cases is *not* actually zero, but only to the degree of accuracy quoted, i.e. it is less than 0·05.

0·0 means (without*) that there were in fact *no cases.*

— in the Survival Rate column means that no survival rate can be calculated because there were no cases in that category. This might not accord with the figure given in the Distribution column, which may indicate a non-zero number of cases; the reason for such apparent discrepancies is that the survival rates are based on a fewer number of years than that used as the base of the Distribution figures.

LEUKAEMIAS, ETC. ICD (8th) **204–208**

INCIDENCE RATE (per 100,000)

Male —— *Female* ----

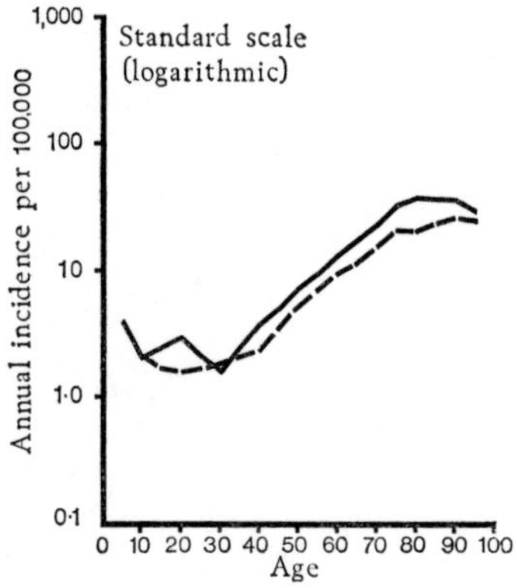

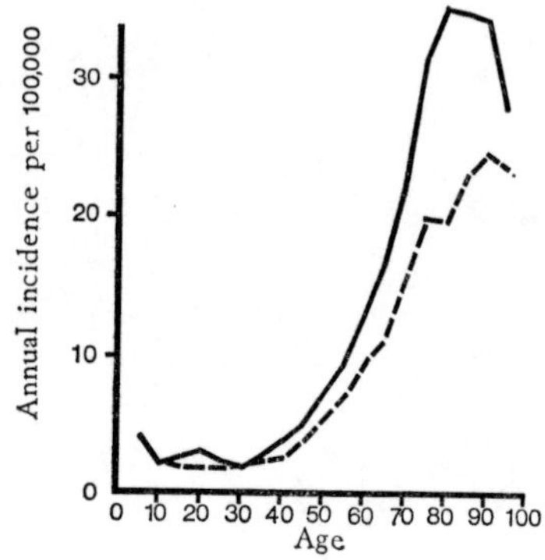

INCIDENCE RATES (per 100,000) by Age

Total cases 876 *males*; 757 *females* (of which age not stated for 2 *males* and 2 *females*)

Age	M	F	Age	M	F	Age	M	F
0–4	5·1	4·7	*35–39*	3·4	2·2	*70–74*	28·8	20·8
5–9	2·3	2·4	*40–44*	3·5	2·3	*75–79*	35·0	18·2
10–14	1·5	1·6	*45–49*	5·9	4·4	*80–84*	34·7	21·8
15–19	3·3	1·6	*50–54*	8·1	6·1	*85–89*	34·6	24·9
20–24	2·2	1·4	*55–59*	10·1	7·4	*90–94*	30·8	21·9
25–29	1·8	1·8	*60–64*	15·9	11·3	*95+*	0·0	32·2
30–34	1·3	1·8	*65–69*	17·0	10·6	*All ages*	6·2	5·2

SEX AND AGE DISTRIBUTION

	Male	*Female*
Mean age (*years*)	51·6	53·9
95% between ages	2 & 84	2 & 87
Children under 15 (%)	11·9	12·6
Median age (*years*)	57·2	60·4
Proportion by sex (%)	53·6	46·4
Proportion of all cancers by sex (%)	2·0	1·9
Trend over 10 years	(+)	(−)

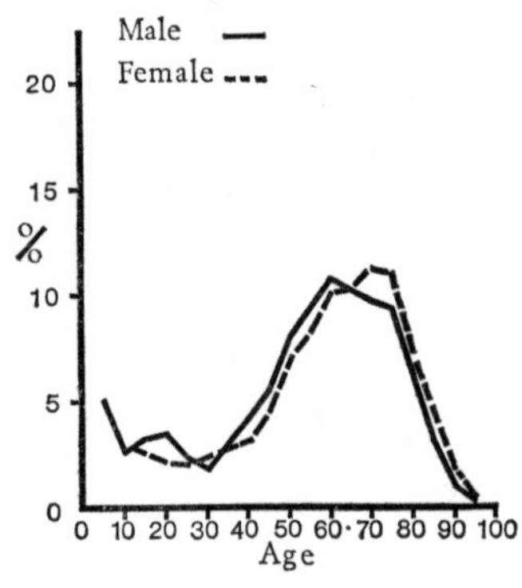

NOTES

Includes: Thrombocythaemia (289.9 in 8th revision; 299 in 7th) and polycythaemia (208 in 8th; 294 in 7th), which are sometimes classed as benign conditions.

5-YEAR SURVIVAL RATES BY AGE

Crude ——— *Corrected* - - - -

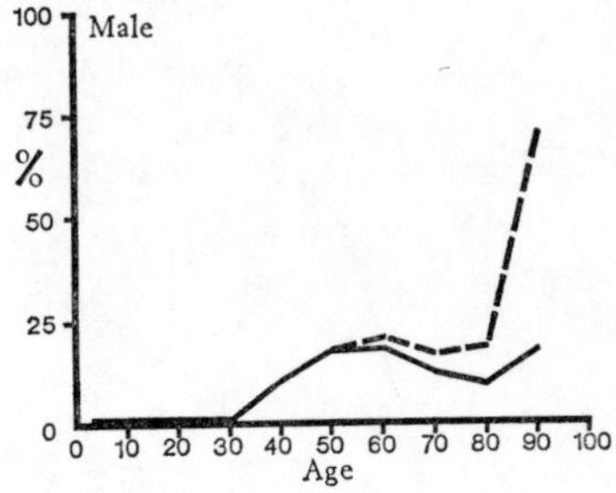

ALL CASES

Total 860
Male 453
Female 407

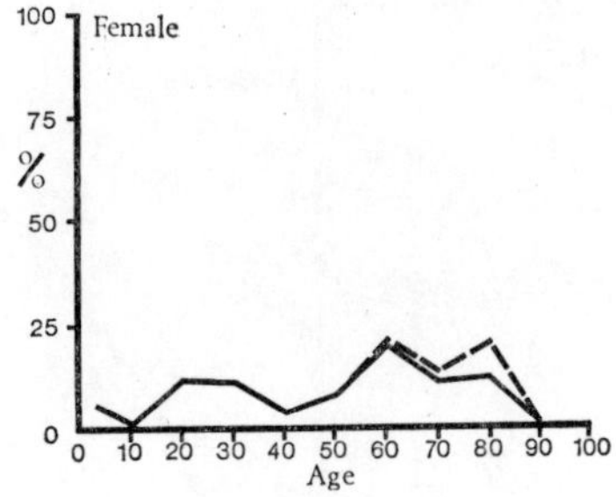

RADICAL TREATMENT

(0·5% of total)
0·2% *male*
0·7% *female*

INDICES OF SURVIVAL

	All cases *Male*	All cases *Female*	Radical Treatment *Male*	Radical Treatment *Female*
FIVE YEAR SURVIVAL RATE (%)				
Crude	10·8	10·3	100·0	0·0
Corrected	*12·9*	*11·7*	*100·0*	*0·0*
Total cases†	453	407	1	3
TEN YEAR SURVIVAL RATE (%)				
Crude	4·1	4·8	50·0	0·0
Corrected	*5·3*	*6·0*	*100·0*	*0·0*
Total cases†	245	207	2	1

†Number of cases on which survival rate is based

SURVIVAL TIME (*months*)				
First quartile (75% S.R.)	1·0	0·9	>60	4·5
Median (50% S.R.)	**14·6**	**6·1**	**>60**	**15·5**
Third quartile (25% S.R.)	24·0	22·5	>60	34·5

ANNUAL SURVIVAL RATES

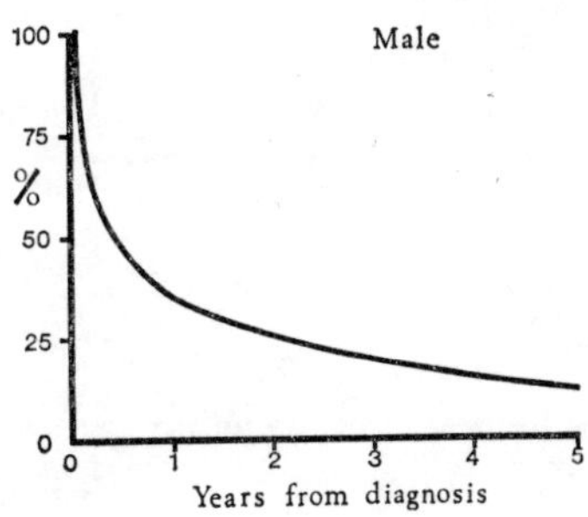

All cases ———
Radical treatment - - - -

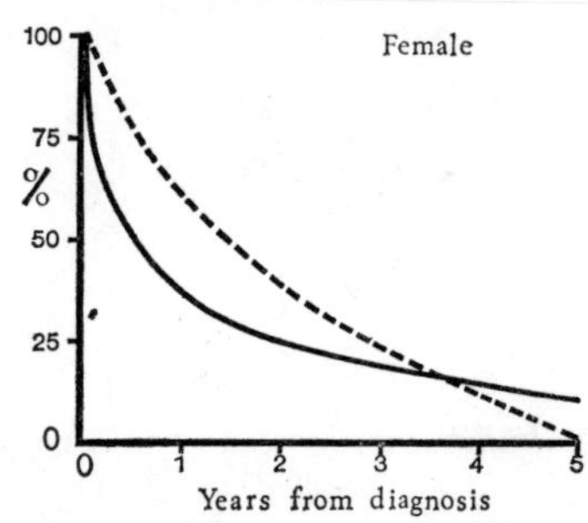

UNKNOWN PRIMARY ICD (8th) **159, 163.9, 195, 196, 197, 198, 199**

INCIDENCE RATE (per 100,000)

Male —— *Female* - - - -

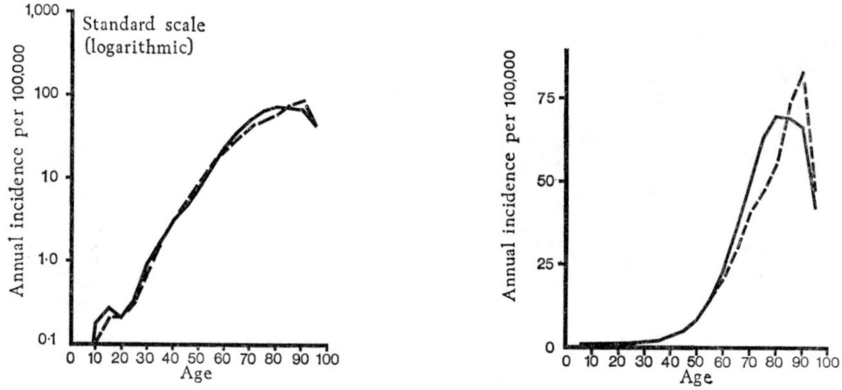

INCIDENCE RATES (per 100,000) by Age

Total cases 1181 *males*; 1395 *females* (of which age not stated for 0 *males* and 1 *female*)

Age	M	F	Age	M	F	Age	M	F
0–4	0·0	0·0	*35–39*	2·0	2·2	*70–74*	58·5	45·7
5–9	0·1	0·1	*40–44*	3·9	4·1	*75–79*	69·6	47·3
10–14	0·2	0·2	*45–49*	4·8	6·1	*80–84*	68·4	66·5
15–19	0·3	0·3	*50–54*	10·5	11·5	*85–89*	69·3	89·7
20–24	0·1	0·1	*55–59*	16·9	16·5	*90–94*	46·1	49·3
25–29	0·5	0·5	*60–64*	29·8	23·3	*95+*	0·0	32·2
30–34	1·2	0·8	*65–69*	42·3	35·2	*All ages*	8·4	9·7

SEX AND AGE DISTRIBUTION

	Male	*Female*
Mean age (*years*)	64·5	66·6
95% between ages	36 & 85	38 & 88
Children under 15 (%)	0·4	0·2
Median age (*years*)	65·6	67·8
Proportion by sex (%)	45·9	54·1
Proportion of all cancers by sex (%)	2·7	3·4
Trend over 10 years	(+)	(+)

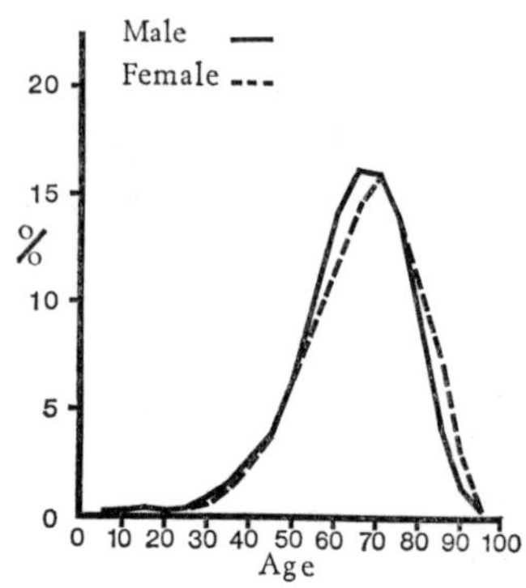

NOTES

Includes: All cases of malignant disease in which it has not been possible to identify the site of the primary tumour.

ICD (7th) **156, 159, 163, 165, 198, 199** **UNKNOWN PRIMARY**

5-YEAR SURVIVAL RATES BY AGE

Crude —— *Corrected* ----

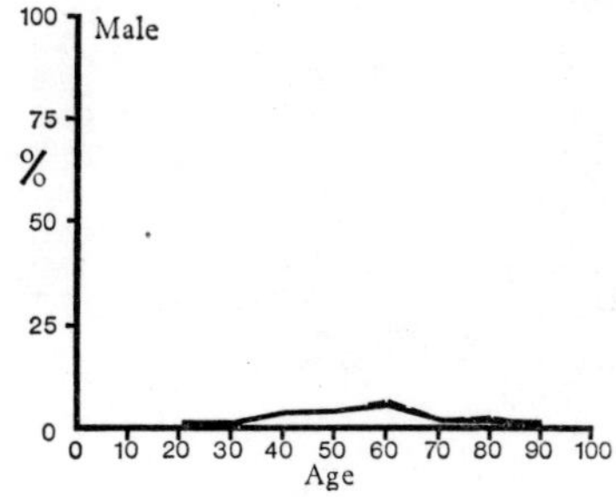

ALL CASES

Total 1283
Male 579
Female 704

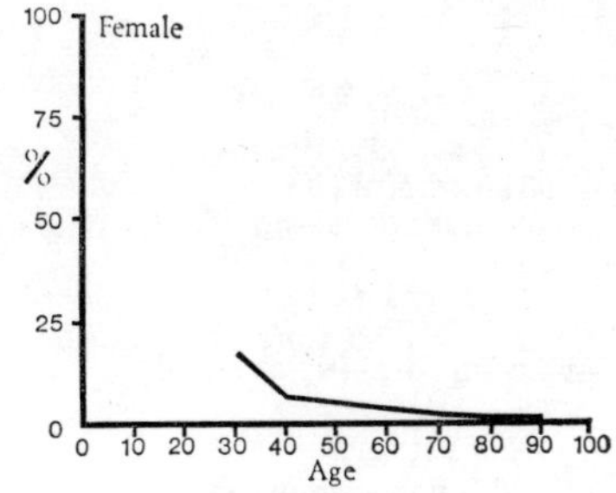

RADICAL TREATMENT

(1·0% of total)
0·7% *male*
1·3% *female*

INDICES OF SURVIVAL

	All cases *Male*	All cases *Female*	Radical Treatment *Male*	Radical Treatment *Female*
FIVE YEAR SURVIVAL RATE (%)				
Crude	2·8	2·1	0·0	11·1
Corrected	*3·6*	*2·5*	*0·0*	*12·4*
Total cases†	579	704	4	9
TEN YEAR SURVIVAL RATE (%)				
Crude	1·9	3·4	25·0	16·7
Corrected	*3·2*	*5·1*	*44·4*	*23·4*
Total cases†	303	322	4	6
SURVIVAL TIME (*months*)				
First quartile (75% S.R.)	0·8	0·9	4·8	1·5
Median (50% S.R.)	**1·8**	**2·3**	**7·0**	**6·5**
Third quartile (25% S.R.)	4·6	5·5	9·3	23·0

†Number of cases on which survival rate is based

ANNUAL SURVIVAL RATES

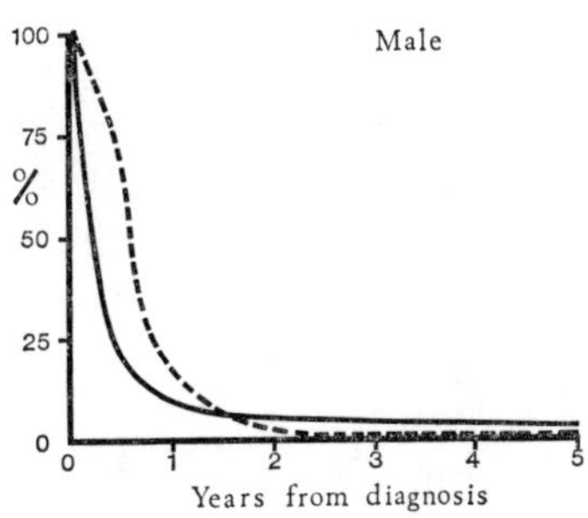

All cases ——
Radical treatment ----

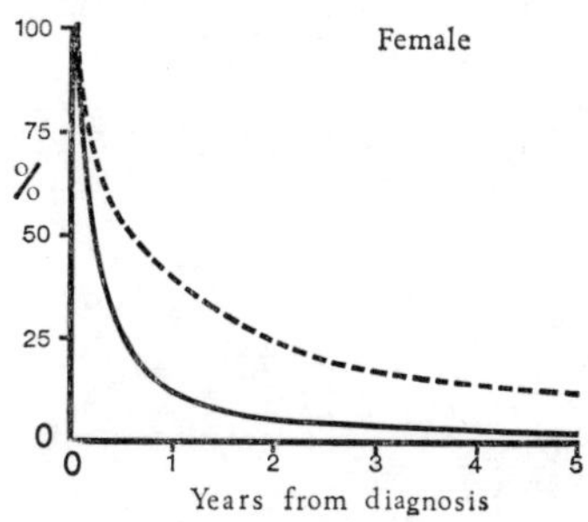

UNKNOWN PRIMARY

	Distribution (%) of System				5-Year Survival Rate (%)	
	Male		*Female*		*Male*	*Female*
Site of Secondary						
Alimentary tract		0·5		1·4	*0·0*	*0·0*
Liver		38·8		37·4	0·0	0·7
Lung		7·1		5·8	3·1	0·0
Bone		18·4		13·2	0·0	0·0
Skin		2·3		2·5	*16·7*	10·0
Reproductive organs		0·2		1·9	—	18·2
Brain		3·4		2·6	0·0	*0·0*
Lymph nodes—auxillary, cervical or inguinal		17·0		10·7	8·0	12·2
—other		3·9		2·7	7·1	0·0
Other specified		8·4		21·8	13·8	2·2
Total with specified secondary	70·6	**100·0**	59·0	**100·0**	3·4	2·9
Generalised	29·4		41·0		0·5	0·3
Total with unknown primary	**100·0**		**100·0**		**2·8**	**2·1**
Total cases	1,794		2,126		579	704

Rates printed in italics are based on less than ten cases

0·0* means (with*) that the number of cases is *not* actually zero, but only to the degree of accuracy quoted, i.e. it is less than 0·05.

0·0 means (without*) that there were in fact *no cases.*

— in the Survival Rate column means that no survival rate can be calculated because there were no cases in that category. This might not accord with the figure given in the Distribution column, which may indicate a non-zero number of cases; the reason for such apparent discrepancies is that the survival rates are based on a fewer number of years than that used as the base of the Distribution figures.

BLADDER—PAPILLOMA ICD (8th) **223.3**

INCIDENCE RATE (per 100,000)

Male —— *Female* ----

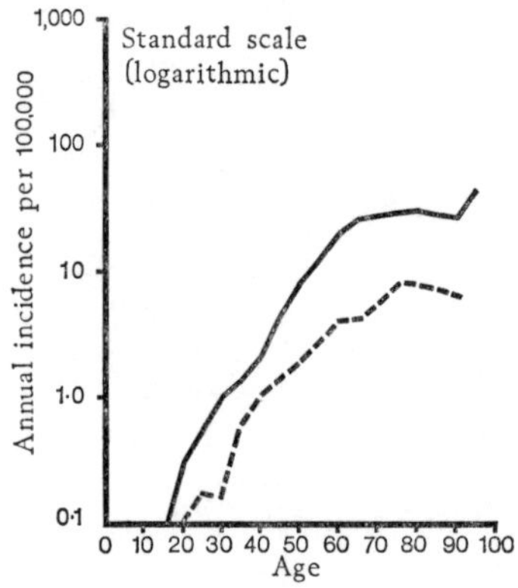

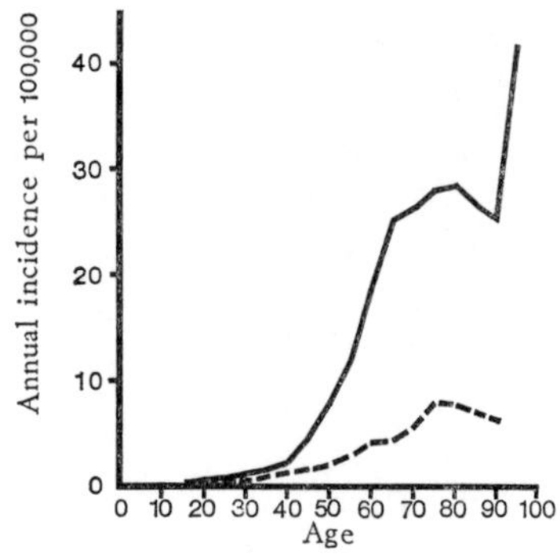

INCIDENCE RATES (per 100,000) by Age

Total cases 792 *males*; 228 *females* (of which age not stated for 6 *males* and 0 *females*)

Age	M	F	Age	M	F	Age	M	F
0–4	0·0	0·0	*35–39*	1·2	1·1	*70–74*	27·2	7·2
5–9	0·0	0·0	*40–44*	2·8	0·9	*75–79*	28·5	8·1
10–14	0·0	0·0	*45–49*	5·7	1·8	*80–84*	27·2	6·5
15–19	0·1	0·0	*50–54*	9·7	1·8	*85–89*	24·0	7·5
20–24	0·5	0·2	*55–59*	13·8	3·5	*90–94*	30·8	0·0
25–29	0·5	0·1	*60–64*	24·6	4·3	*95+*	135·5	0·0
30–34	1·4	0·2	*65–69*	25·1	3·7	*All ages*	5·6	1·6

SEX AND AGE DISTRIBUTION

	Male	*Female*
Mean age (*years*)	61·3	62·8
95% between ages	34 & 84	36 & 86
Children under 15 (%)	0·0	0·0
Median age (*years*)	61·9	63·6
Proportion by sex (%)	77·6	22·4

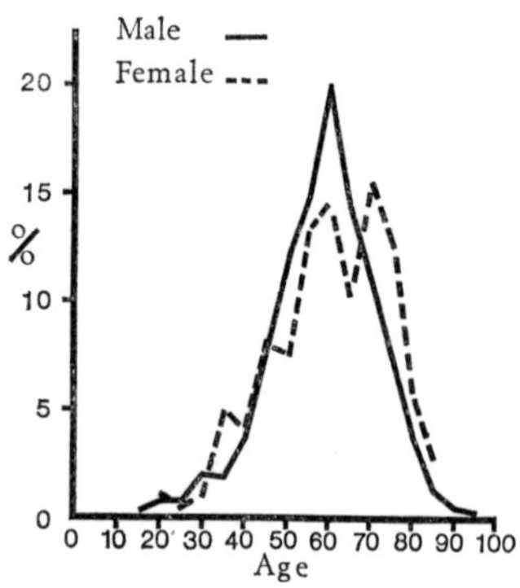

5-YEAR SURVIVAL RATES BY AGE

Crude ——— *Corrected* - - - -

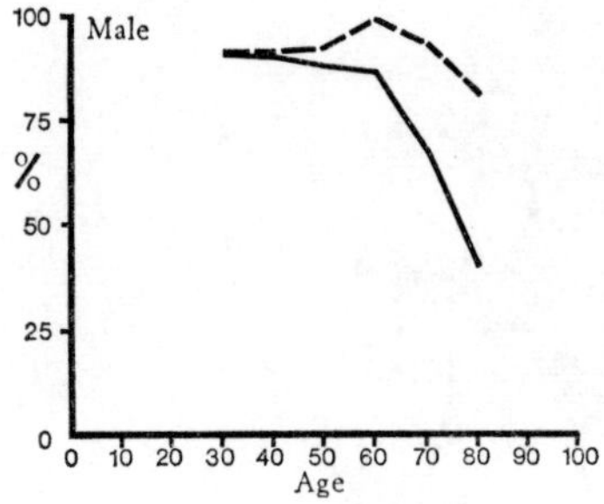

ALL CASES

Total 460
Male 347
Female 113

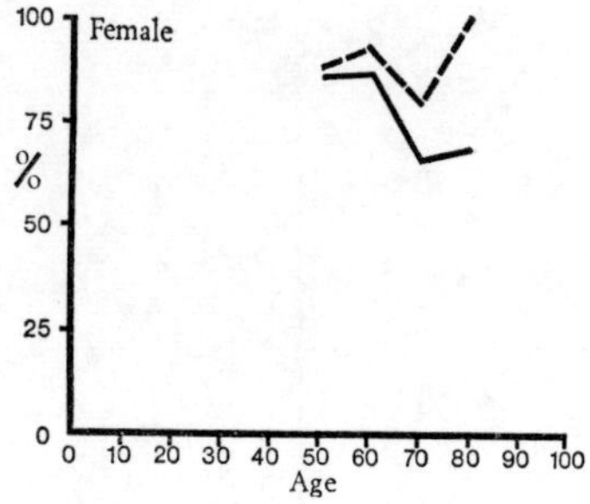

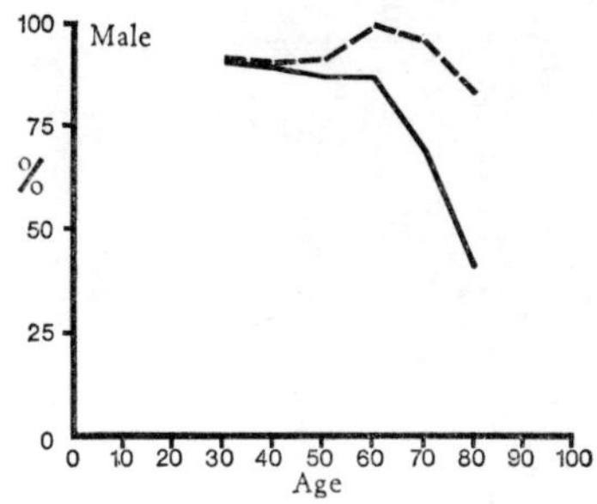

RADICAL TREATMENT

(94·8 % of total)
93·9 % *male*
97·3% *female*

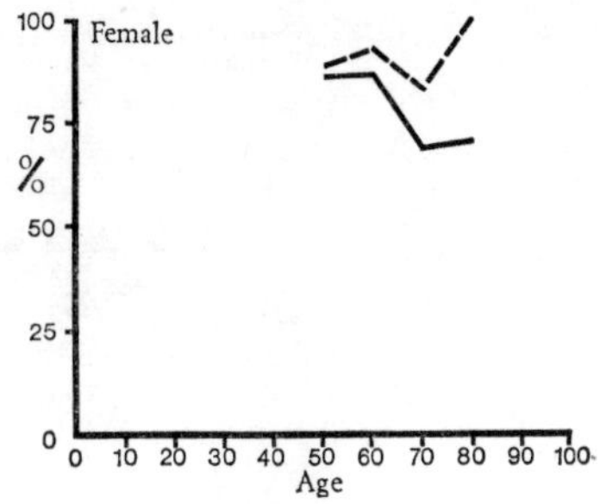

INDICES OF SURVIVAL

	All cases		Radical Treatment	
	Male	*Female*	*Male*	*Female*
FIVE YEAR SURVIVAL RATE (%)				
Crude	76·9	76·1	77·9	77·3
Corrected	*93·0*	*92·1*	*93·8*	*93·1*
Total cases†	347	113	326	110
TEN YEAR SURVIVAL RATE (%)				
Crude	67·5	72·0	68·8	72·6
Corrected	*99·2*	*100·0*	*99·7*	*100·0*
Total cases†	212	75	205	73

†Number of cases on which survival rate is based

SURVIVAL TIME (*months*)				
First quartile (75% S.R.)	>60	>60	>60	>60
Median (50% S.R.)	**>60**	**>60**	**>60**	**>60**
Third quartile (25% S.R.)	>60	>60	>60	>60

ANNUAL SURVIVAL RATES

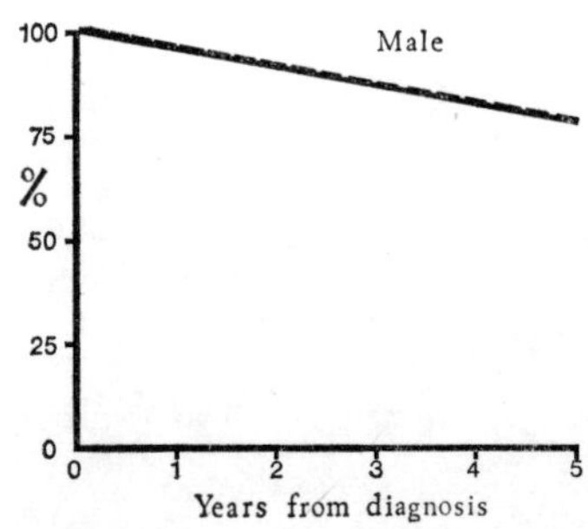

All cases ———
Radical treatment - - - -

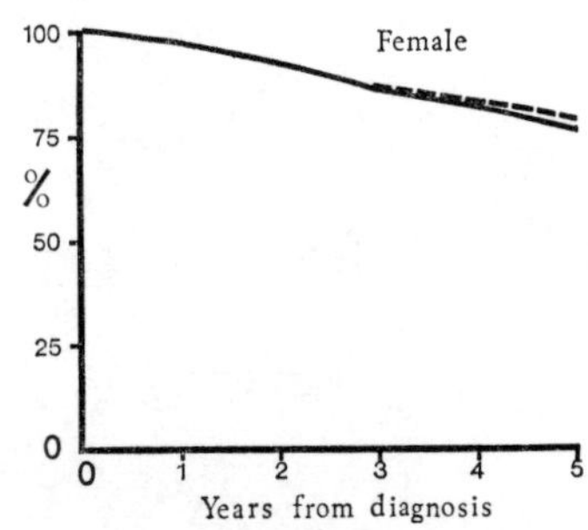

RISK

CERVIX: CARCINOMA-IN-SITU — ICD (8th) **234.0**

INCIDENCE RATE (per 100,000)

Female ----

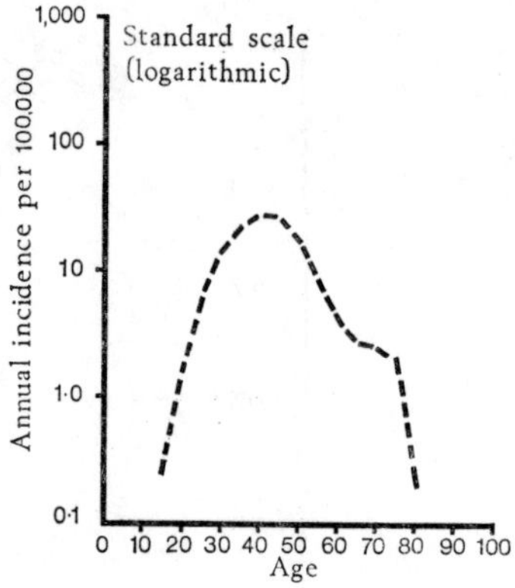

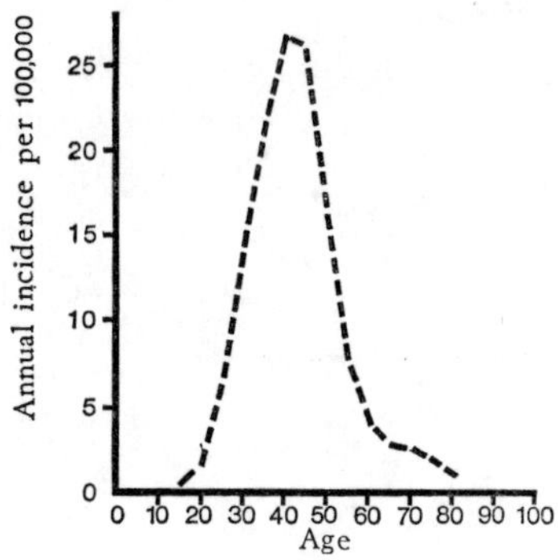

INCIDENCE RATES (per 100,000) by Age

Total cases 1212 *females* (of which age not stated for 2 *females*)

Age	F	Age	F	Age	F
0–4	0·0	*35–39*	23·6	*70–74*	2·2
5–9	0·0	*40–44*	29·0	*75–79*	1·4
10–14	0·0	*45–49*	22·5	*80–84*	0·0
15–19	0·4	*50–54*	10·2	*85–89*	0·0
20–24	2·7	*55–59*	5·0	*90–94*	0·0
25–29	9·7	*60–64*	2·6	*95+*	0·0
30–34	18·0	*65–69*	2·5	*All ages*	8·1

SEX AND AGE DISTRIBUTION

	Female
Mean age (*years*)	42·0
95% between ages	25 & 66
Children under 15(%)	0·0
Median age (*years*)	41·8

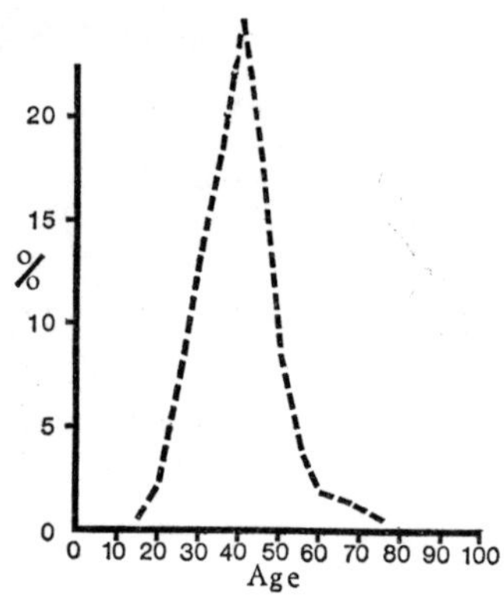

5-YEAR SURVIVAL RATES BY AGE

Crude —— *Corrected* ----

ALL CASES

Total 106

Female 106

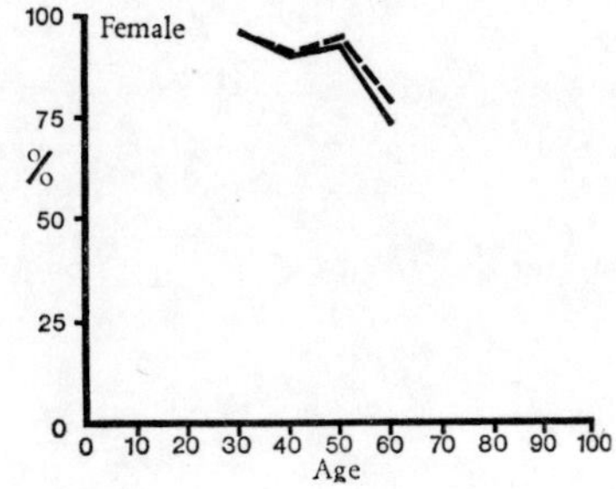

RADICAL TREATMENT

(97·2% of total)

97·2% *female*

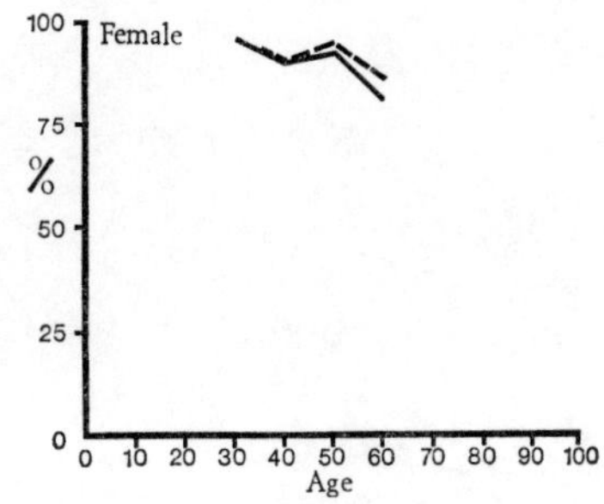

INDICES OF SURVIVAL

	All cases *Female*	Radical Treatment *Female*
FIVE YEAR SURVIVAL RATE (%)		
Crude	88·7	89·3
Corrected	*90·7*	*91·3*
Total cases†	106	103
TEN YEAR SURVIVAL RATE (%)		
Crude	78·9	78·9
Corrected	*87·1*	*87·1*
Total cases†	57	57
†Number of cases on which survival rate is based		
SURVIVAL TIME (*months*)		
First quartile (75% S.R.)	>60	>60
Median (50% S.R.)	**>60**	**>60**
Third quartile (25% S.R.)	>60	>60

ANNUAL SURVIVAL RATES

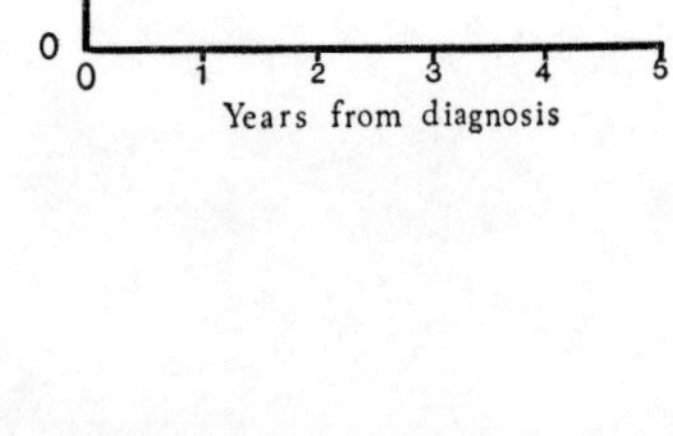

TUMOURS OF CHILDHOOD

The distribution by site of malignant disease in childhood differs widely from that seen in the adult. The preponderant tumours are those of the reticulo-endothelial system and of the nervous system, which together constitute nearly two-thirds of all cases, followed by embryonic tumours. The classification adopted here is based on that of Powell (1973), and is shown in the table below.

DISTRIBUTION BY SITE (%)

	Male	*Female*	*Persons*
Leukaemia	30.1	29.9	30.0
Lymphoma	13.7	7.9	11.0
Embryonic	21.5	22.9	22.2
Nervous system	21.7	22.1	21.9
Mesenchymal	5.8	6.4	6.1
Epithelial	2.7	4.9	3.7
Vestigial	2.4	2.8	2.6
Remainder	2.1	3.1	2.5
All sites	100.0	100.0	100.0
Number of cases	1,083	921	2,004

Only two of the major groups in the table show evidence of a sizeable sex difference, the Lymphomas and the Epithelial tumours. It is consistently shown among the lymphosarcomas, reticulosarcomas, Hodgkin's disease and the small remainder which make up the Lymphoma group, but only by the melanomas of skin and by the ovarian tumours included in the Epithelial group. Some other sex differences are concealed within other groups, such as the male excess of embryonic sarcomas and of the medulloblastomas, but otherwise the incidence by sex is substantially similar. The overall excess of males amounts to a ratio of about 7:6. Thus in terms of actual numbers rather than proportions, the Leukaemia group shows a ratio of 323:266 cases of acute leukaemia, and 3:9 of chronic myelocytic leukaemia. But the ratio shows no statistically significant difference from the sex ratio at birth, while in terms of proportionate contribution the table above shows the remarkable similarity between the sexes for the Leukaemia group.

Relationship to Age

It is perhaps in their relationship to age that the tumours of childhood display most clearly their differences of incidence. The Figure on the opposite page shows for each of the tumour groups the distribution by age at onset. The graphs refer to all cases, male and female combined, and are drawn on a logarithmic scale in order to validate the direct comparison of their slopes. Probably most striking is the rapid decrease in incidence of the Embryonic tumours which cuts across many of the others. Both Leukaemia and Nervous system show a falling rate after an initial rise to a peak at about the age of three years. Lymphomas and Mesenchymal tumours show a steady rise in incidence over the whole age-range, while Epithelial and Vestigial tumours rise in the second half of the range after some hesitation initially. Although the overall behaviour of these latter groups is similar they have not been combined because of the dissimilarities of the subgroups composing them. In the Vestigial group for instance, there are more than twice as many female cases of appendix tumours as male, while it is almost the reverse with the craniopharyngiomas. Three quarters of the Teratomas occur under the age of three, and they account for the shape of the first section of the Remainder group, the rest of which consists mainly of cases where the site of the primary growth was not known.

A fuller discussion and analysis of behaviour of this series of tumours of childhood will be found in the paper by Powell (1973), on which much of this section has been based.

INCIDENCE RATE (per 100,000)

Male —— *Female* ----

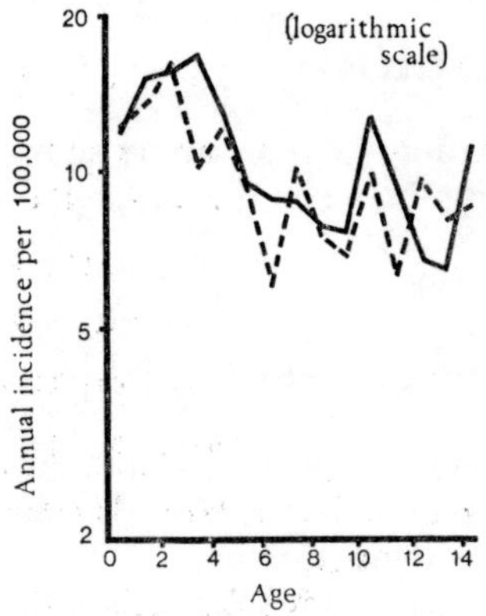

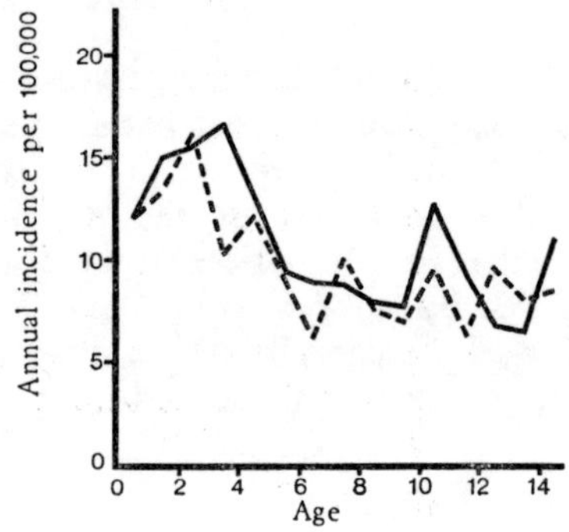

INCIDENCE RATES (per 100,000) by Age

Total cases 658 *males*; 566 *females* (of which age was not stated for 1 *male* and 0 *females*)

Age	M	F	Age	M	F	Age	M	F
0	11·9	12·0	*5*	9·4	9·2	*10*	12·6	9·5
1	15·0	13·4	*6*	8·8	6·0	*11*	9·1	6·3
2	15·5	16·1	*7*	8·7	10·0	*12*	6·7	9·5
3	16·6	10·2	*8*	7·8	7·5	*13*	6·4	8·0
4	13·0	12·1	*9*	7·6	6·9	*14*	11·1	8·5

SEX AND AGE DISTRIBUTION

	Male	*Female*
Mean age (*years*)	6·2	6·4
95% *between ages*	0·2 & 13·6	0·2 & 13·5
Median age (*years*)	4·1	4·2
Proportion by sex (%)	53·8	46·2
Proportion of all cancers by sex (%)	0·9	0·8

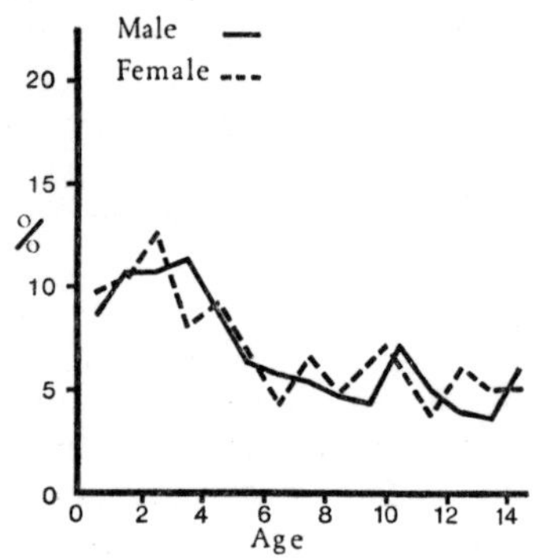

NOTES

Includes: All malignant tumours occurring under the age of 15 years.

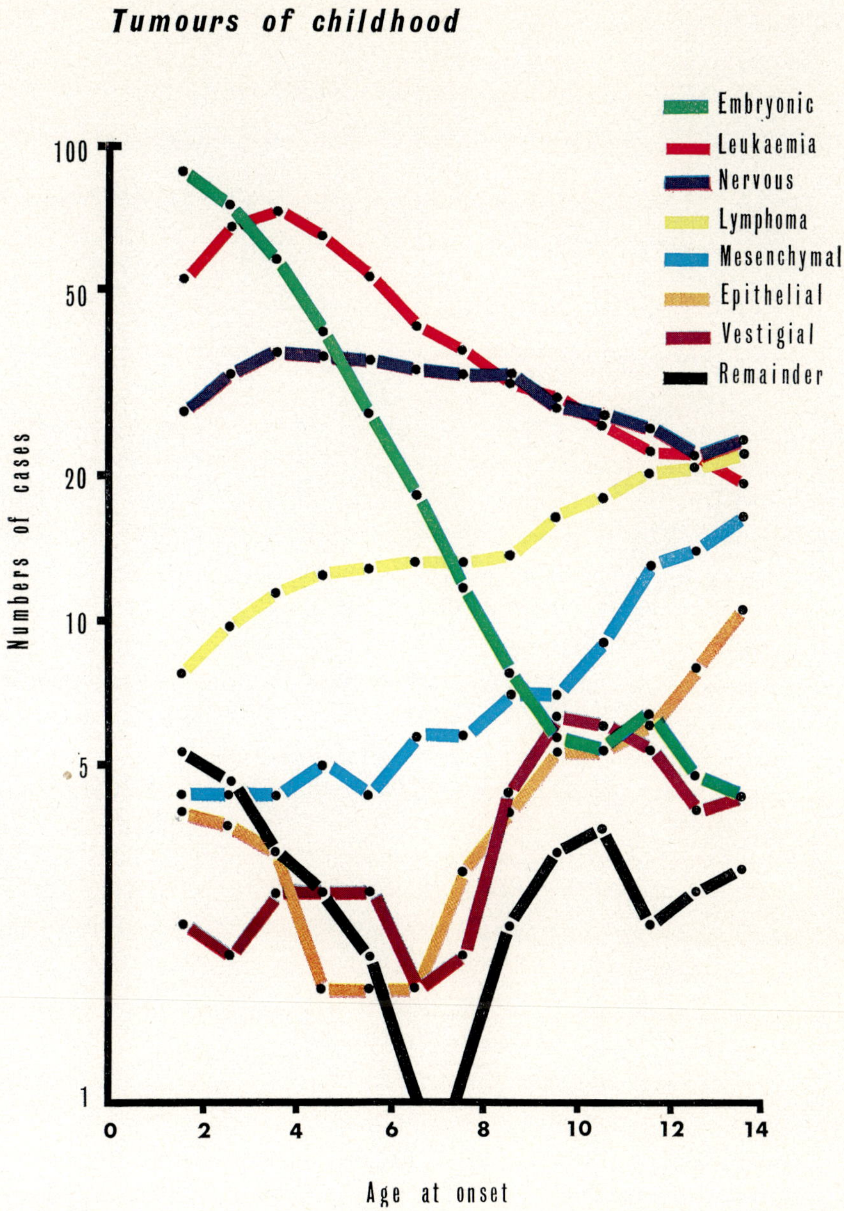
Tumours of childhood
Embryonic
Leukaemia
Nervous
Lymphoma
Mesenchymal
Epithelial
Vestigial
Remainder
100
50
20
10
5
1
Numbers of cases
0
2
4
6
8
10
12
14
Age at onset

Facing p. 92

ANNUAL SURVIVAL RATE

Note: The graphs of survival rates on this page differ in two important respects from those presented elsewhere in this book on the FATE page of a page-pair. First, they give the percentage survival in relation, not to age, which ranges over only three quinquennial groups, but to successive years after treatment or diagnosis. Secondly, no age-correction of the survival rates is made, since mortality rates are at their lowest in this period of life and the adjustment is therefore irrelevant.

All cases —— *Radically treated cases* ----

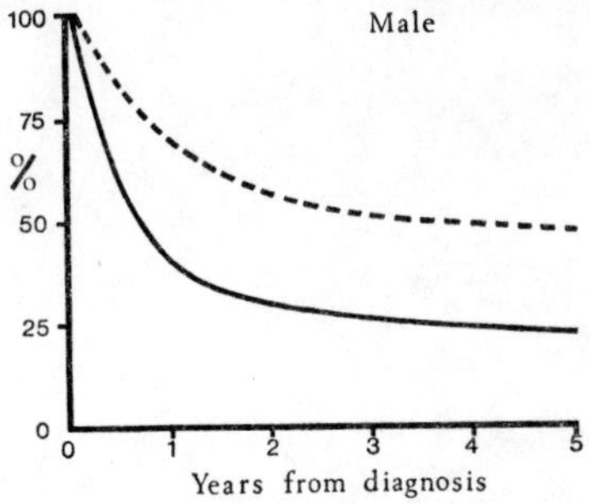

ALL CASES

Total 1314
Male 704
Female 610

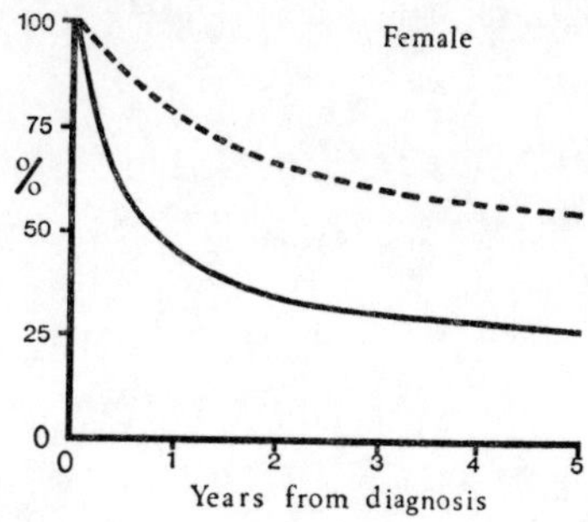

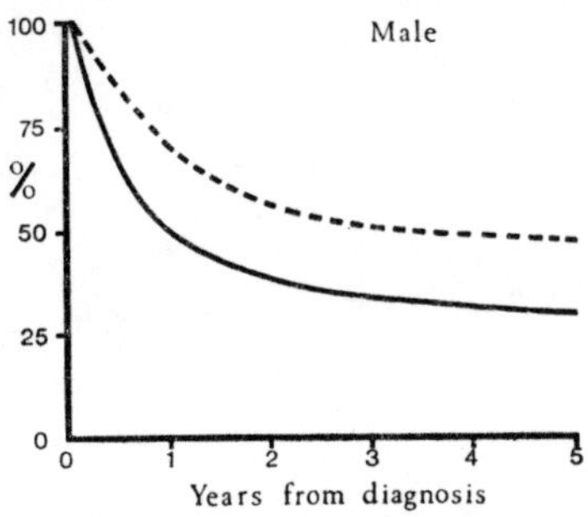

ALL SITES EXCEPT LEUKAEMIA

Radical Treatment

(50·5% of total)
48·2% *male*
53·0% *female*

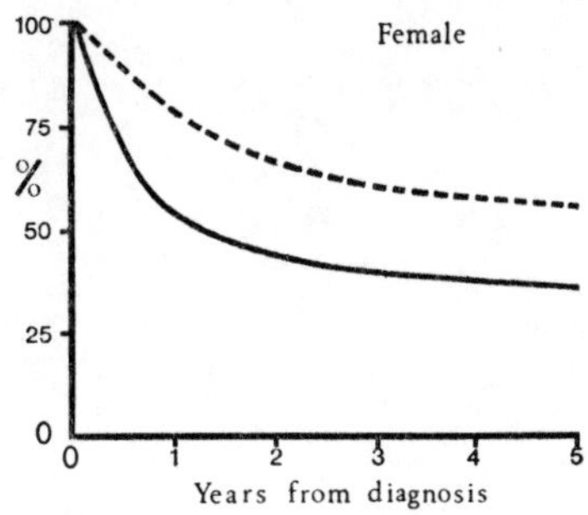

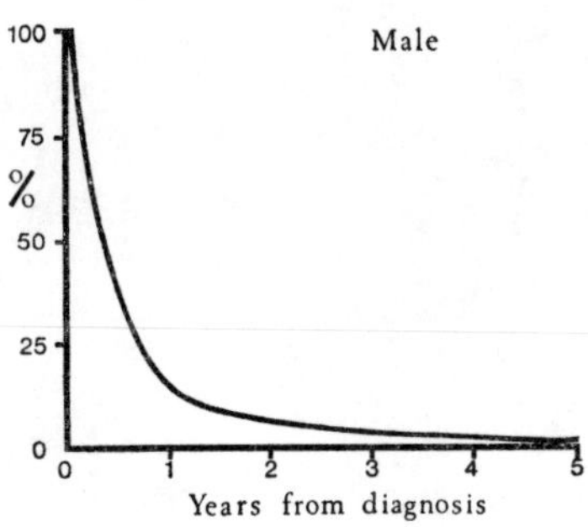

LEUKAEMIA

Total 349
Male 192
Female 157

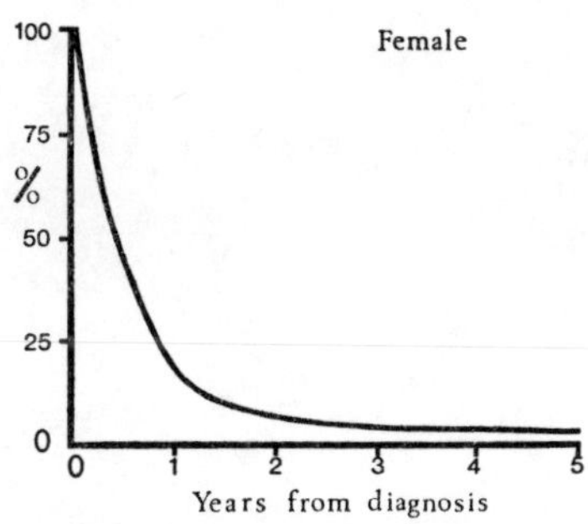

INDICES OF SURVIVAL

	All cases		Radical Treatment		Leukaemia	
	Male	*Female*	*Male*	*Female*	*Male*	*Female*
FIVE YEAR SURVIVAL RATE (%)	21·9	26·7	46·2	54·2	1·6	3·8
Total cases†	704	610	247	240	192	157
TEN YEAR SURVIVAL RATE (%)	22·2	24·8	42·6	45·5	0·0	1·3
Total cases†	333	298	141	143	108	76
SURVIVAL TIME (*months*)						
First quartile	3·4	4·1	7·9	13·6	1·4	1·4
Median	**8·0**	**9·6**	**36·0**	**>60**	**4·6**	**4·6**
Third quartile	36·0	>60	>60	>60	8·2	8·6

†Number of cases on which survival rate is based

PART III

GENERAL SITE DATA

LIP VERMILION
(Squamous cell carcinoma)

ICD (8th) 140

INCIDENCE RATE (per 100,000)

Male —— *Female* - - - -

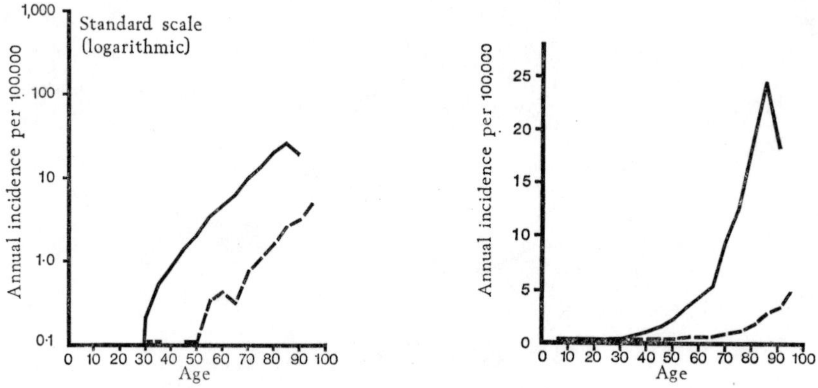

INCIDENCE RATES (per 100,000) by Age

Total cases 258 *males*; 29 *females* (of which age not stated for 1 *male* and 0 *females*)

Age	M	F	Age	M	F	Age	M	F
0–4	0·0	0·0	*35–39*	0·7	0·0	*70–74*	11·1	1·0
5–9	0·0	0·0	*40–44*	0·9	0·1	*75–79*	15·0	0·9
10–14	0·0	0·0	*45–49*	1·7	0·1	*80–84*	25·3	2·5
15–19	0·0	0·0	*50–54*	2·2	0·1	*85–89*	21·3	2·5
20–24	0·0	0·0	*55–59*	4·3	0·6	*90–94*	0·0	5·5
25–29	0·0	0·0	*60–64*	4·3	0·1	*95+*	0·0	0·0
30–34	0·3	0·1	*65–69*	8·1	0·5	*All ages*	1·8	0·2

SEX AND AGE DISTRIBUTION

	Male	*Female*
Mean age (*years*)	64·9	69·1
95% between ages	37 & 86	34 & 91
Children under 15 (%)	0·0	0·0
Median age (*years*)	66·0	71·5
Proportion by sex (%)	89·9	10·1
Proportion of all cancers by sex (%)	0·6	0·1
Trend over 10 years	(−)	(+)

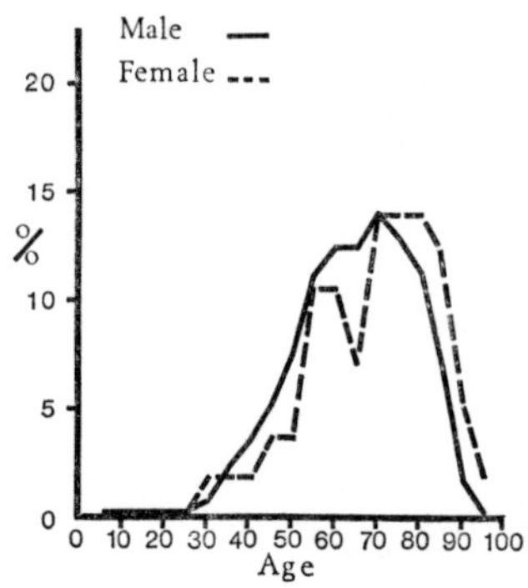

NOTES

Includes: Squamous cell carcinoma of upper lip, lower lip, and commissures, specified as of the vermilion, or not further specified.

Excludes: Skin of lip (classified with SKIN); melanoma of lip; basal cell carcinoma (rodent ulcer) of lip.

 LIP VERMILION (Squamous cell carcinoma)

5-YEAR SURVIVAL RATES BY AGE

Crude ——— *Corrected* - - - -

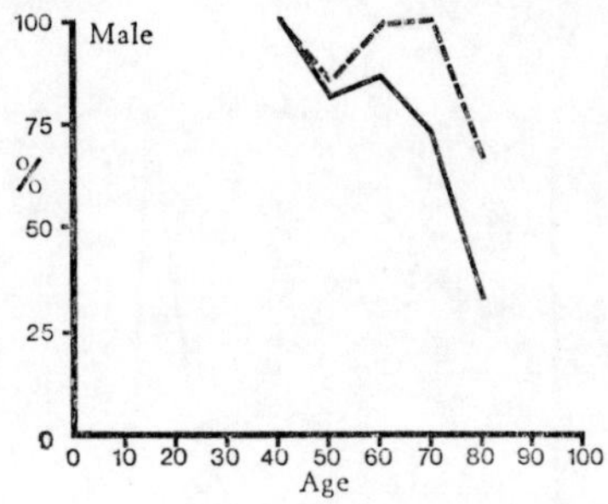

ALL CASES

Total 172
Male 157
Female 15

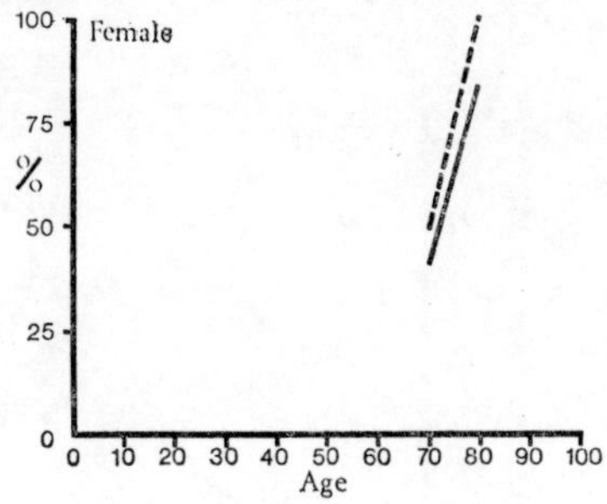

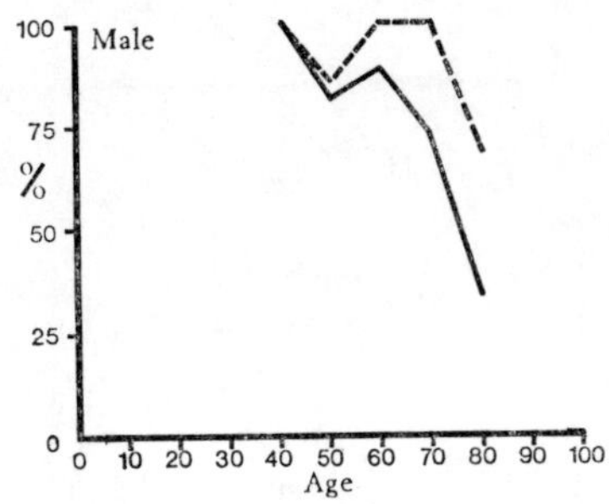

RADICAL TREATMENT

(98·8% of total)
98·7% *male*
100·0% *female*

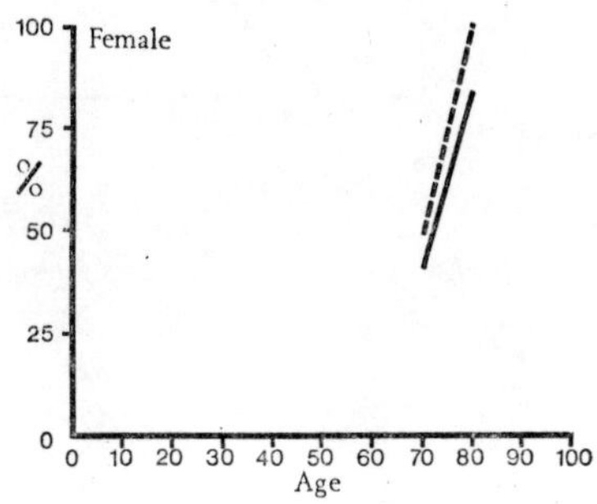

INDICES OF SURVIVAL

	All cases *Male*	All cases *Female*	Radical Treatment *Male*	Radical Treatment *Female*
FIVE YEAR SURVIVAL RATE (%)				
Crude	66·9	53·3	67·7	53·3
Corrected	*91·2*	*79·8*	*92·1*	*79·8*
Total cases†	157	15	155	15
TEN YEAR SURVIVAL RATE (%)				
Crude	40·2	38·1	41·5	44·4
Corrected	*83·1*	*81·5*	*84·4*	*87·4*
Total cases†	169	21	164	18
SURVIVAL TIME (*months*)				
First quartile (75% S.R.)	36·7	36·0	38·0	36·0
Median (50% S.R.)	**>60**	**>60**	**>60**	**>60**
Third quartile (25% S.R.)	>60	>60	>60	>60

† Number of cases on which survival rate is based

ANNUAL SURVIVAL RATES

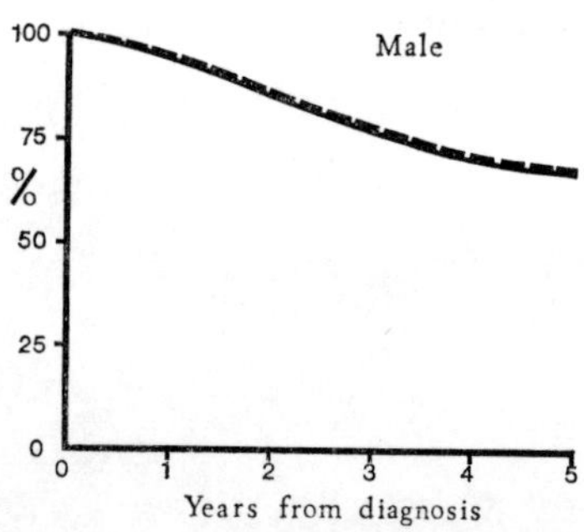

All cases ———
Radical treatment - - - -

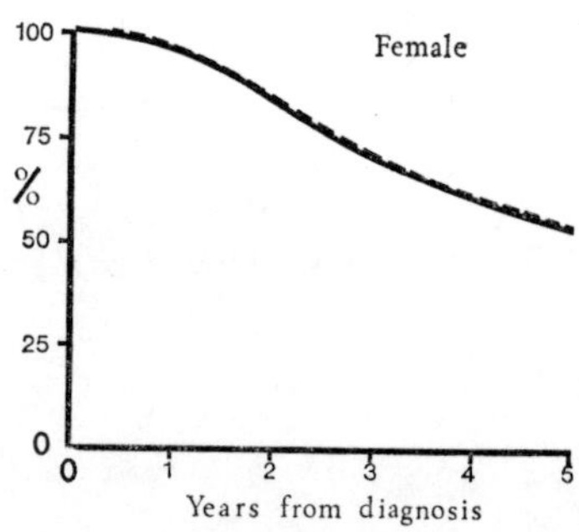

TONGUE ICD (8th) **141**

INCIDENCE RATE (per 100,000)

Male —— *Female* - - - -

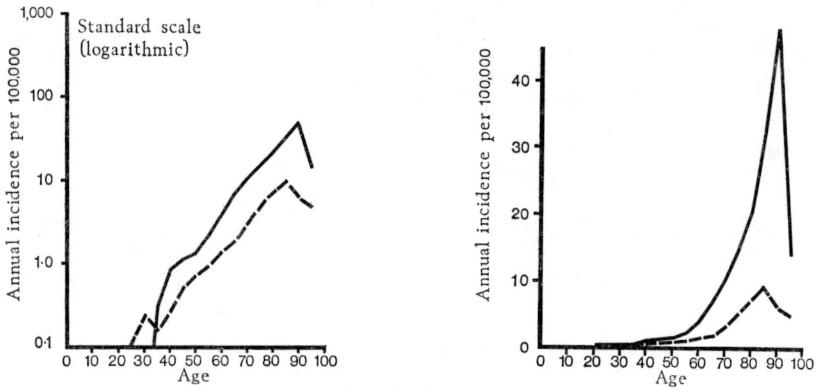

INCIDENCE RATES (per 100,000) by Age

Total cases 261 *males*; 120 *females* (of which age not stated for 1 *male* and 0 *females*)

Age	M	F	Age	M	F	Age	M	F
0–4	0·1	0·0	*35–39*	0·6	0·1	*70–74*	12·3	4·5
5–9	0·0	0·0	*40–44*	1·1	0·4	*75–79*	18·0	5·2
10–14	0·0	0·0	*45–49*	1·0	0·5	*80–84*	24·4	9·9
15–19	0·0	0·0	*50–54*	1·6	0·8	*85–89*	53·3	6·2
20–24	0·1	0·0	*55–59*	2·5	0·9	*90–94*	15·4	5·5
25–29	0·1	0·2	*60–64*	5·4	1·7	*95+*	0·0	0·0
30–34	0·0	0·2	*65–69*	8·5	1·8	*All ages*	1·9	0·8

SEX AND AGE DISTRIBUTION

	Male	*Female*
Mean age (*years*)	67·3	68·1
95% between ages	38 & 89	32 & 88
Children under 15 (%)	0·4	0·0
Median age (*years*)	68·9	71·4
Proportion by sex (%)	68·5	31·5
Proportion of all cancers by sex (%)	0·6	0·3
Trend over 10 years	– –	(+)

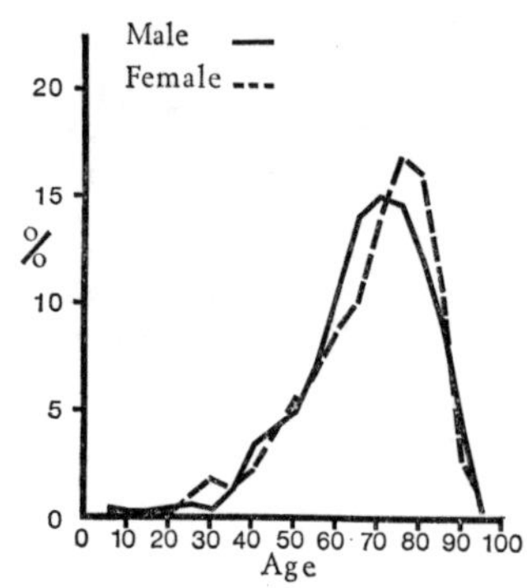

NOTES

Includes: All parts of the tongue. For subdivisions see p. 20.

5-YEAR SURVIVAL RATES BY AGE

Crude —— *Corrected* ----

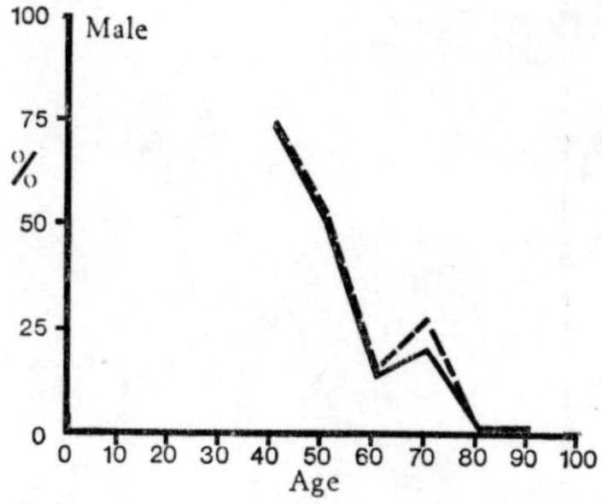

ALL CASES

Total 248
Male 187
Female 61

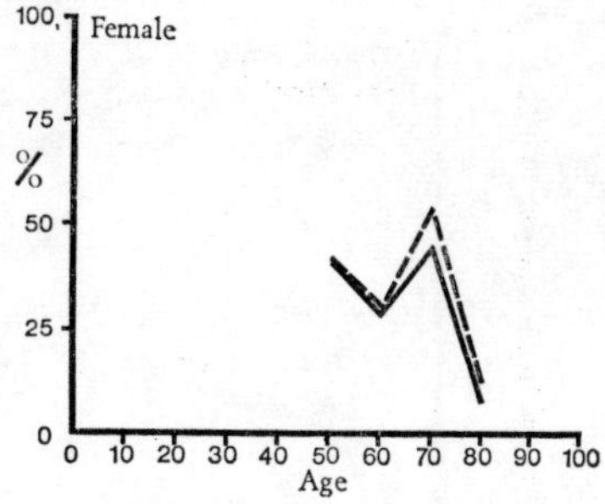

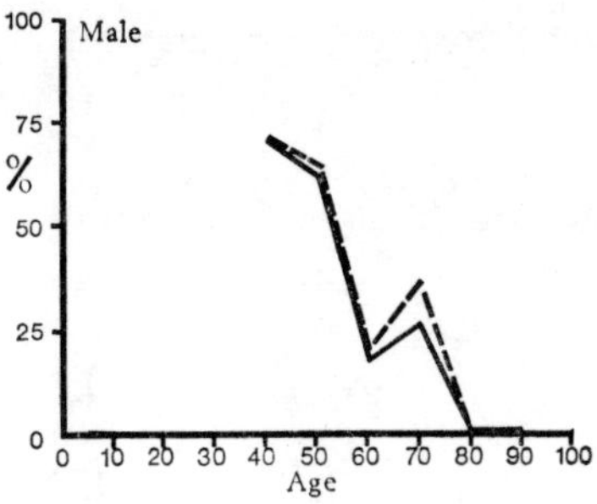

RADICAL TREATMENT

(73·4% of total)
71·1% *male*
80·3% *female*

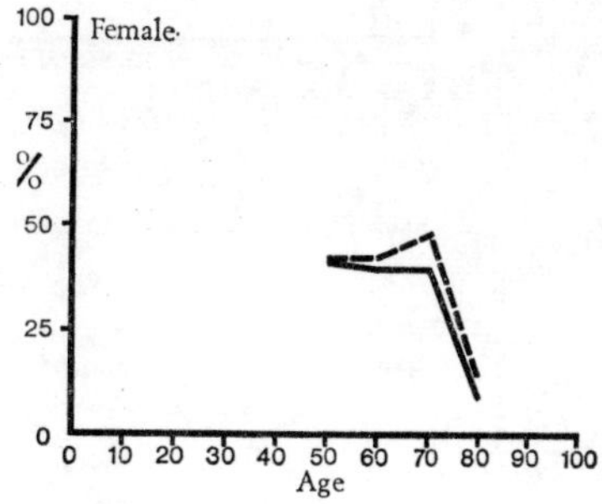

INDICES OF SURVIVAL

	All cases		Radical Treatment	
	Male	*Female*	*Male*	*Female*
FIVE YEAR SURVIVAL RATE (%)				
Crude	18·2	27·9	24·8	30·6
Corrected	*25·8*	*35·0*	*34·0*	*37·8*
Total cases†	187	61	133	49
TEN YEAR SURVIVAL RATE (%)				
Crude	13·7	19·7	24·2	25·0
Corrected	*30·3*	*34·7*	*45·2*	*41·8*
Total cases†	212	66	120	48

† Number of cases on which survival rate is based

SURVIVAL TIME (*months*)				
First quartile (75% S.R.)	4·6	5·4	8·1	6·7
Median (50% S.R.)	**12·0**	**16·5**	**16·0**	**20·0**
Third quartile (25% S.R.)	39·3	>60	>60	>60

ANNUAL SURVIVAL RATES

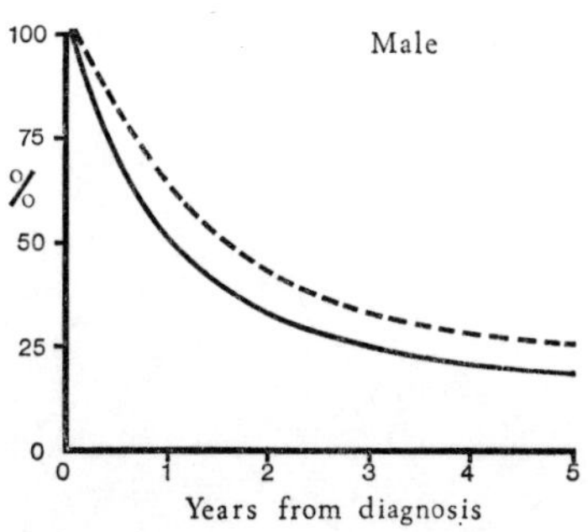

All cases ——
Radical treatment ----

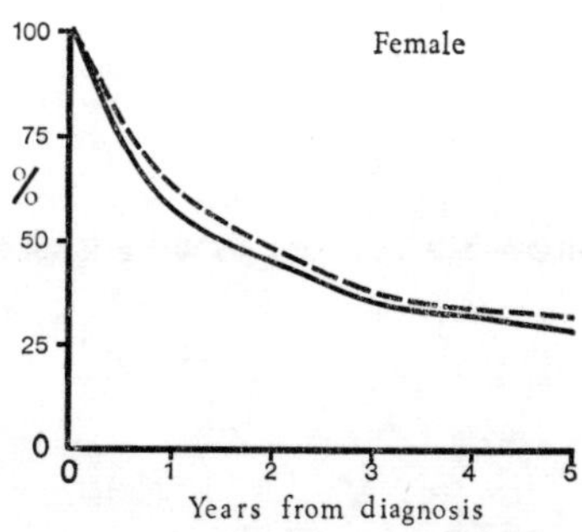

SALIVARY GLANDS

ICD (8th) 142

INCIDENCE RATE (per 100,000)

Male —— *Female* - - - -

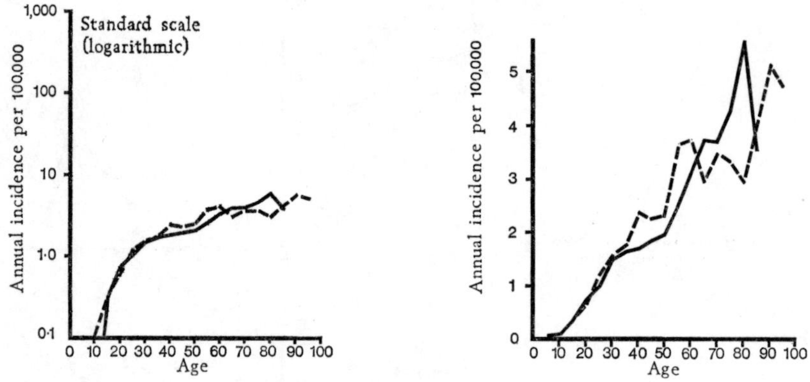

INCIDENCE RATES (per 100,000) by Age

Total cases 205 *males*; 253 *females* (of which age not stated for 0 *males* and 1 *female*)

Age	M	F	Age	M	F	Age	M	F
0–4	0·0	0·0	*35–39*	1·4	1·9	*70–74*	3·2	3·9
5–9	0·0	0·0	*40–44*	1·9	2·8	*75–79*	6·0	2·6
10–14	0·1	0·2	*45–49*	1·7	1·7	*80–84*	4·7	3·5
15–19	0·5	0·5	*50–54*	2·2	2·8	*85–89*	0·0	5·0
20–24	0·9	0·8	*55–59*	2·7	4·5	*90–94*	0·0	5·5
25–29	1·1	1·6	*60–64*	3·5	2·8	*95+*	0·0	0·0
30–34	1·8	1·5	*65–69*	4·0	3·1	*All ages*	1·5	1·8

SEX AND AGE DISTRIBUTION

	Male	*Female*
Mean age (*years*)	50·8	52·2
95% between ages	18 & 80	19 & 84
Children under 15 (%)	0·5	0·8
Median age (*years*)	52·0	53·7
Proportion by sex (%)	44·7	55·2
Proportion of all cancers by sex (%)	0·5	0·6
Trend over 10 years	(–)	(–)

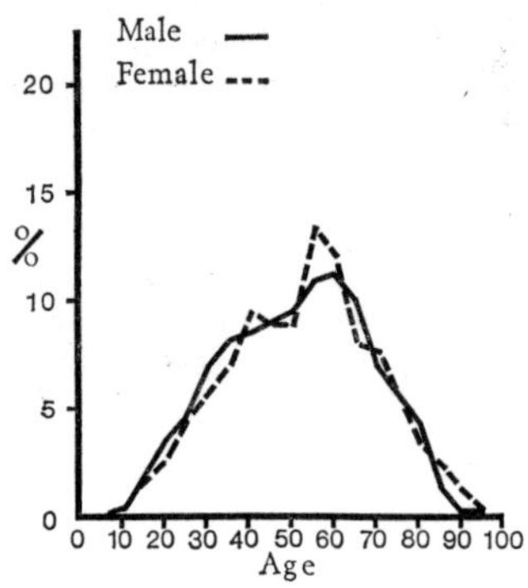

NOTES

Includes: All salivary glands. For subdivisions see p. 20.

5-YEAR SURVIVAL RATES BY AGE

Crude —— *Corrected* ----

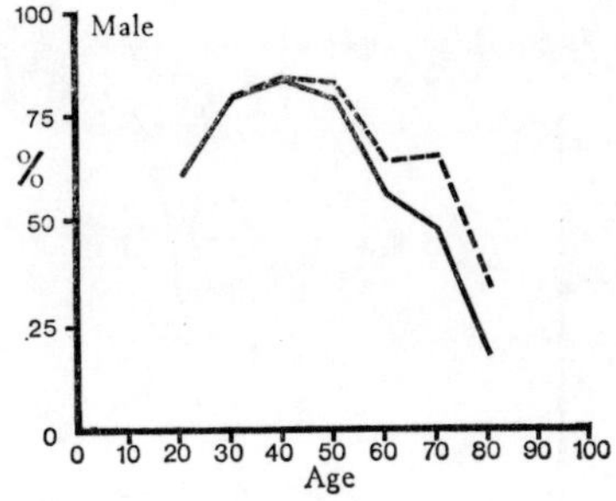

ALL CASES

Total 264
Male 121
Female 143

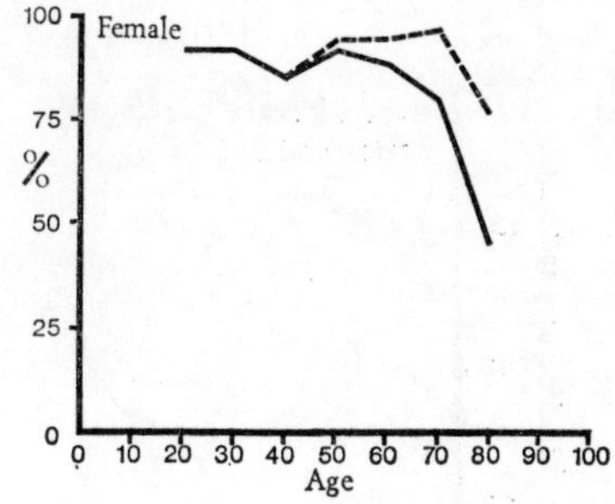

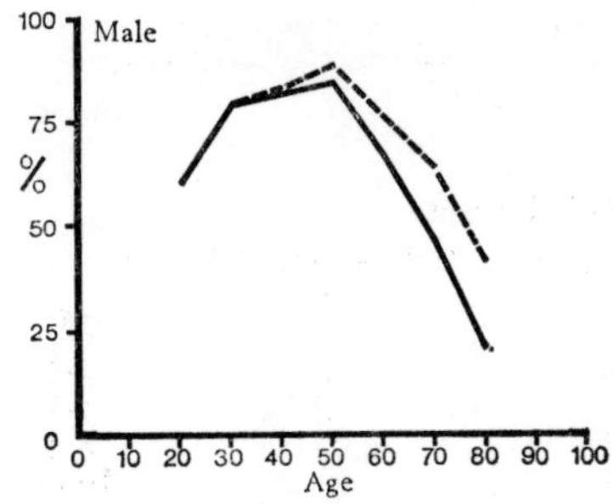

RADICAL TREATMENT

(89·8% of total)
88·4% *male*
90·9% *female*

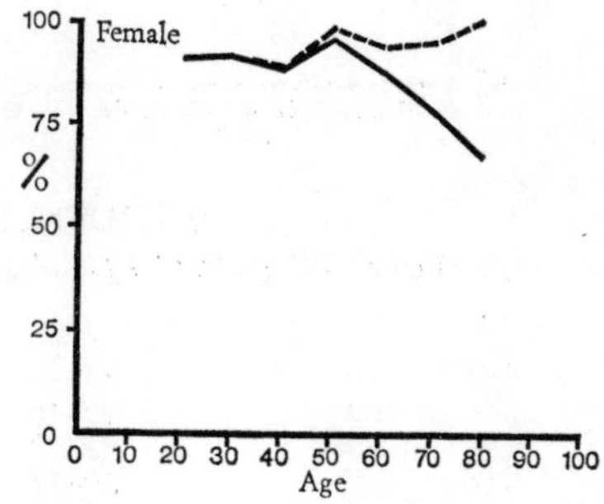

INDICES OF SURVIVAL

	All cases		Radical Treatment	
	Male	*Female*	*Male*	*Female*
FIVE YEAR SURVIVAL RATE (%)				
Crude	65·3	82·5	70·1	86·9
Corrected	*73·5*	*89·8*	*77·9*	*92·8*
Total cases†	121	143	107	130
TEN YEAR SURVIVAL RATE (%)				
Crude	43·8	71·2	57·7	74·5
Corrected	*62·7*	*83·7*	*74·9*	*86·8*
Total cases†	89	104	67	94

† Number of cases on which survival rate is based

SURVIVAL TIME (*months*)				
First quartile (75% S.R.)	33·0	>60	36·8	>60
Median (50% S.R.)	**>60**	**>60**	**>60**	**>60**
Third quartile (25% S.R.)	>60	>60	>60	>60

ANNUAL SURVIVAL RATES

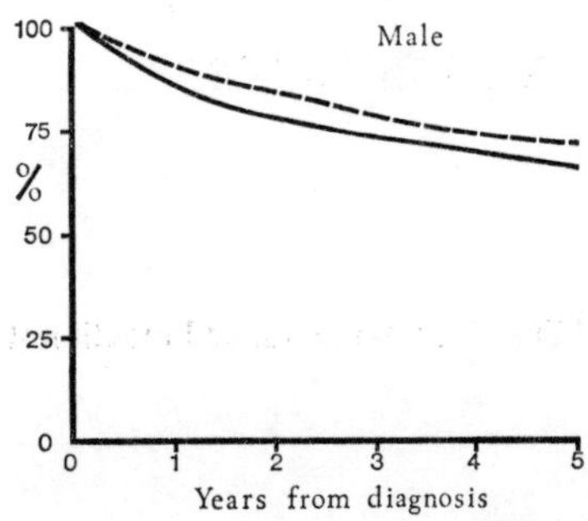

All cases ——
Radical treatment ----

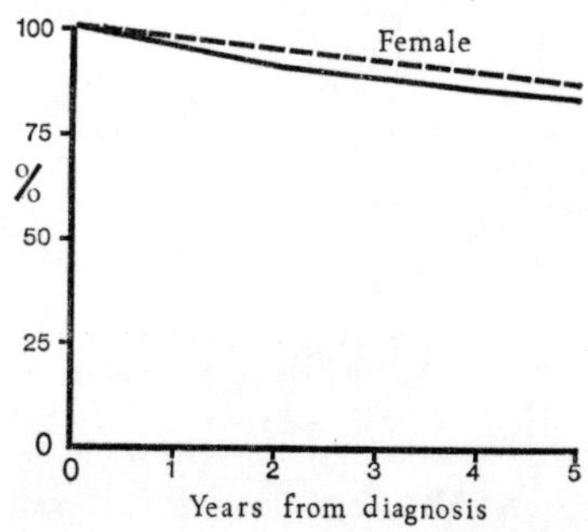

FLOOR OF MOUTH ICD (8th) **144**

INCIDENCE RATE (per 100,000)

Male —— *Female* ----

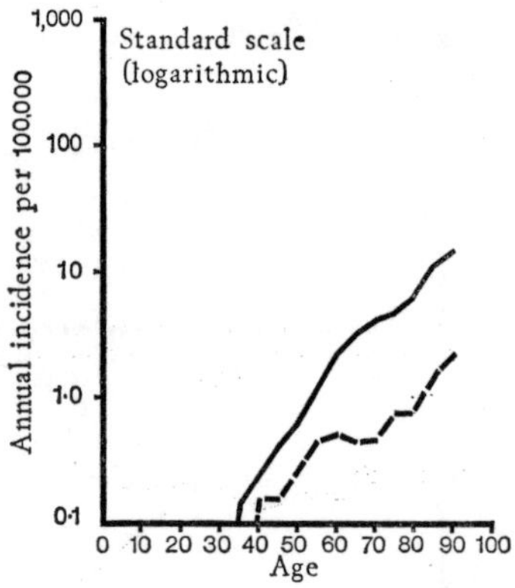

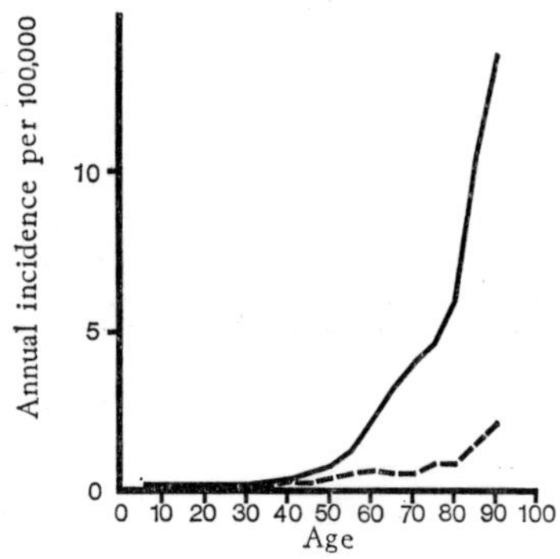

INCIDENCE RATES (per 100,000) by Age

Total cases 102 *males*; 27 *females* (of which age not stated for 0 *males* and 0 *females*)

Age	M	F	Age	M	F	Age	M	F
0–4	0·0	0·0	*35–39*	0·3	0·0	*70–74*	4·4	0·8
5–9	0·0	0·0	*40–44*	0·2	0·3	*75–79*	4·5	0·6
10–14	0·0	0·0	*45–49*	0·6	0·0	*80–84*	8·4	1·0
15–19	0·0	0·0	*50–54*	0·6	0·5	*85–89*	16·0	2·5
20–24	0·0	0·0	*55–59*	1·7	0·3	*90–94*	0·0	0·0
25–29	0·0	0·0	*60–64*	2·7	0·7	*95+*	0·0	0·0
30–34	0·0	0·0	*65–69*	3·6	0·2	*All ages*	0·7	0·2

SEX AND AGE DISTRIBUTION

	Male	*Female*
Mean age (*years*)	65·9	64·0
95% between ages	39 & 88	41 & 88
Children under 15 (%)	0·0	0·0
Median age (*years*)	65·9	62·5
Proportion by sex (%)	79·1	20·9
Proportion of all cancers by sex (%)	0·2	0·1
Trend over 10 years	–	(–)

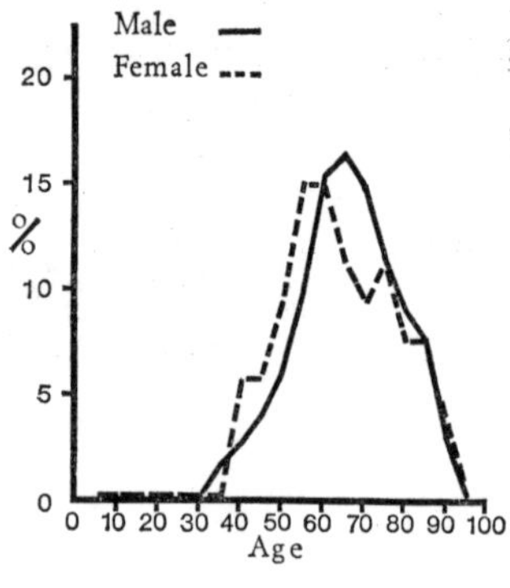

NOTES

Includes: Upper and lower alveolus, hard palate, buccal aspect of cheek and lips, floor of mouth, and mouth not further specified. For details of subdivisions see p. 20.

5-YEAR SURVIVAL RATES BY AGE

Crude —— *Corrected* ----

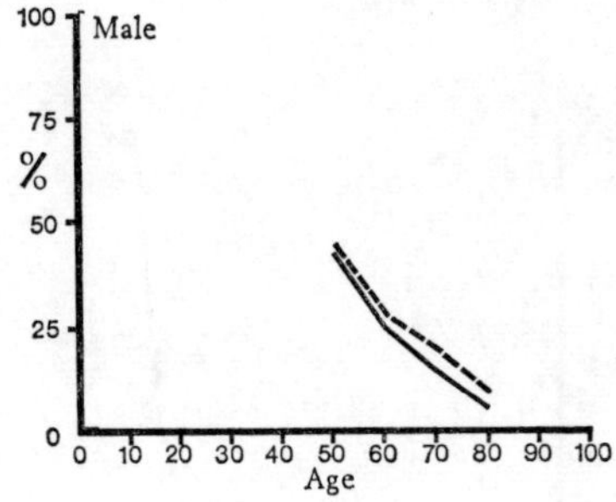

ALL CASES

Total	98
Male	82
Female	16

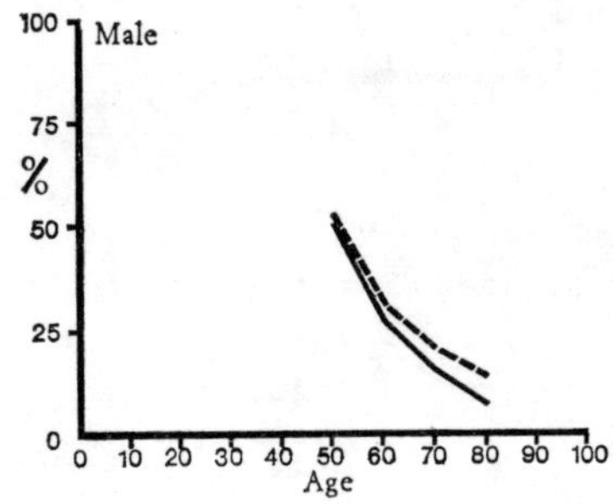

RADICAL TREATMENT

(75·5% of total)
80·5% *male*
50·0% *female*

INDICES OF SURVIVAL

	All cases *Male*	All cases *Female*	Radical Treatment *Male*	Radical Treatment *Female*
FIVE YEAR SURVIVAL RATE (%)				
Crude	17·1	18·8	19·7	37·5
Corrected	*24·3*	*25·7*	*27·3*	*46·9*
Total cases†	82	16	66	8
TEN YEAR SURVIVAL RATE (%)				
Crude	10·9	16·7	16·1	50·0
Corrected	*24·2*	*22·1*	*32·7*	*59·6*
Total cases†	92	6	62	2
SURVIVAL TIME (*months*)				
First quartile (75% S.R.)	6·9	1·3	11·3	1·8
Median (50% S.R.)	**17·0**	**5·7**	**21·5**	**13·0**
Third quartile (25% S.R.)	38·8	13·3	32·8	>60

† Number of cases on which survival is based

ANNUAL SURVIVAL RATES

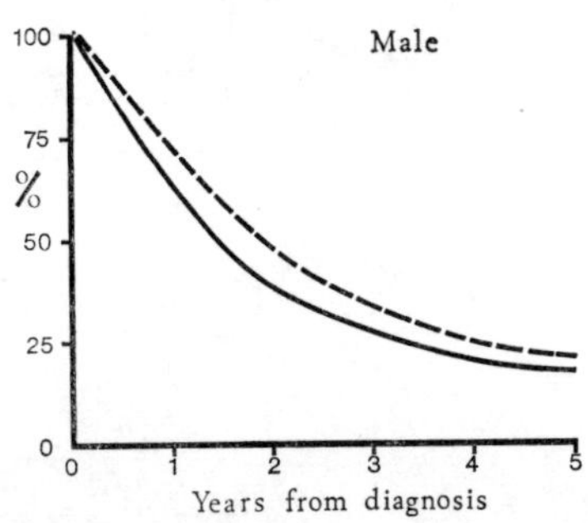

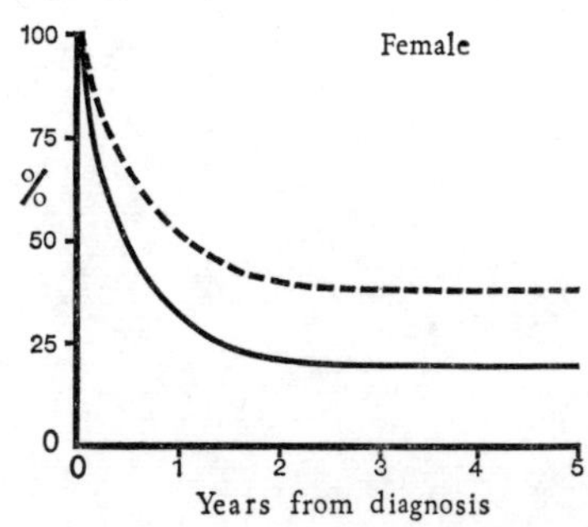

MOUTH OTHER ICD (8th) **143, 145**

INCIDENCE RATE (per 100,000)

Male —— *Female* - - - -

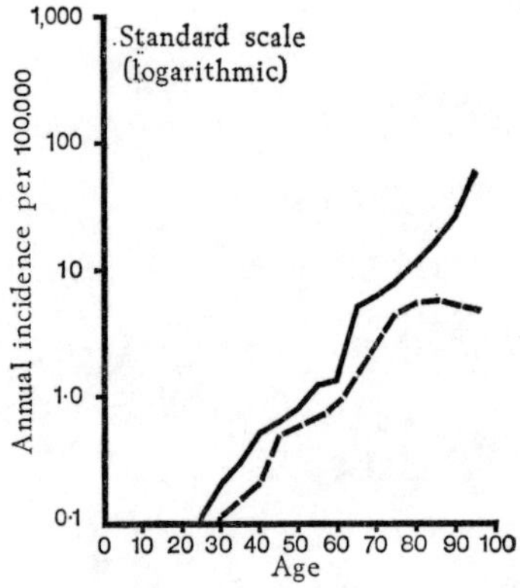

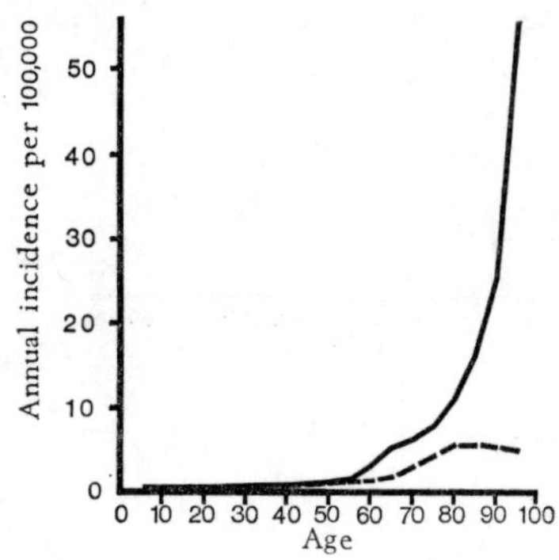

INCIDENCE RATES (per 100,000) by Age

Total cases 161 *males*; 97 *females* (of which age not stated for 0 *males* and 1 *female*)

Age	M	F	Age	M	F	Age	M	F
0–4	0·0	0·0	*35–39*	0·4	0·2	*70–74*	7·0	3·3
5–9	0·1	0·0	*40–44*	0·6	0·2	*75–79*	8·5	5·5
10–14	0·0	0·0	*45–49*	0·6	0·7	*80–84*	15·0	5·0
15–19	0·0	0·1	*50–54*	0·9	0·4	*85–89*	18·6	6·2
20–24	0·0	0·0	*55–59*	1·4	0·9	*90–94*	61·5	0·0
25–29	0·2	0·1	*60–64*	4·7	0·8	*95+*	0·0	32·2
30–34	0·2	0·1	*65–69*	5·2	2·1	*All ages*	1·1	0·7

SEX AND AGE DISTRIBUTION

	Male	*Female*
Mean age (*years*)	66·0	67·6
95% between ages	33 & 90	32 & 89
Children under 15 (%)	0·6	0·0
Median age (*years*)	66·8	70·9
Proportion by sex (%)	62·4	37·6
Proportion of all cancers by sex (%)	0·4	0·2
Trend over 10 years	(–)	(–)

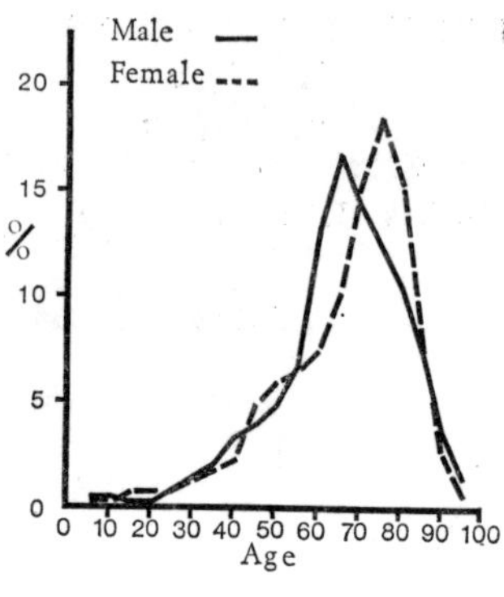

5-YEAR SURVIVAL RATES BY AGE

Crude ——— *Corrected* ----

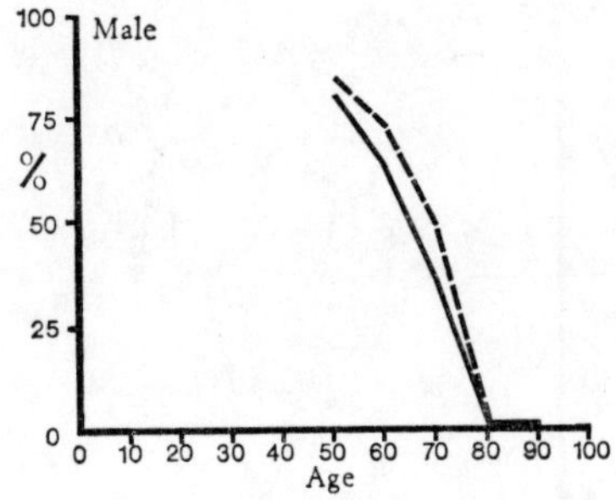

ALL CASES

Total 164
Male 100
Female 64

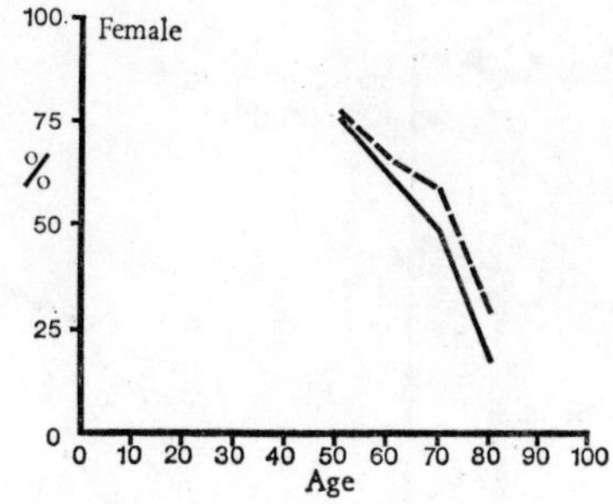

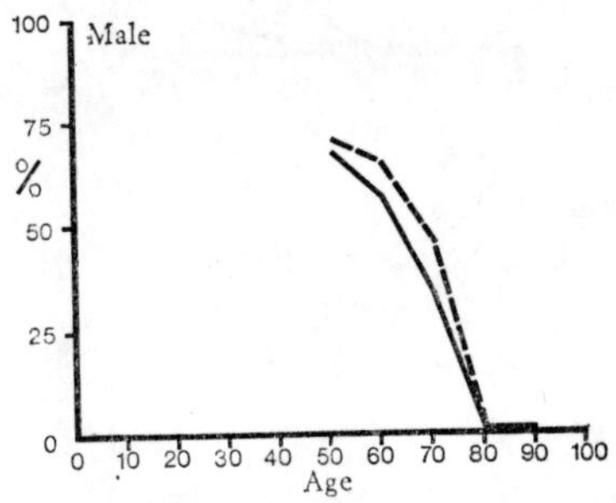

RADICAL TREATMENT

(80·5% of total)
76·0% *male*
87·5% *female*

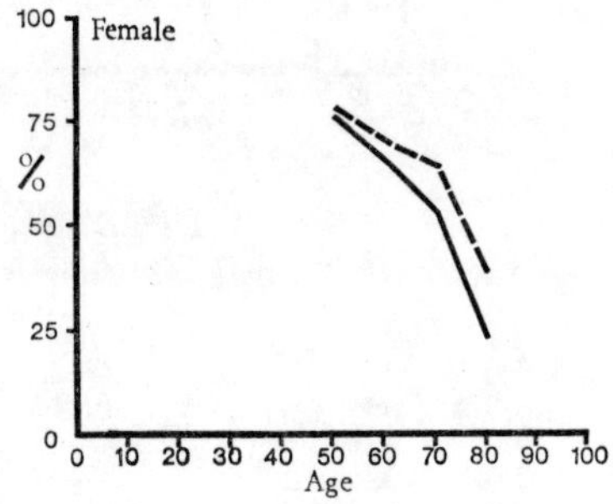

INDICES OF SURVIVAL

	All cases		Radical Treatment	
	Male	*Female*	*Male*	*Female*
FIVE YEAR SURVIVAL RATE (%)				
Crude	27·0	48·4	32·9	55·4
Corrected	*41·7*	*58·9*	*48·3*	*65·2*
Total cases†	100	64	76	56
TEN YEAR SURVIVAL RATE (%)				
Crude	22·3	24·7	28·2	28·9
Corrected	*47·8*	*42·2*	*56·8*	*44·7*
Total cases†	130	57	103	45

† Number of cases on which survival rate is based

SURVIVAL TIME (*months*)				
First quartile (75% S.R.)	6·4	7·9	8·2	*10·9*
Median (50% S.R.)	**14·3**	**39·0**	**16·0**	**>60**
Third quartile (25% S.R.)	>60	>60	>60	>60

ANNUAL SURVIVAL RATES

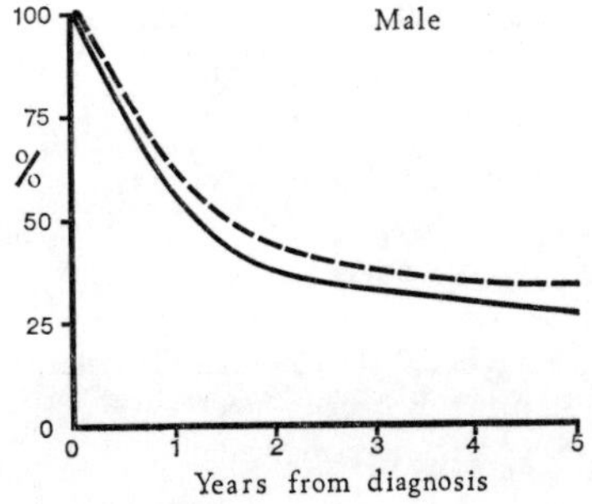

All cases ———
Radical treatment ----

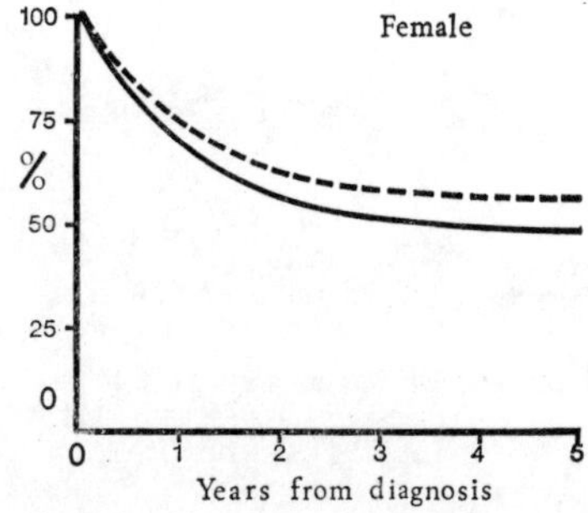

FAUCES ICD (8th) **146 (part)**

INCIDENCE RATE (per 100,000)

Male —— *Female* ----

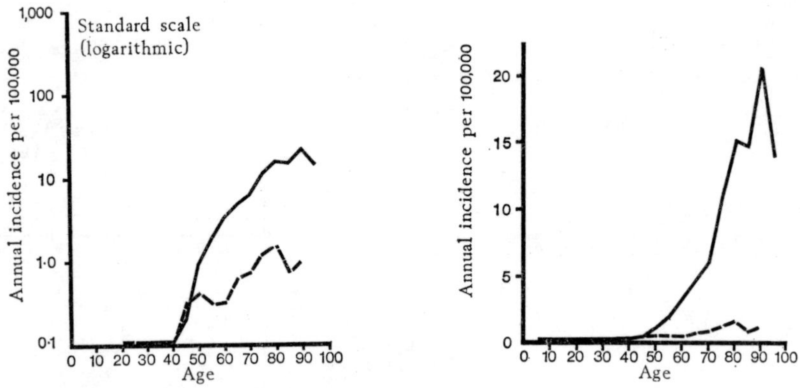

INCIDENCE RATES (per 100,000) by Age

Total cases 168 *males*; 33 *females* (of which age not stated for 0 *males* and 0 *females*)

Age	M	F	Age	M	F	Age	M	F
0–4	0·0	0·0	*35–39*	0·1	0·0	*70–74*	7·3	0·6
5–9	0·0	0·0	*40–44*	0·1	0·3	*75–79*	16·5	2·0
10–14	0·0	0·0	*45–49*	0·4	0·3	*80–84*	12·2	0·5
15–19	0·0	0·0	*50–54*	1·3	0·4	*85–89*	21·3	1·2
20–24	0·1	0·1	*55–59*	2·4	0·2	*90–94*	15·4	0·0
25–29	0·0	0·0	*60–64*	4·3	0·4	*95+*	0·0	0·0
30–34	0·1	0·0	*65–69*	4·9	0·8	*All ages*	1·2	0·2

SEX AND AGE DISTRIBUTION

	Male	*Female*
Mean age (*years*)	68·0	62·8
95% between ages	45 & 88	24 & 86
Children under 15 (%)	0·0	0·0
Median age (*years*)	68·6	65·5
Proportion by sex (%)	83·6	16·4
Proportion of all cancers by sex (%)	0·4	0·1
Trend over 10 years	– –	(–)

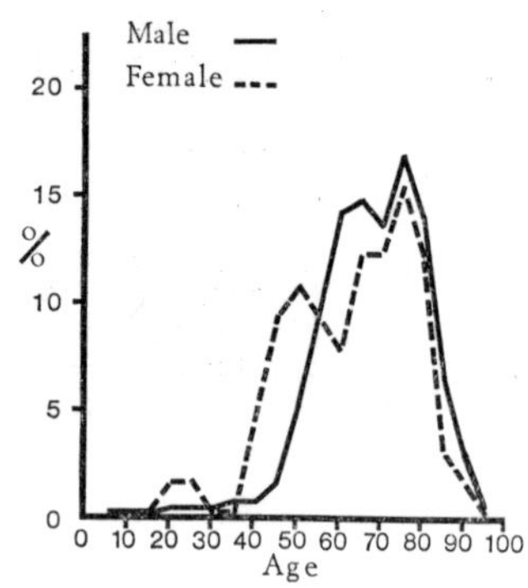

NOTES

Includes: Tonsil, pillar of fauces, soft palate and uvula. Soft palate and uvula are included under rubric 145 in 8th revision and under rubric 144 in the 7th.

Excludes: Branchial cleft (146·8 in 8th revision) which is classified with extra-gonadal developmental tumours (see ENDOCRINE GLANDS, ETC., p. 72); Epiglottis (146·8 in 8th) which is classified with LARYNX (as in 7th).

5-YEAR SURVIVAL RATES BY AGE

Crude ——— *Corrected* - - - -

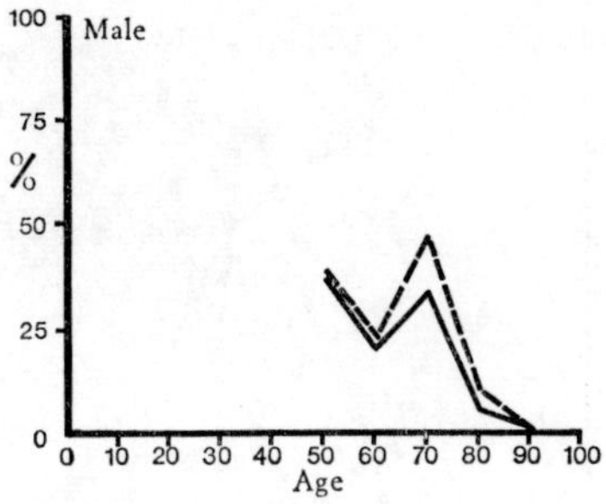

ALL CASES

Total 161
Male 140
Female 21

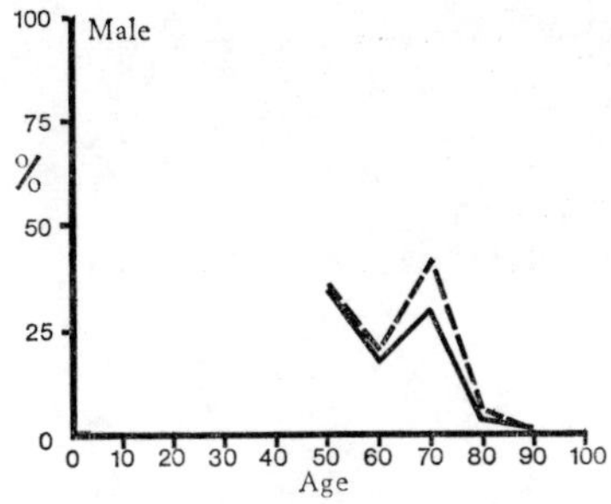

RADICAL TREATMENT

(75·2% of total)
76·4% *male*
66·7% *female*

INDICES OF SURVIVAL

	All cases *Male*	All cases *Female*	Radical Treatment *Male*	Radical Treatment *Female*
FIVE YEAR SURVIVAL RATE (%)				
Crude	15·7	42·9	20·6	57·1
Corrected	*23·0*	*53·6*	*28·5*	*64·1*
Total cases†	140	21	107	14
TEN YEAR SURVIVAL RATE (%)				
Crude	9·6	14·3	14·1	25·0
Corrected	*21·9*	*25·3*	*29·3*	*37·8*
Total cases†	157	28	99	16
SURVIVAL TIME (*months*)				
First quartile (75% S.R.)	5·3	9·0	6·7	9·6
Median (50% S.R.)	**11·2**	**13·8**	**17·8**	**>60**
Third quartile (25% S.R.)	32·6	>60	45·5	>60

† Number of cases on which survival rate is based

ANNUAL SURVIVAL RATES

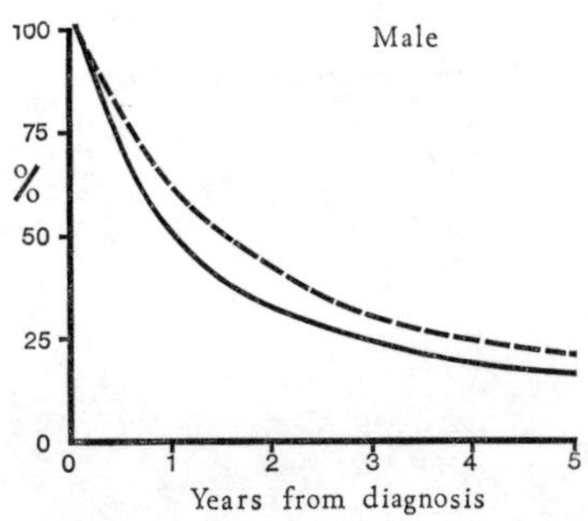

All cases ———
Radical Treatment - - - -

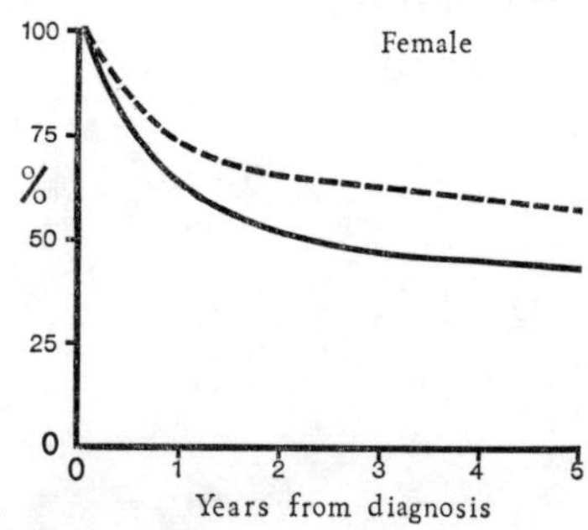

NASOPHARYNX **ICD (8th) 147**

INCIDENCE RATE (per 100,000)

Male —— *Female* ----

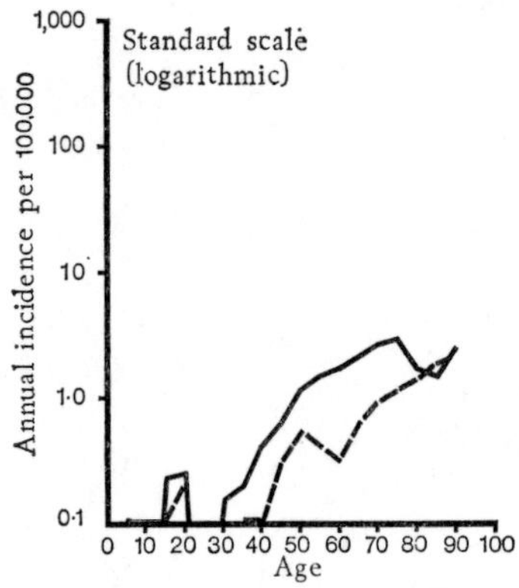

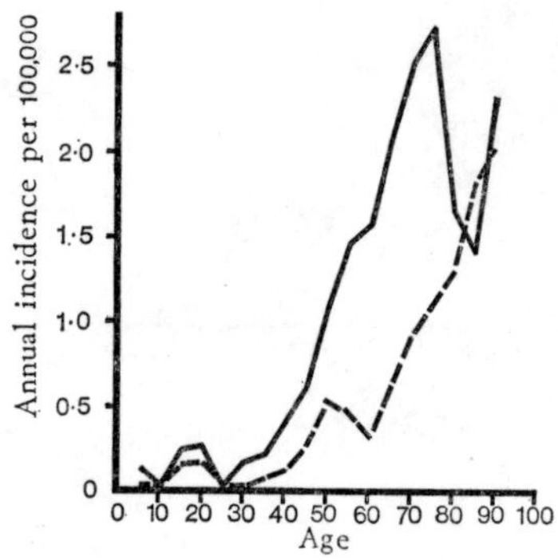

INCIDENCE RATES (per 100,000) by Age

Total cases 87 *males*; 39 *females* (of which age not stated for 0 *males* and 0 *females*)

Age	M	F	Age	M	F	Age	M	F
0–4	0·2	0·0	*35–39*	0·1	0·1	*70–74*	3·2	1·0
5–9	0·0	0·0	*40–44*	0·7	0·1	*75–79*	2·0	1·2
10–14	0·0	0·0	*45–49*	0·5	0·4	*80–84*	0·9	1·5
15–19	0·5	0·3	*50–54*	1·7	0·6	*85–89*	2·7	2·5
20–24	0·0	0·0	*55–59*	1·2	0·2	*90–94*	0·0	0·0
25–29	0·0	0·0	*60–64*	2·1	0·4	*95+*	0·0	0·0
30–34	0·3	0·0	*65–69*	2·0	0·8	*All ages*	0·6	0·3

SEX AND AGE DISTRIBUTION

	Male	*Female*
Mean age (*years*)	55·2	60·8
95% between ages	15 & 80	17 & 88
Children under 15 (%)	2·3	0·0
Median age (*years*)	57·3	64·2
Proportion by sex (%)	69·0	31·0
Proportion of all cancers by sex (%)	0·2	0·1
Trend over 10 years	(–)	(–)

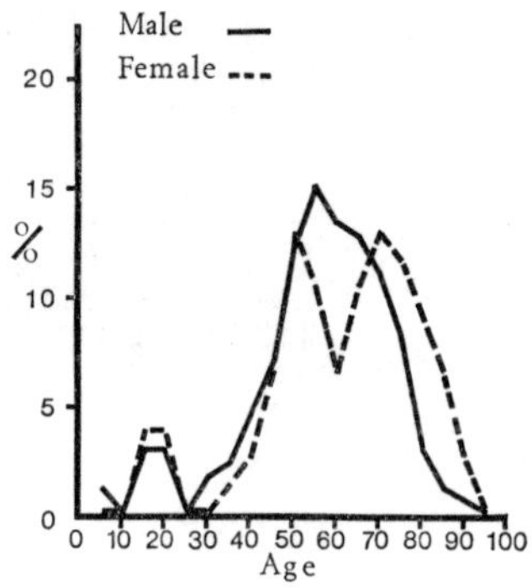

5-YEAR SURVIVAL RATES BY AGE

Crude—— *Corrected* ----

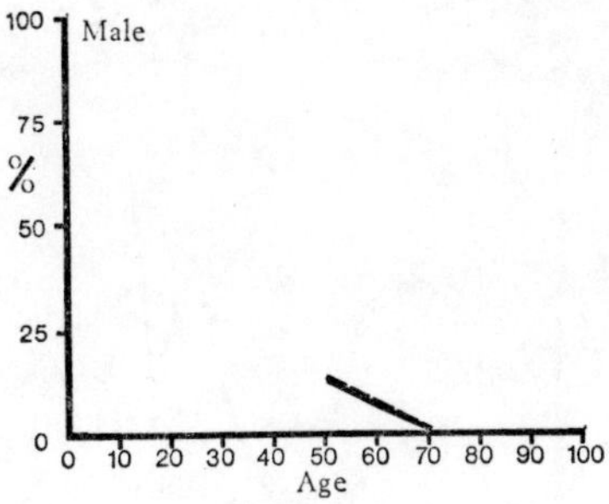

ALL CASES

Total 81
Male 52
Female 29

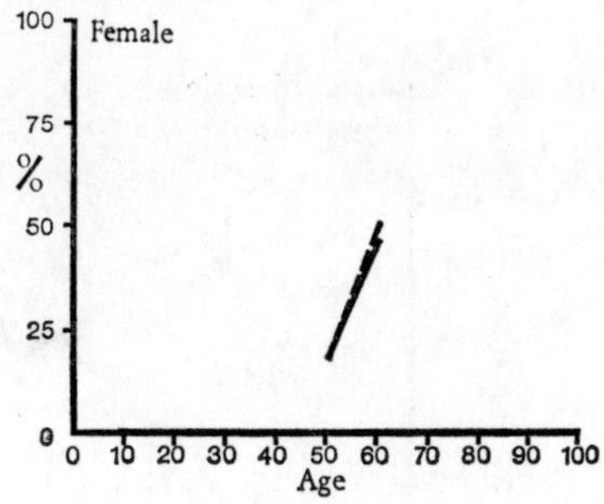

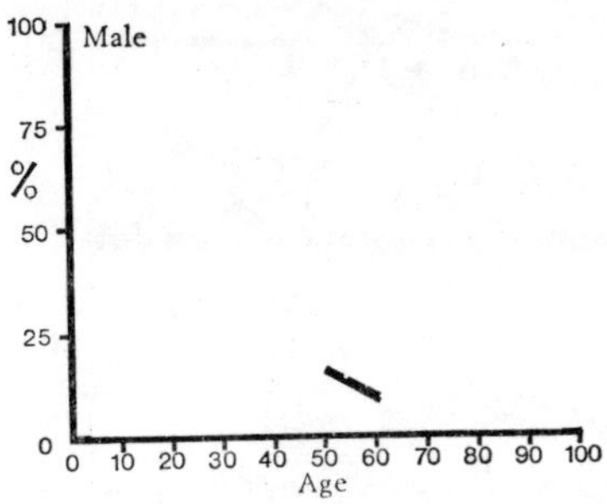

RADICAL TREATMENT

(79·0% of total)
76·9% *male*
82·8% *female*

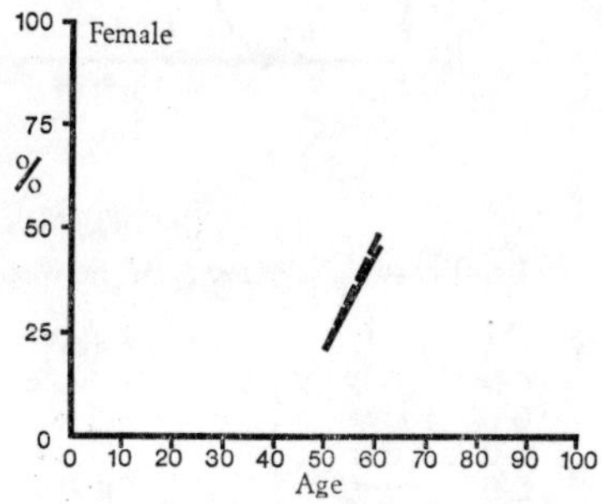

INDICES OF SURVIVAL

	All cases		Radical Treatment	
	Male	*Female*	*Male*	*Female*
FIVE YEAR SURVIVAL RATE (%)				
Crude	9·6	34·5	12·5	37·5
Corrected	*10·7*	*37·8*	*13·7*	*41·0*
Total cases†	52	29	40	24
TEN YEAR SURVIVAL RATE (%)				
Crude	4·2	20·0	7·4	26·7
Corrected	*5·5*	*24·0*	*9·8*	*30·7*
Total cases†	48	25	27	15
SURVIVAL TIME (*months*)				
First quartile (75% S.R.)	5·2	8·0	5·9	12·8
Median (50% S.R.)	**11·0**	**30·5**	**12·3**	**31·0**
Third quartile (25% S.R.)	16·1	>60	21·3	>60

† Number of cases on which survival is based

ANNUAL SURVIVAL RATES

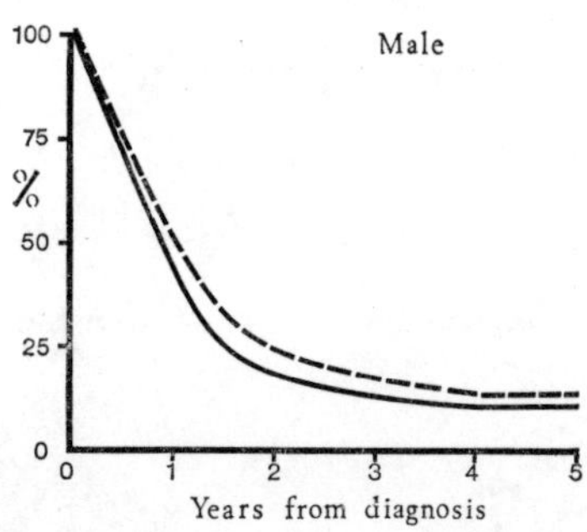

All cases ——
Radical treatment ----

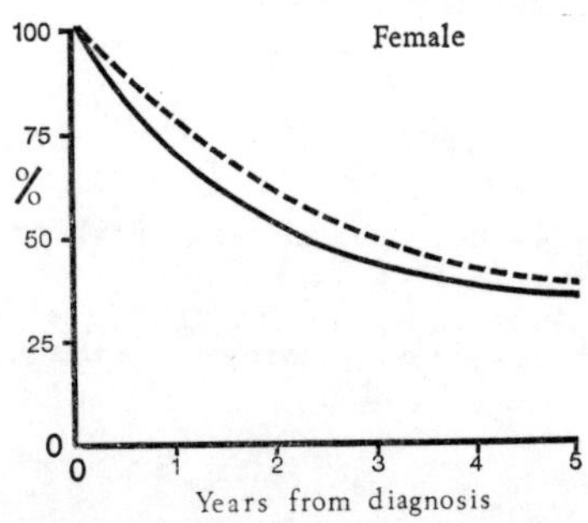

INCIDENCE RATE (per 100,000)

Male —— *Female* ----

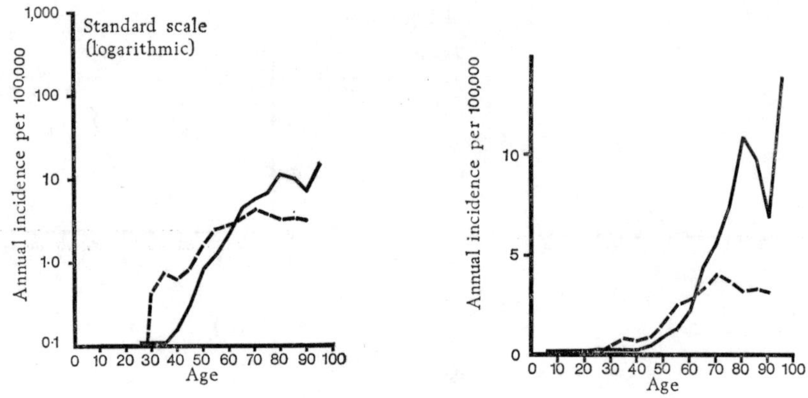

INCIDENCE RATES (per 100,000) by Age

Total cases 130 *males*; 155 *females* (of which age not stated for 0 *males* and 0 *females*)

Age	M	F	Age	M	F	Age	M	F
0–4	0·0	0·0	*35–39*	0·1	0·6	*70–74*	5·4	3·9
5–9	0·0	0·0	*40–44*	0·2	0·6	*75–79*	10·5	3·2
10–14	0·0	0·0	*45–49*	0·4	1·0	*80–84*	11·2	3·0
15–19	0·0	0·0	*50–54*	1·2	2·0	*85–89*	5·3	3·7
20–24	0·0	0·0	*55–59*	1·2	2·8	*90–94*	15·4	0·0
25–29	0·1	0·0	*60–64*	3·3	2·5	*95+*	0·0	0·0
30–34	0·1	0·7	*65–69*	5·6	4·0	*All ages*	0·9	1·1

SEX AND AGE DISTRIBUTION

	Male	*Female*
Mean age (*years*)	66·9	60·8
95% between ages	41 & 85	33 & 84
Children under 15 (%)	0·0	0·0
Median age (*years*)	67·6	61·4
Proportion by sex (%)	45·6	54·4
Proportion of all cancers by sex (%)	0·3	0·4
Trend over 10 years	(–)	(–)

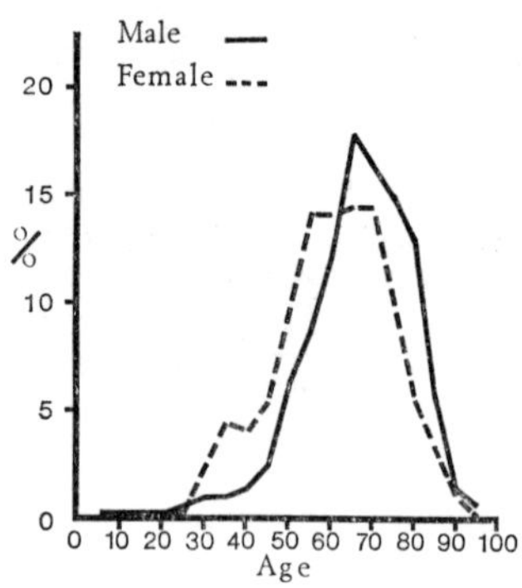

NOTES

Includes: Postcricoid region, pyriform fossa, and hypopharynx not further specified. For details of subdivisions see p. 20.

Pharynx, not further specified (149, and part of 146·9 in 8th revision; 148 in 7th), amounts to too few cases and is not sufficiently homogeneous to warrant analysis in page-pair form.

5-YEAR SURVIVAL RATES BY AGE

Crude ——— *Corrected* ----

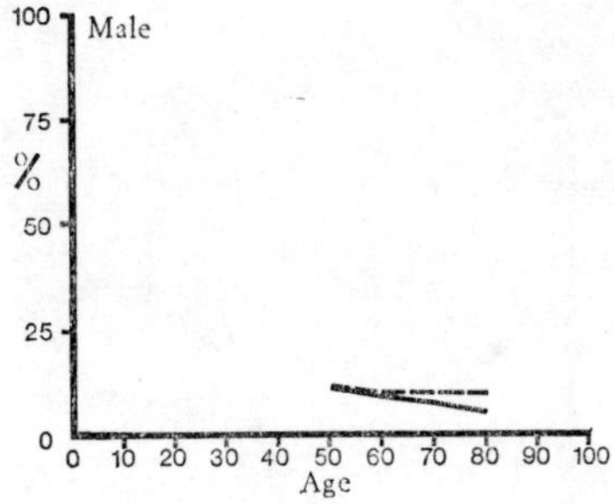

ALL CASES

Total 191
Male 94
Female 97

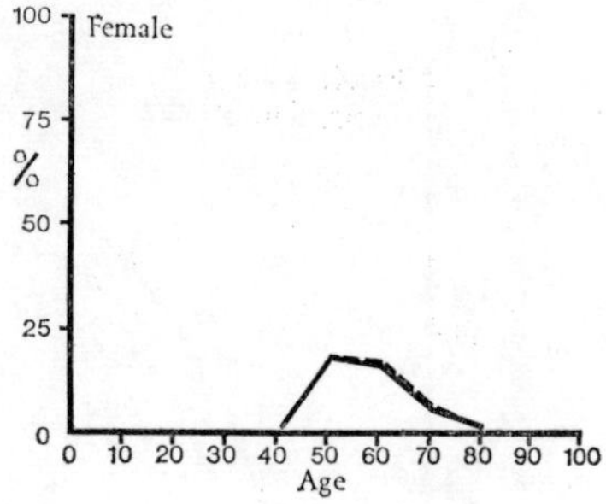

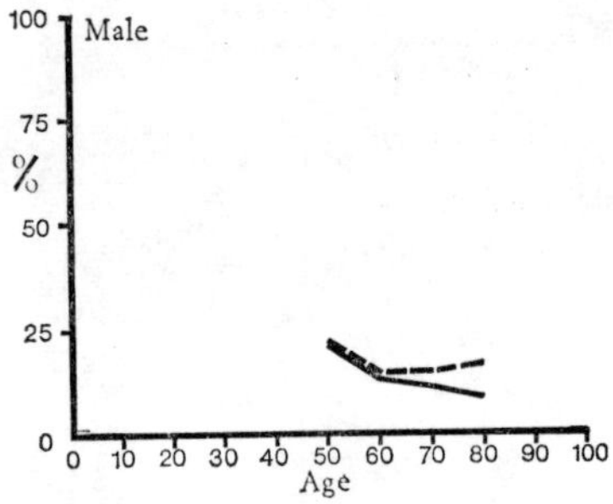

RADICAL TREATMENT

(56·5% of total)
52·1% *male*
60·8% *female*

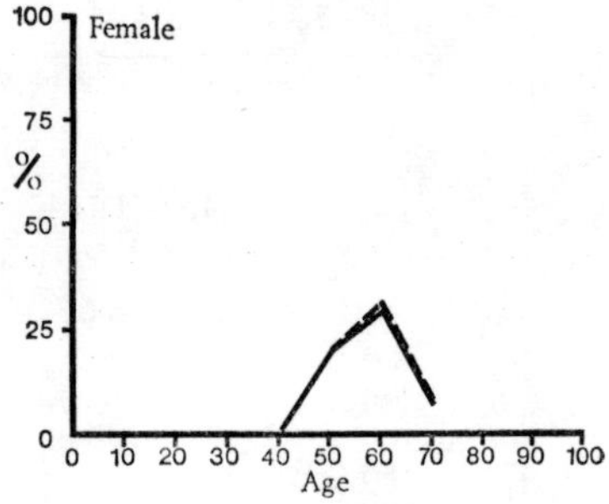

INDICES OF SURVIVAL

	All cases *Male*	All cases *Female*	Radical Treatment *Male*	Radical Treatment *Female*
FIVE YEAR SURVIVAL RATE (%)				
Crude	6·4	10·3	10·2	15·3
Corrected	*8·8*	*11·5*	*13·8*	*17·0*
Total cases†	94	97	49	59
TEN YEAR SURVIVAL RATE (%)				
Crude	1·1	7·0	3·3	13·3
Corrected	*2·3*	*9·7*	*6·3*	*17·2*
Total cases†	92	71	30	30

† Number of cases on which survival rate is based

SURVIVAL TIME (*months*)				
First quartile (75% S.R.)	2·2	2·3	6·6	5·4
Median (50% S.R.)	**7·0**	**6·4**	**9·9**	**10·5**
Third quartile (25% S.R.)	13·3	15·8	25·0	30·5

ANNUAL SURVIVAL RATES

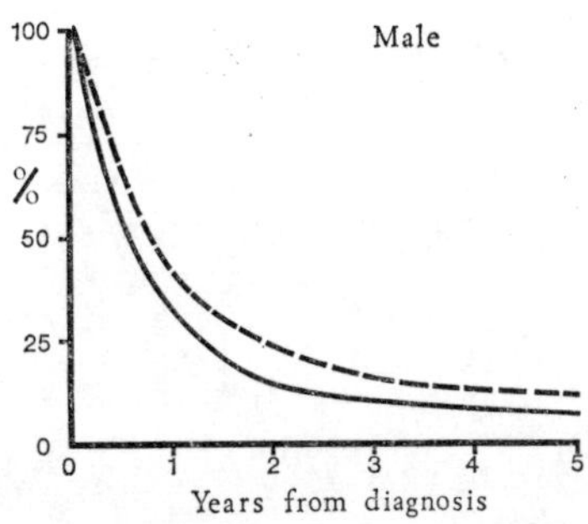

All cases ———
Radical treatment ----

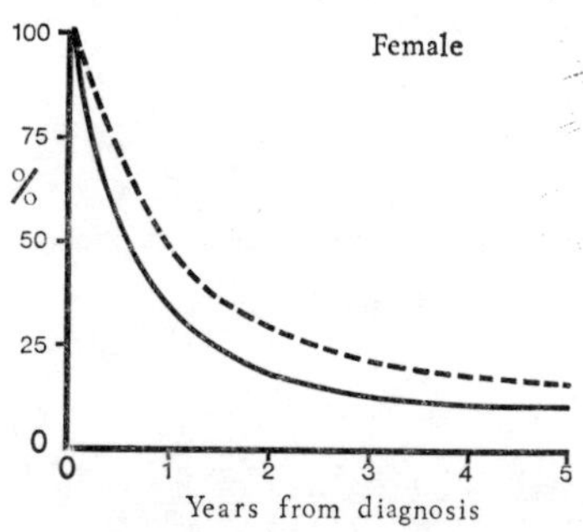

OESOPHAGUS **ICD (8th) 150**

INCIDENCE RATE (per 100,000)

Male —— *Female* - - - -

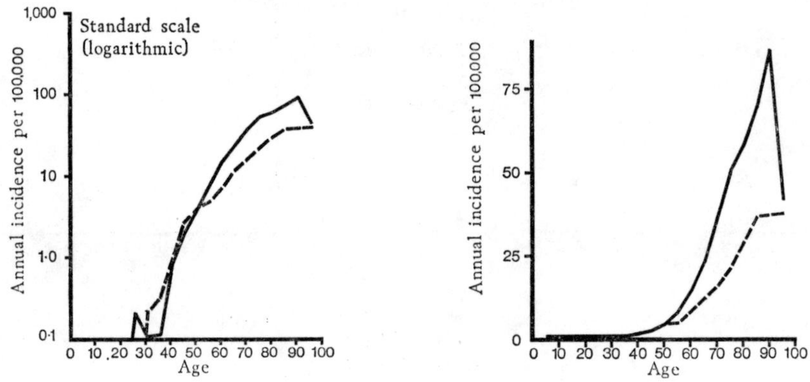

INCIDENCE RATES (per 100,000) by Age

Total cases 789 *males*; 591 *females* (of which age not stated for 0 *males* and 0 *females*)

Age	M	F	Age	M	F	Age	M	F
0–4	0·0	0·0	*35–39*	0·3	0·3	*70–74*	46·2	18·9
5–9	0·0	0·0	*40–44*	1·4	1·5	*75–79*	56·0	24·2
10–14	0·0	0·0	*45–49*	2·4	3·9	*80–84*	60·9	36·2
15–19	0·0	0·0	*50–54*	5·0	3·7	*85–89*	93·2	36·1
20–24	0·1	0·0	*55–59*	10·5	5·5	*90–94*	46·1	38·3
25–29	0·2	0·0	*60–64*	19·1	10·7	*95+*	0·0	32·2
30–34	0·0	0·3	*65–69*	28·2	13·0	*All ages*	5·6	4·1

SEX AND AGE DISTRIBUTION

	Male	*Female*
Mean age (*years*)	67·9	68·2
95% between ages	45 & 88	43 & 89
Children under 15 (%)	0·0	0·0
Median age (*years*)	68·7	69·4
Proportion by sex (%)	57·1	42·9
Proportion of all cancers by sex (%)	1·8	1·5
Trend over 10 years	(+)	(+)

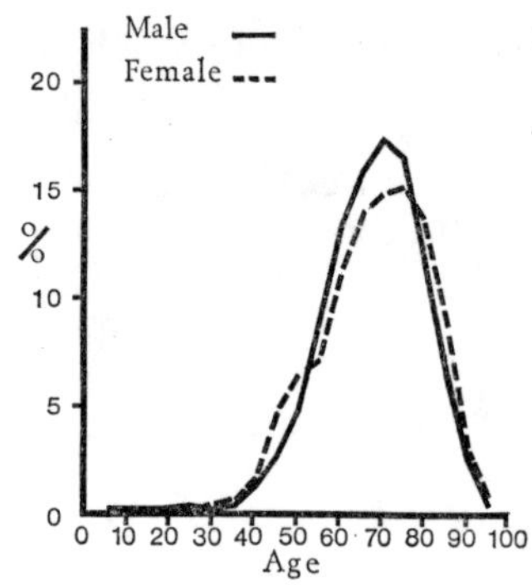

NOTES

Includes: Gastro-oesophageal junction, unless histologically adenocarcinoma, when classified with STOMACH.

5-YEAR SURVIVAL RATES BY AGE

Crude ——— *Corrected* ----

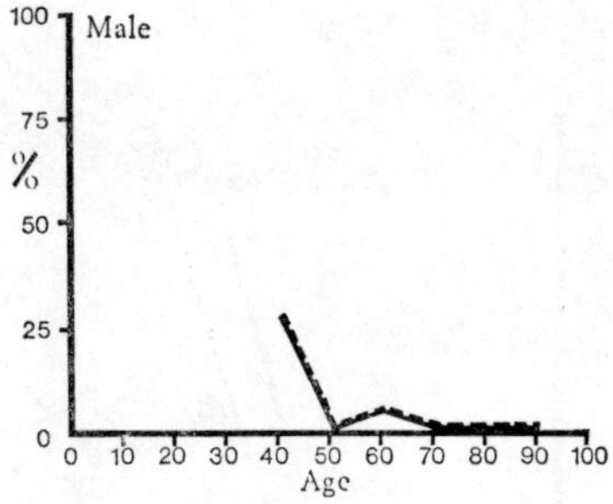

ALL CASES

Total 683
Male 401
Female 282

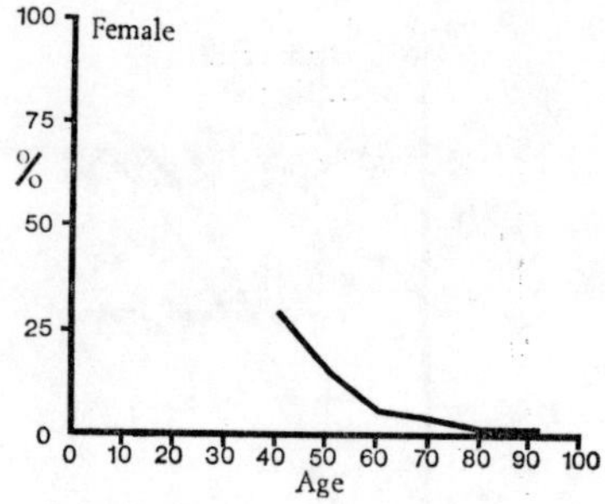

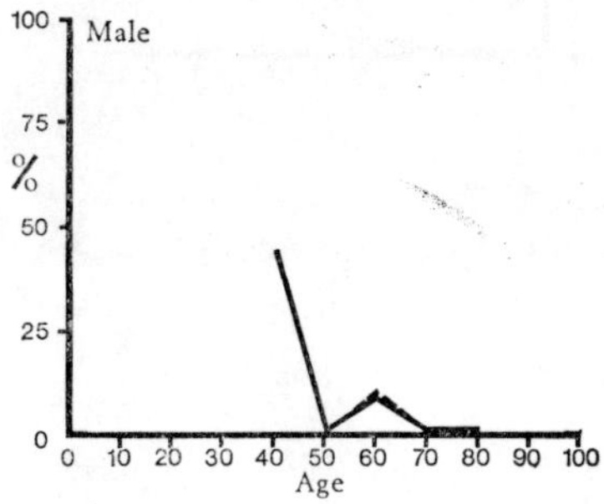

RADICAL TREATMENT

(27·8% of total)
26·7% *male*
29·4% *female*

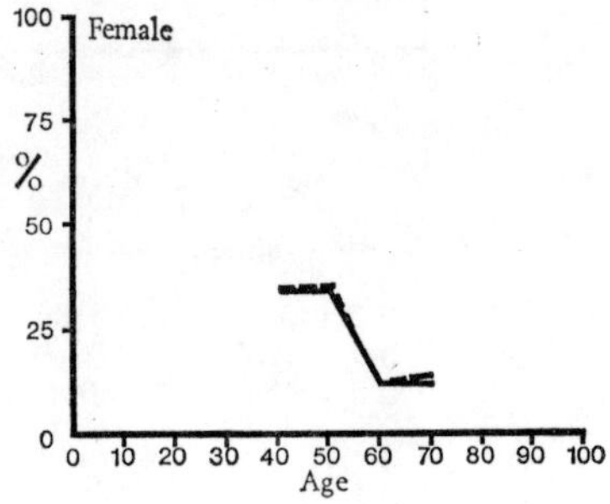

INDICES OF SURVIVAL

	All cases *Male*	All cases *Female*	Radical Treatment *Male*	Radical Treatment *Female*
FIVE YEAR SURVIVAL RATE (%)				
Crude	2·0	4·6	5·6	15·7
Corrected	*2·2*	*5·9*	*6·9*	*17·7*
Total cases†	401	282	107	83
TEN YEAR SURVIVAL RATE (%)				
Crude	1·3	1·7	4·4	3·6
Corrected	*2·6*	*2·9*	*8·0*	*5·3*
Total cases†	313	170	91	56
SURVIVAL TIME (*months*)				
First quartile (75% S.R.)	0·8	0·7	1·0	1·8
Median (50% S.R.)	**2·6**	**2·8**	**7·2**	**9·5**
Third quartile (25% S.R.)	6·1	7·1	20·2	19·5

† Number of cases on which survival rate is based

ANNUAL SURVIVAL RATES

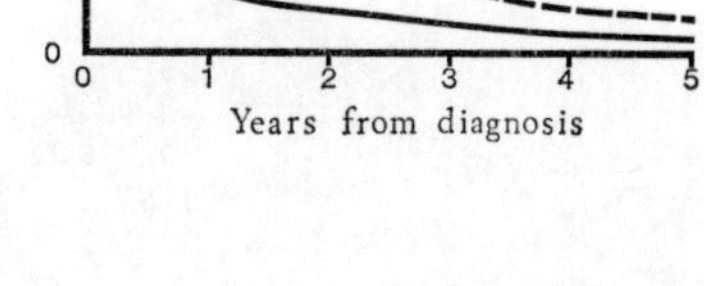

All cases ———
Radical treatment ----

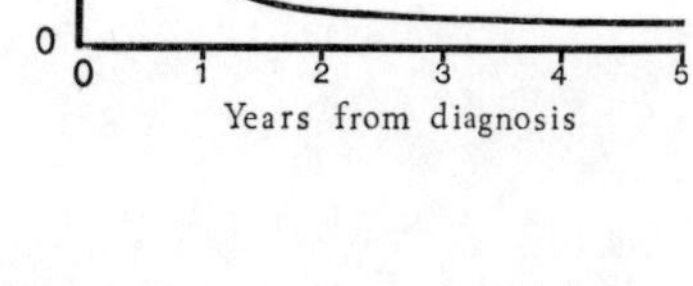

STOMACH **ICD (8th) 151**

INCIDENCE RATE (per 100,000)

Male —— *Female* ----

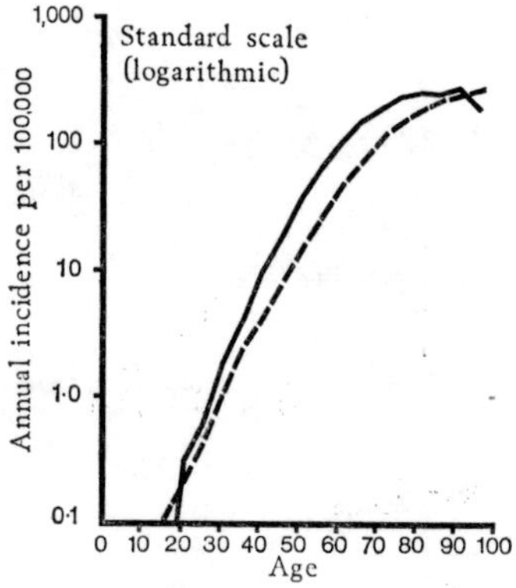

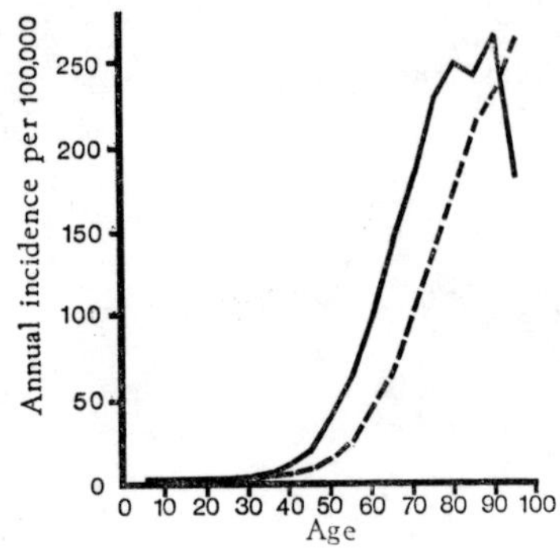

INCIDENCE RATES (per 100,000) by Age

Total cases 4641 *males*; 3346 *females* (of which age not stated for 5 *males* and 19 *females*)

Age	M	F	Age	M	F	Age	M	F
0–4	0·0	0·0	*35–39*	4·6	2·9	*70–74*	206·8	121·7
5–9	0·0	0·0	*40–44*	14·3	5·1	*75–79*	258·2	159·0
10–14	0·0	0·0	*45–49*	20·5	9·6	*80–84*	225·7	204·5
15–19	0·0	0·2	*50–54*	51·5	17·9	*85–89*	277·1	220·6
20–24	0·6	0·1	*55–59*	74·2	30·3	*90–94*	184·5	279·1
25–29	0·6	0·7	*60–64*	129·1	51·8	*95+*	135·5	160·9
30–34	2·9	1·4	*65–69*	163·0	83·1	*All ages*	32·9	23·2

SEX AND AGE DISTRIBUTION

	Male	*Female*
Mean age (*years*)	64·5	69·8
95% between ages	41 & 85	43 & 89
Children under 15 (%)	0·0	0·0
Median age (*years*)	64·6	71·1
Proportion by sex (%)	58·1	41·9
Proportion of all cancers by sex (%)	10·8	8·2
Trend over 10 years	(−)	(+)

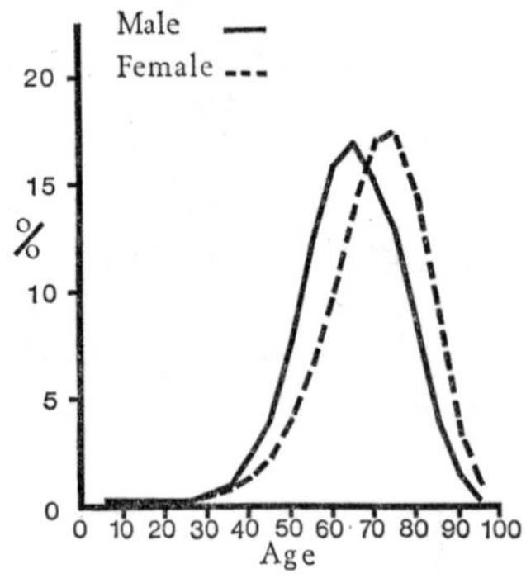

5-YEAR SURVIVAL RATES BY AGE

Crude —— *Corrected* - - - -

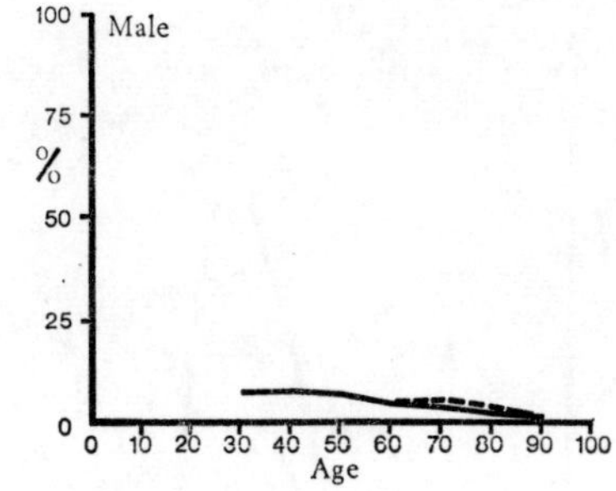

ALL CASES

Total 4180

Male 2500
Female 1680

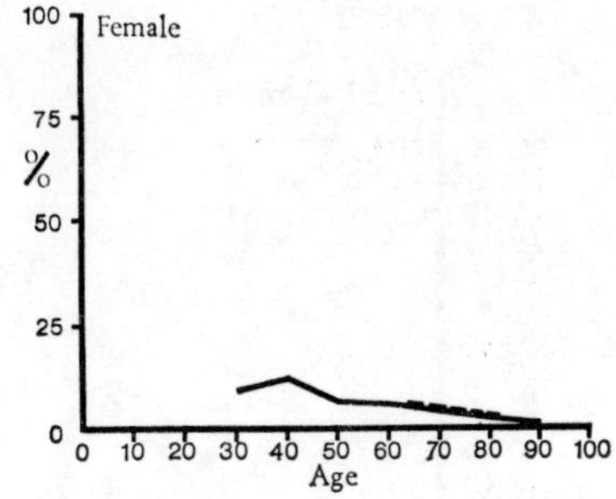

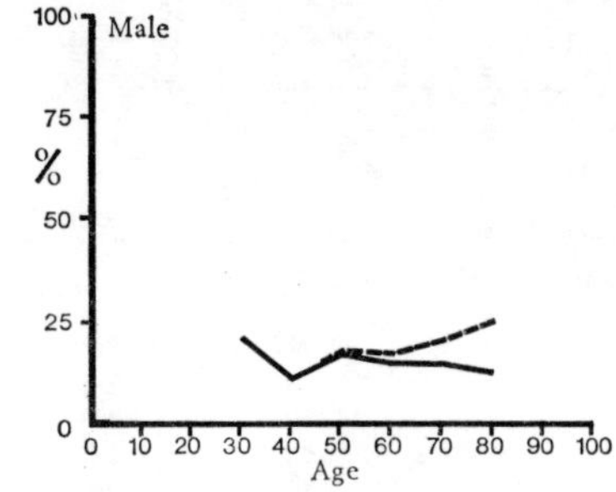

RADICAL TREATMENT

(22·8% of total)
24·0% *male*
21·0% *female*

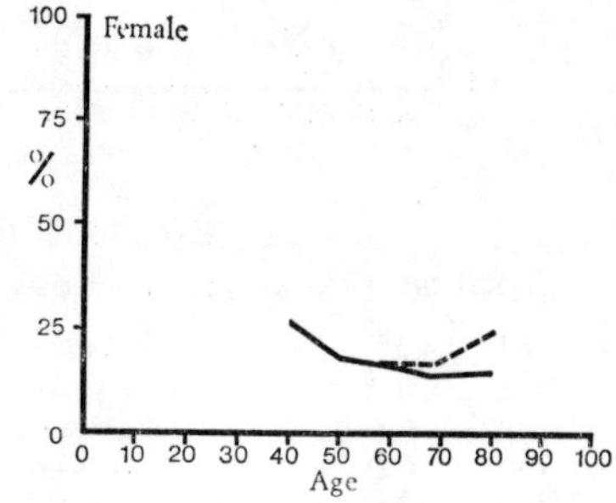

INDICES OF SURVIVAL

	All cases		Radical Treatment	
	Male	*Female*	*Male*	*Female*
FIVE YEAR SURVIVAL RATE (%)				
Crude	3·9	3·3	14·3	15·1
Corrected	*5·0*	*4·3*	*17·2*	*17·7*
Total cases†	2500	1680	601	352
TEN YEAR SURVIVAL RATE (%)				
Crude	3·4	2·6	10·9	9·7
Corrected	*5·6*	*3·9*	*16·2*	*13·1*
Total cases†	1316	804	374	216

†Number of cases on which survival rate is based

SURVIVAL TIME (*months*)				
First quartile (75% S.R.)	0·7	0·8	3·1	4·4
Median (50% S.R.)	**2·3**	**2·4**	**12·4**	**12·6**
Third quartile (25% S.R.)	7·4	7·1	31·0	34·4

ANNUAL SURVIVAL RATES

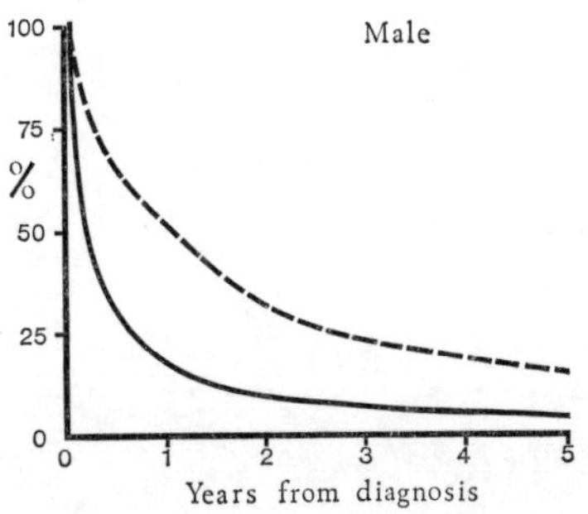

All cases ——————

Radical treatment - - - -

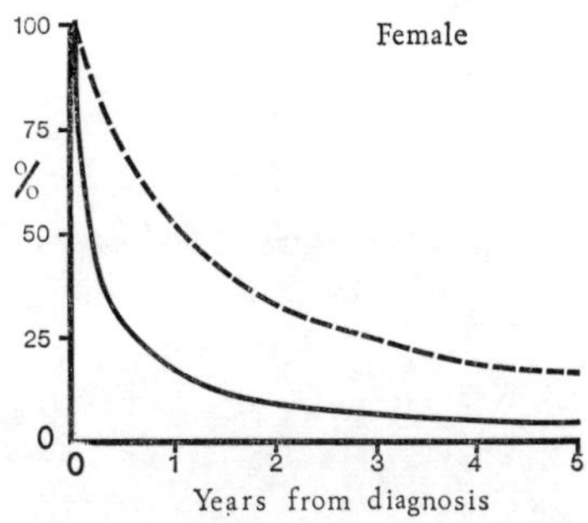

INCIDENCE RATE (per 100,000)

Male —— *Female* - - - -

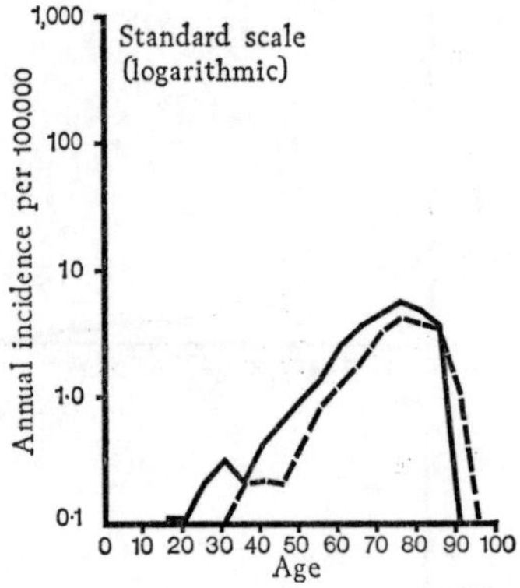

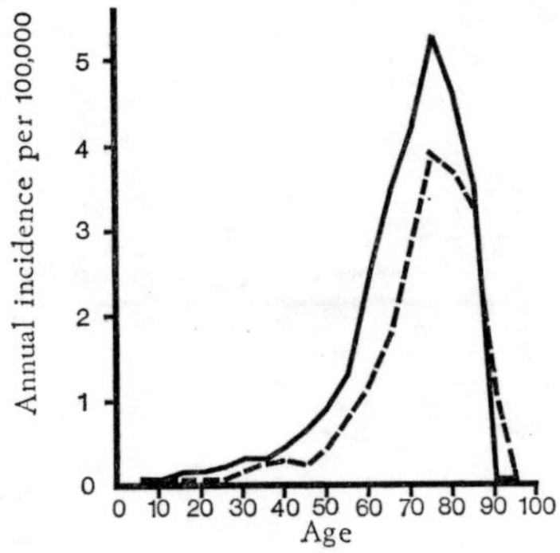

INCIDENCE RATES (per 100,000) by Age

Total cases 114 *males*; 87 *females* (of which age not stated for 0 *males* and 0 *females*)

Age	M	F	Age	M	F	Age	M	F
0–4	0·0	0·0	*35–39*	0·3	0·2	*70–74*	5·7	4·1
5–9	0·0	0·0	*40–44*	0·5	0·3	*75–79*	4·5	3·5
10–14	0·0	0·0	*45–49*	0·7	0·1	*80–84*	4·7	4·0
15–19	0·2	0·0	*50–54*	1·0	0·7	*85–89*	0·0	1·2
20–24	0·0	0·0	*55–59*	1·5	0·8	*90–94*	0·0	0·0
25–29	0·3	0·0	*60–64*	3·6	1·6	*95+*	0·0	0·0
30–34	0·2	0·2	*65–69*	3·1	1·9	*All ages*	0·8	0·6

SEX AND AGE DISTRIBUTION

	Male	*Female*
Mean age (*years*)	60·6	66·4
95% between ages	26 & 82	35 & 84
Children under 15 (%)	0·0	0·0
Median age (*years*)	62·6	69·0
Proportion by sex (%)	56·7	43·3
Proportion of all cancers by sex (%)	0·3	0·2
Trend over 10 years	(+)	(−)

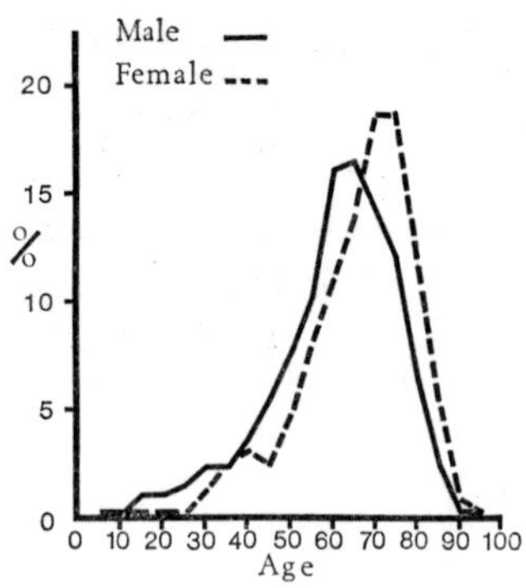

NOTES

Includes: Duodenum, jejunum and ileum. For details of subdivisions see p. 26.

5-YEAR SURVIVAL RATES BY AGE

Crude —— *Corrected* ----

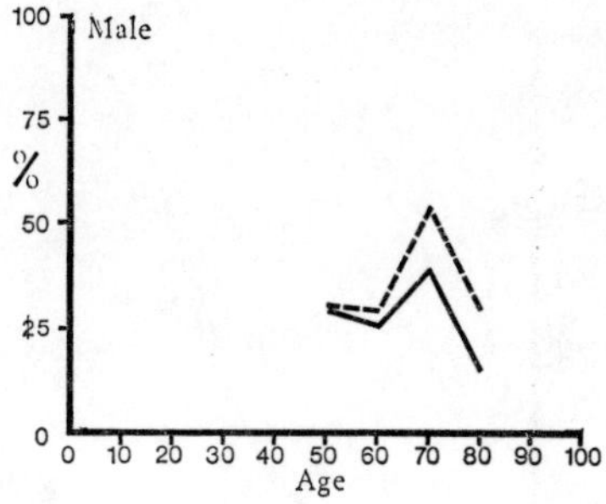

ALL CASES

Total	94
Male	44
Female	50

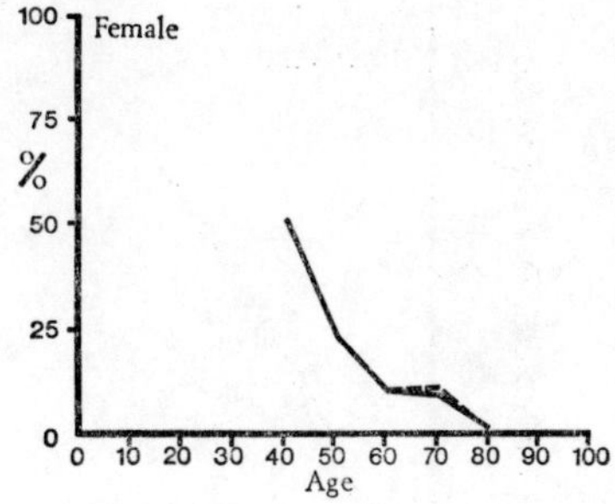

RADICAL TREATMENT

(42·6% of total)
45·5% *male*
40·0% *female*

INDICES OF SURVIVAL

	All cases *Male*	All cases *Female*	Radical Treatment *Male*	Radical Treatment *Female*
FIVE YEAR SURVIVAL RATE (%)				
Crude	31·8	16·0	45·0	25·0
Corrected	*40·3*	*19·0*	*57·9*	*28·4*
Total cases†	44	50	20	20
TEN YEAR SURVIVAL RATE (%)				
Crude	27·9	16·7	71·4	33·3
Corrected	*46·3*	*22·2*	*100·0*	*41·2*
Total cases†	18	36	7	18
SURVIVAL TIME (*months*)				
First quartile (75% S.R.)	0·8	0·8	6·8	2·8
Median (50% S.R.)	**13·0**	**8·0**	**43·0**	**20·0**
Third quartile (25% S.R.)	>60	31·8	>60	>60

† Number of cases on which survival rate is based

ANNUAL SURVIVAL RATES

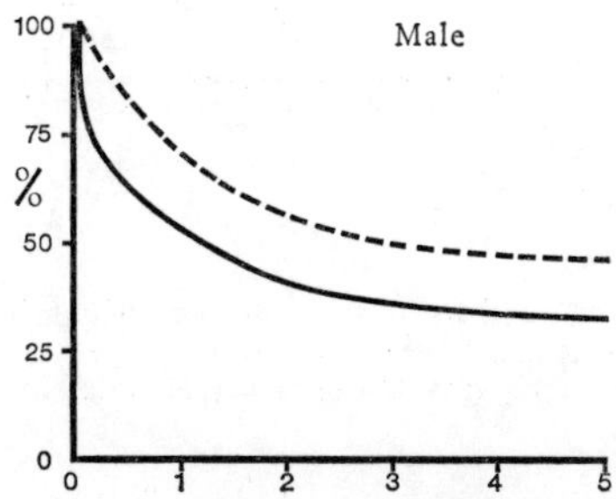

All cases ——
Radical treatment ----

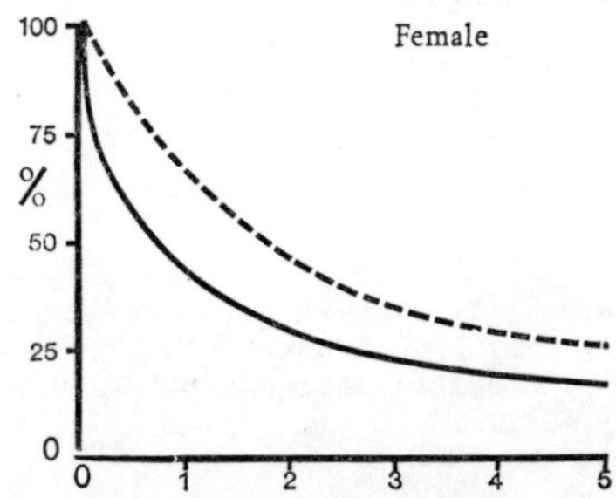

INCIDENCE RATE (per 100,000)

Male —— *Female* ----

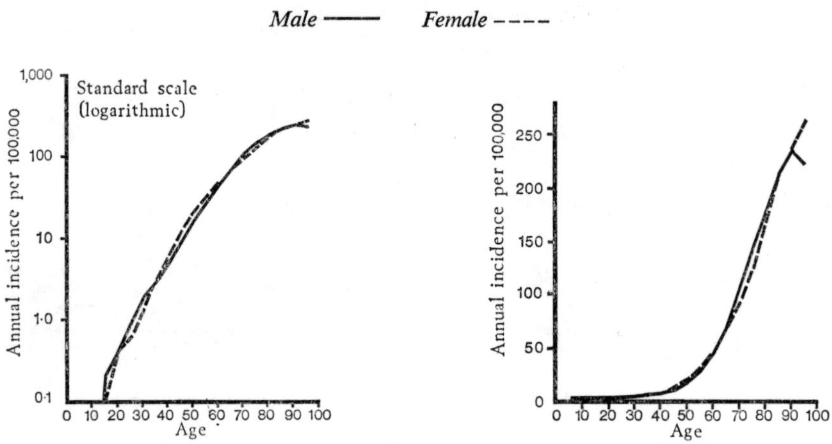

INCIDENCE RATES (per 100,000) by Age

Total cases 2508 *males*; 3438 *females* (of which age not stated for 1 *male* and 3 *females*)

Age	M	F	Age	M	F	Age	M	F
0–4	0·0	0·0	*35–39*	3·2	4·0	*70–74*	129·3	106·7
5–9	0·0	0·0	*40–44*	6·4	7·8	*75–79*	160·6	144·9
10–14	0·1	0·0	*45–49*	11·3	15·9	*80–84*	203·2	200·1
15–19	0·3	0·2	*50–54*	20·3	24·2	*85–89*	234·4	225·6
20–24	0·5	0·5	*55–59*	32·4	38·7	*90–94*	230·6	273·7
25–29	1·3	0·7	*60–64*	56·3	55·0	*95+*	135·5	193·1
30–34	2·4	2·0	*65–69*	83·5	77·9	*All ages*	17·8	23·8

SEX AND AGE DISTRIBUTION

	Male	*Female*
Mean age (*years*)	66·1	68·2
95% between ages	38 & 87	41 & 89
Children under 15 (%)	0·0	0·0
Median age (*years*)	67·3	69·4
Proportion by sex (%)	42·2	57·8
Proportion of all cancers by sex (%)	5·8	8·5
Trend over 10 years	(−)	(−)

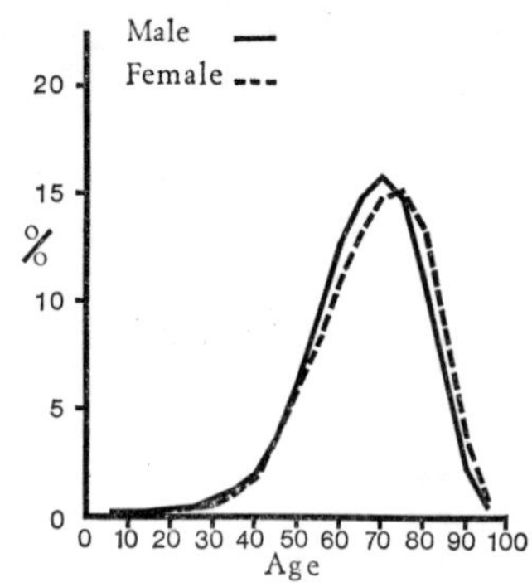

NOTES

Excludes: Appendix. Both in its incidence by age (which is relatively flat) and in its survival rate (which is very good) it is different from the rest of the large intestine. It was originally intended to form the subject of a separate page-pair, but the numbers proved inadequate to justify this course. Further details will be found on p. 26.

5-YEAR SURVIVAL RATES BY AGE

Crude —— *Corrected* ----

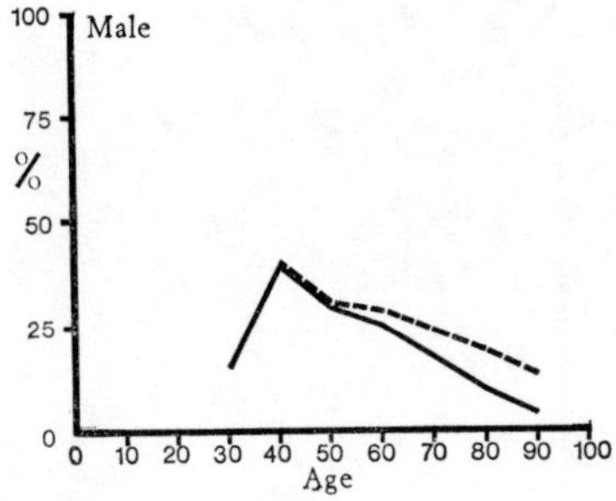

ALL CASES

Total 3242

Male 1398
Female 1844

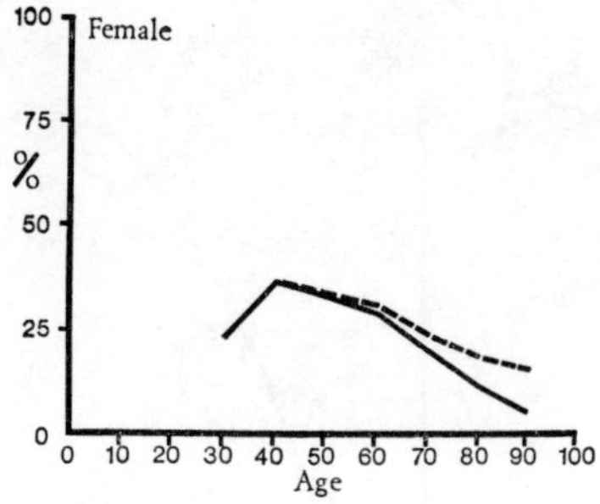

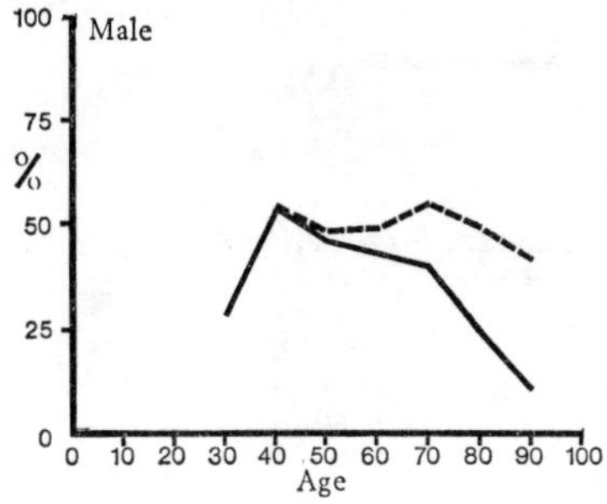

RADICAL TREATMENT

(46·0% of total)
46·4% *male*
45·7% *female*

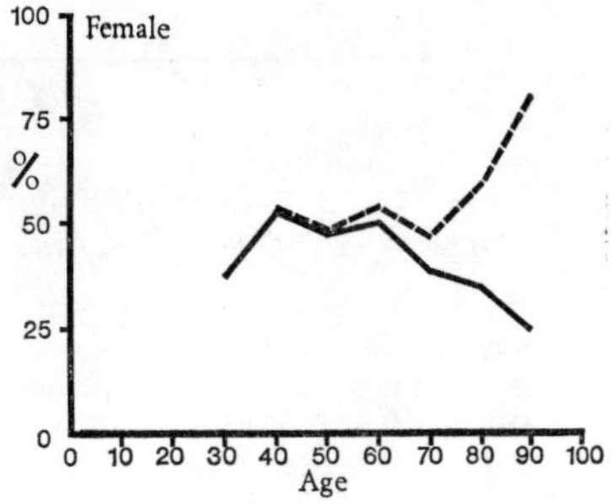

INDICES OF SURVIVAL

	All cases *Male*	All cases *Female*	Radical Treatment *Male*	Radical Treatment *Female*
FIVE YEAR SURVIVAL RATE (%)				
Crude	18·8	20·6	39·2	42·8
Corrected	*25·6*	*26·2*	*50·0*	*50·1*
Total cases†	1398	1844	648	842
TEN YEAR SURVIVAL RATE (%)				
Crude	10·7	15·2	21·9	29·7
Corrected	*19·5*	*23·8*	*37·5*	*42·7*
Total cases†	807	1089	384	525

† Number of cases on which survival rate is based

SURVIVAL TIME (*months*)				
First quartile (75% S.R.)	0·0	1·3	11·8	13·8
Median (50% S.R.)	**6·8**	**8·7**	**35·1**	**41·5**
Third quartile (25% S.R.)	33·4	38·8	>60	>60

ANNUAL SURVIVAL RATES

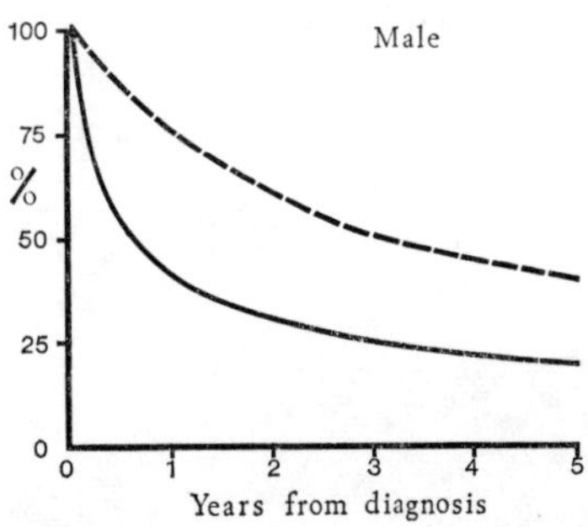

All cases ——
Radical treatment ----

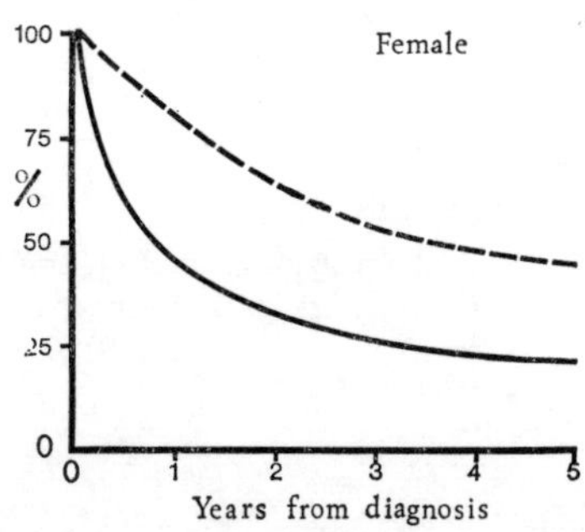

INCIDENCE RATE (per 100,000)

Male ——— *Female* - - - -

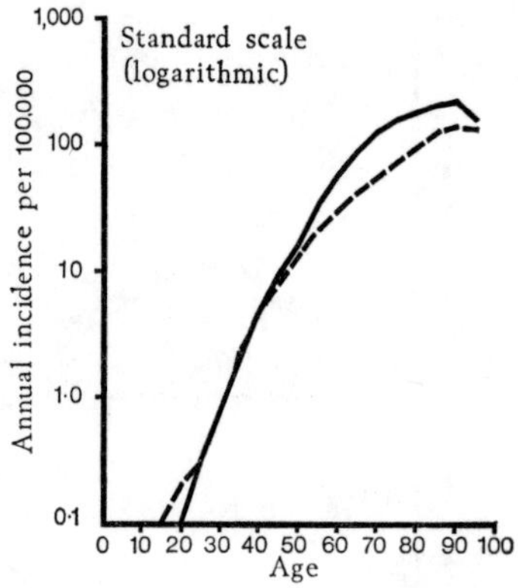

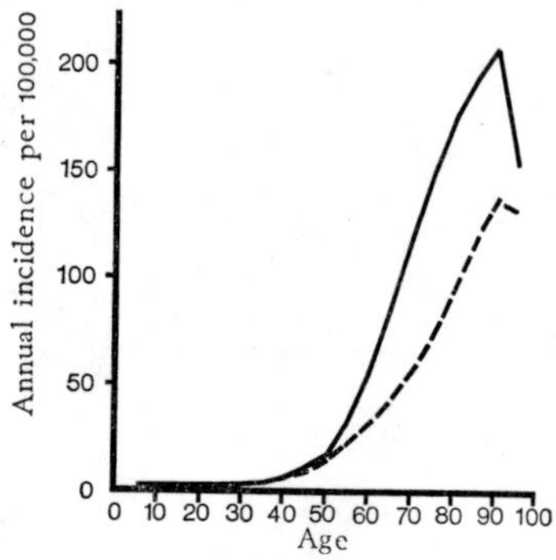

INCIDENCE RATES (per 100,000) by Age

Total cases 2743 *males*; 2103 *females* (of which age not stated for 2 *males* and 4 *females*)

Age	M	F	Age	M	F	Age	M	F
0–4	0·0	0·0	*35–39*	2·3	3·4	*70–74*	136·3	62·6
5–9	0·0	0·0	*40–44*	6·7	5·6	*75–79*	170·1	83·6
10–14	0·1	0·1	*45–49*	10·8	9·1	*80–84*	184·5	110·2
15–19	0·0	0·2	*50–54*	19·2	16·8	*85–89*	215·8	134·6
20–24	0·2	0·1	*55–59*	43·7	25·1	*90–94*	153·8	136·8
25–29	0·3	0·5	*60–64*	68·2	35·7	*95+*	135·5	96·5
30–34	1·0	0·9	*65–69*	107·3	48·4	*All ages*	19·4	14·6

SEX AND AGE DISTRIBUTION

	Male	*Female*
Mean age (*years*)	66·3	67·4
95% between ages	42 & 86	40 & 89
Children under 15 (%)	0·0	0·0
Median age (*years*)	66·8	68·4
Proportion by sex (%)	56·6	43·4
Proportion of all cancers by sex (%)	6·4	5·2
Trend over 10 years	(–)	(–)

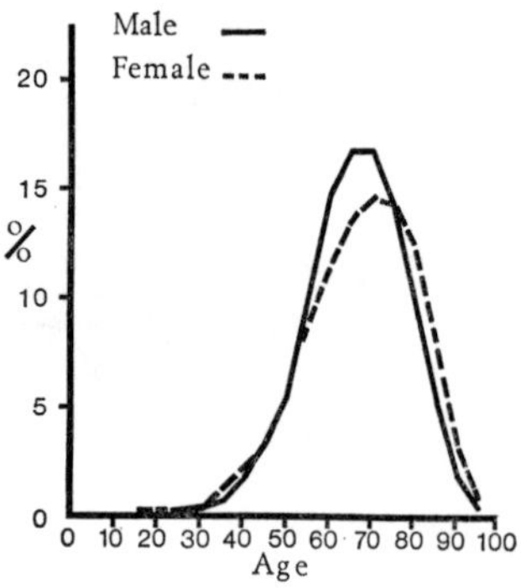

NOTES

Includes: Rectosigmoid junction and anal canal.

Excludes: Anus, which is classified with SKIN.

5-YEAR SURVIVAL RATES BY AGE

Crude —— *Corrected* - - - -

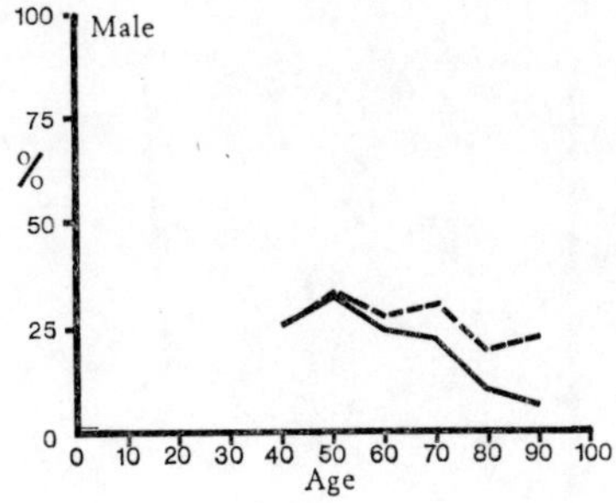

ALL CASES

Total 2692

Male 1546
Female 1146

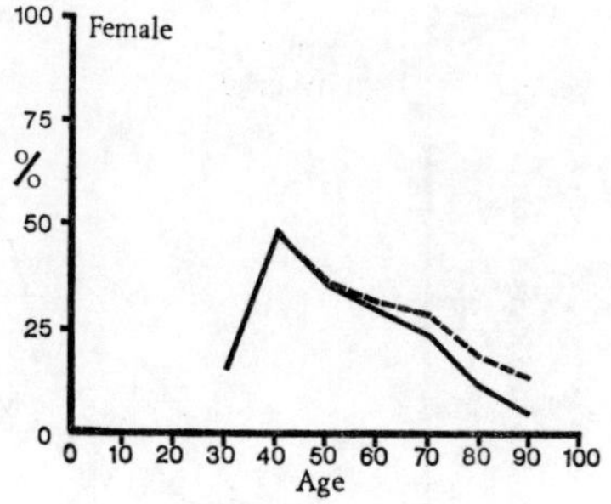

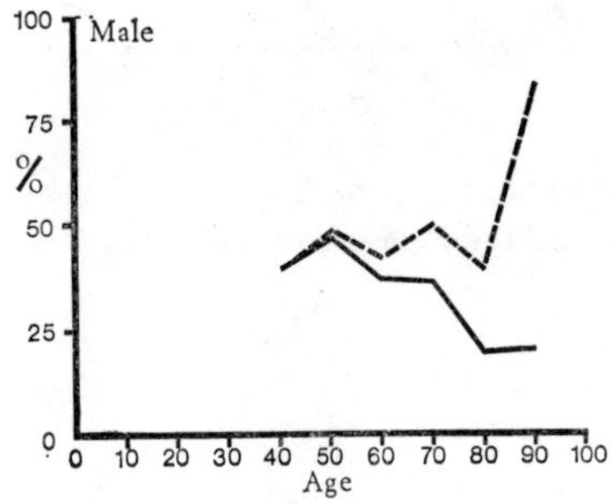

RADICAL TREATMENT

(51·9% of total)
53·3% *male*
50·0% *female*

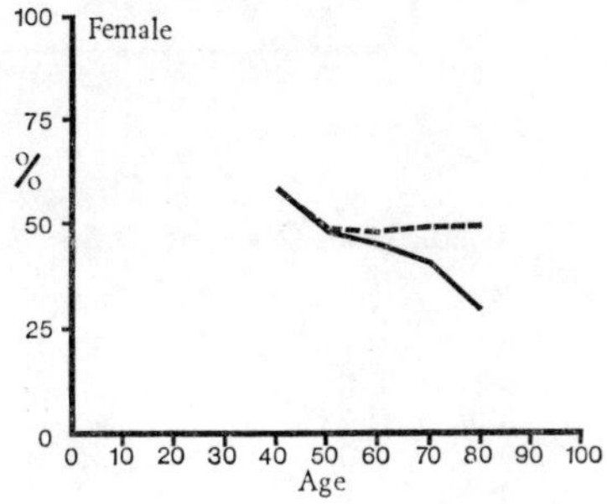

INDICES OF SURVIVAL

	All cases		Radical Treatment	
	Male	*Female*	*Male*	*Female*
FIVE YEAR SURVIVAL RATE (%)				
Crude	20·3	22·9	35·9	41·9
Corrected	*27·5*	*28·7*	*45·8*	*48·5*
Total cases†	1546	1146	824	573
TEN YEAR SURVIVAL RATE (%)				
Crude	13·7	15·5	25·6	28·9
Corrected	*25·4*	*23·6*	*41·4*	*39·1*
Total cases†	1090	729	570	387
SURVIVAL TIME (*months*)				
First quartile (75% S.R.)	2·1	2·7	13·0	16·4
Median (50% S.R.)	**13·1**	**13·8**	**34·1**	**43·7**
Third quartile (25% S.R.)	44·3	52·5	>60	>60

† Number of cases on which survival rate is based

ANNUAL SURVIVAL RATES

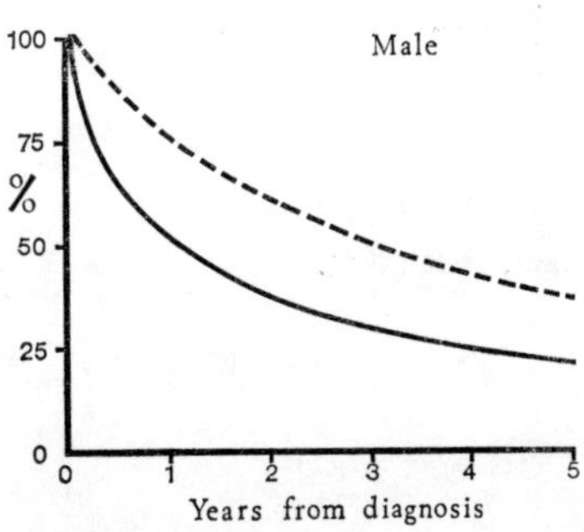

All cases ——
Radical treatment - - - -

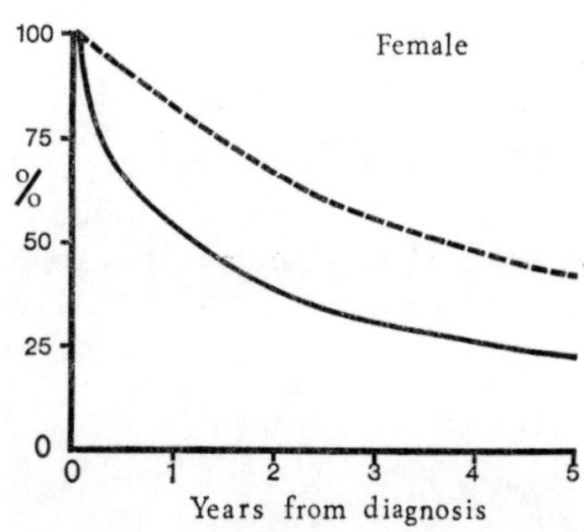

INCIDENCE RATE (per 100,000)

Male —— *Female* ----

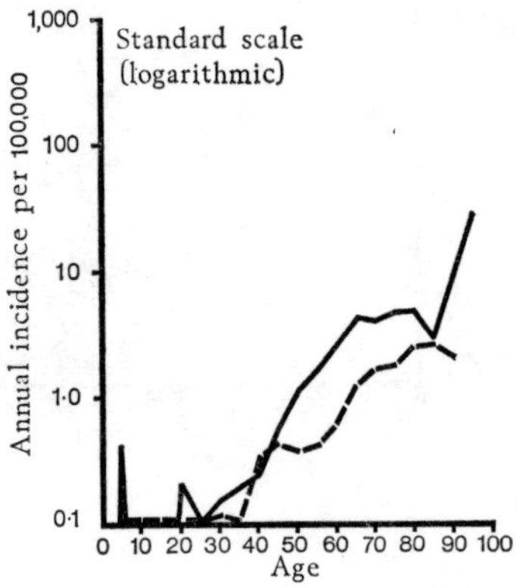

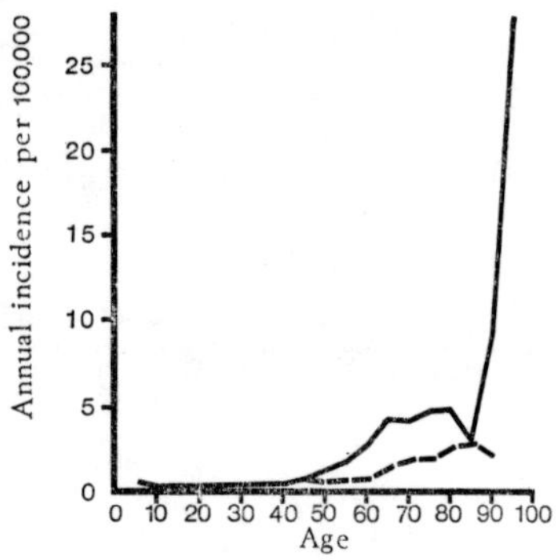

INCIDENCE RATES (per 100,000) by Age

Total cases 127 *males*; 59 *females* (of which age not stated for 0 *males* and 0 *females*)

Age	M	F	Age	M	F	Age	M	F
0–4	0·6	0·1	*35–39*	0·1	0·0	*70–74*	3·5	1·2
5–9	0·1	0·0	*40–44*	0·4	0·5	*75–79*	6·0	2·3
10–14	0·0	0·1	*45–49*	0·7	0·3	*80–84*	1·9	2·5
15–19	0·1	0·0	*50–54*	1·5	0·4	*85–89*	5·3	2·5
20–24	0·2	0·1	*55–59*	1·7	0·5	*90–94*	30·8	0·0
25–29	0·0	0·0	*60–64*	3·9	0·7	*95+*	0·0	0·0
30–34	0·3	0·2	*65–69*	4·3	1·9	*All ages*	0·9	0·4

SEX AND AGE DISTRIBUTION

	Male	*Female*
Mean age (*years*)	58·0	62·1
95% between ages	2 & 87	12 & 86
Children under 15 (%)	6·3	3·4
Median age (*years*)	61·9	66·5
Proportion by sex (%)	68·3	31·7
Proportion of all cancers by sex (%)	0·3	0·1
Trend over 10 years	(+)	(−)

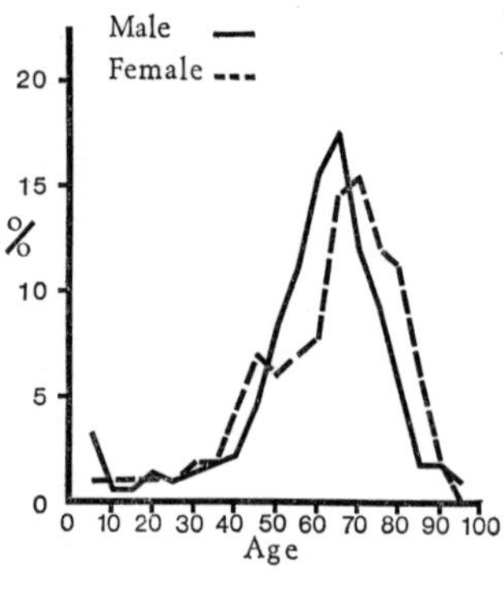

NOTES

Includes: Only tumours of liver specified as primary; and tumours of intrahepatic bile ducts.

5-YEAR SURVIVAL RATES BY AGE

Crude —— *Corrected* - - - -

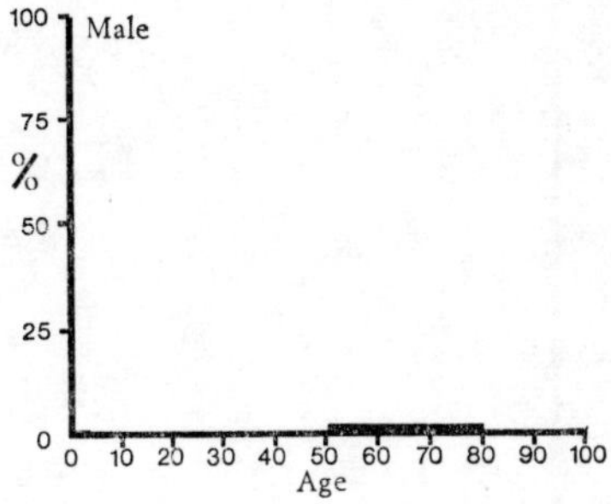

ALL CASES

Total	81
Male	56
Female	25

RADICAL TREATMENT

(6·2% of total)
1·8% *male*
16·0% *female*

INDICES OF SURVIVAL

	All cases *Male*	All cases *Female*	Radical Treatment *Male*	Radical Treatment *Female*
FIVE YEAR SURVIVAL RATE (%)				
Crude	0·0	0·0	0·0	0·0
Corrected	*0·0*	*0·0*	*0·0*	*0·0*
Total cases†	56	25	1	4
TEN YEAR SURVIVAL RATE (%)				
Crude	0·0	0·0	0·0	0·0
Corrected	*0·0*	*0·0*	*0·0*	*0·0*
Total cases†	15	7	1	0
† Number of cases on which survival rate is based				
SURVIVAL TIME (*months*)				
First quartile (75% S.R.)	0·4	0·5	15·0	0·8
Median (50% S.R.)	**0·8**	**1·1**	**15·5**	**2·0**
Third quartile (25% S.R.)	2·1	3·0	16·0	21·3

ANNUAL SURVIVAL RATES

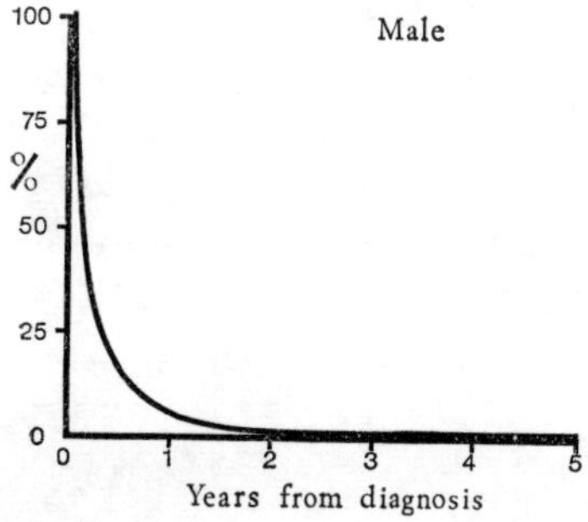

All cases ——
Radical treatment - - - -

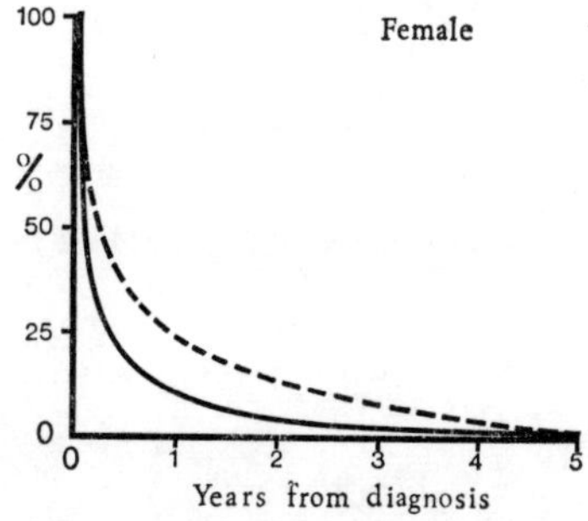

INCIDENCE RATE (per 100,000)

Male —— *Female* ----

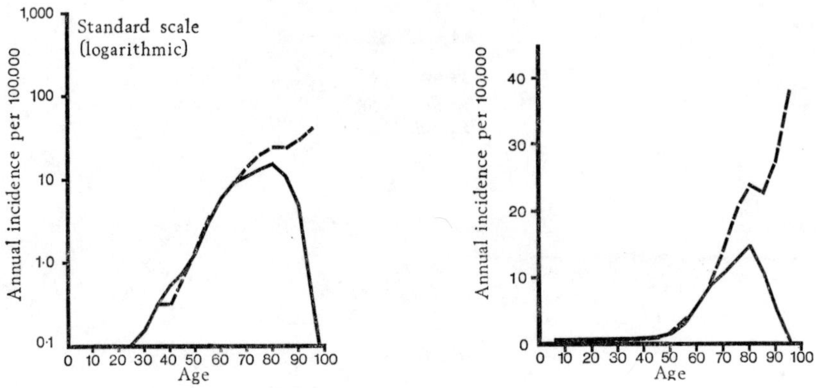

INCIDENCE RATES (per 100,000) by Age

Total cases 243 *males*; 436 *females* (of which age not stated for 0 *males* and 0 *females*)

Age	M	F	Age	M	F	Age	M	F
0–4	0·0	0·0	*35–39*	0·4	0·4	*70–74*	10·4	16·7
5–9	0·0	0·0	*40–44*	0·6	0·2	*75–79*	15·5	24·5
10–14	0·0	0·0	*45–49*	0·8	0·9	*80–84*	12·2	21·8
15–19	0·0	0·0	*50–54*	1·7	2·0	*85–89*	5·3	23·7
20–24	0·0	0·0	*55–59*	4·0	4·7	*90–94*	0·0	43·8
25–29	0·1	0·1	*60–64*	7·6	6·3	*95+*	0·0	0·0
30–34	0·2	0·2	*65–69*	10·1	11·7	*All ages*	1·7	3·0

SEX AND AGE DISTRIBUTION

	Male	*Female*
Mean age (*years*)	64·8	70·0
95% between ages	39 & 83	46 & 89
Children under 15 (%)	0·0	0·0
Median age (*years*)	65·3	71·2
Proportion by sex (%)	35·8	64·2
Proportion of all cancers by sex (%)	0·6	1·1
Trend over 10 years	(+)	(−)

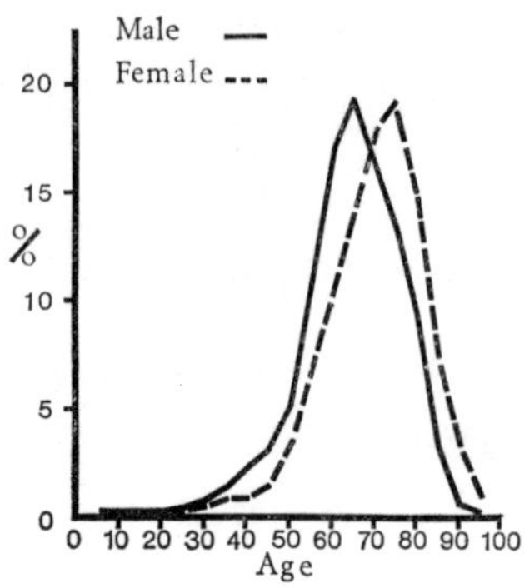

NOTES

Excludes: Ampulla of Vater (156·2 in 8th revision, and included in 155·1 in the 7th), which is classified with PANCREAS.

5-YEAR SURVIVAL RATES BY AGE

Crude ——— *Corrected* - - - -

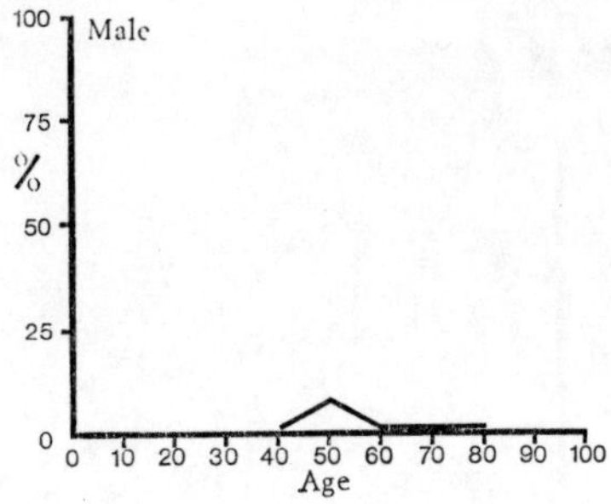

ALL CASES

Total 321
Male 105
Female 216

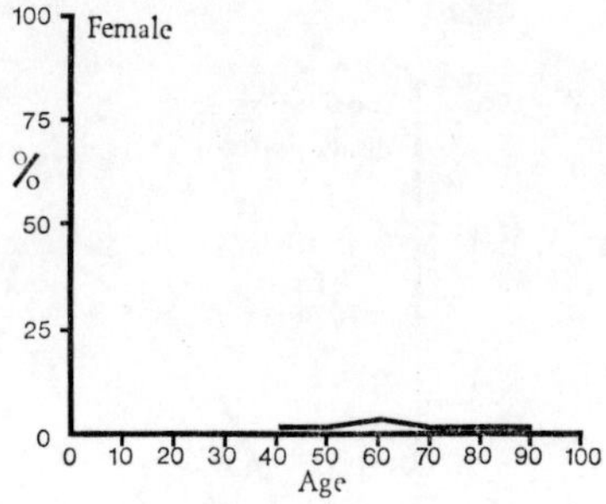

RADICAL TREATMENT

(10·3% of total)
9·5% *male*
10·6% *female*

INDICES OF SURVIVAL

	All cases *Male*	All cases *Female*	Radical Treatment *Male*	Radical Treatment *Female*
FIVE YEAR SURVIVAL RATE (%)				
Crude	0·9	0·5	10·0	4·3
Corrected	*1·3*	*0·6*	*12·1*	*5·2*
Total cases†	105	216	10	23
TEN YEAR SURVIVAL RATE (%)				
Crude	0·0	0·0	0·0	0·0
Corrected	*0·0*	*0·0*	*0·0*	*0·0*
Total cases†	69	129	5	23
SURVIVAL TIMES (*months*)				
First quartile (75% S.R.)	0·6	0·5	0·8	4·5
Median (50% S.R.)	**1·5**	**1·2**	**14·0**	**7·8**
Third quartile (25% S.R.)	4·3	4·3	32·8	10·8

† Number of cases on which survival rate is based

ANNUAL SURVIVAL RATES

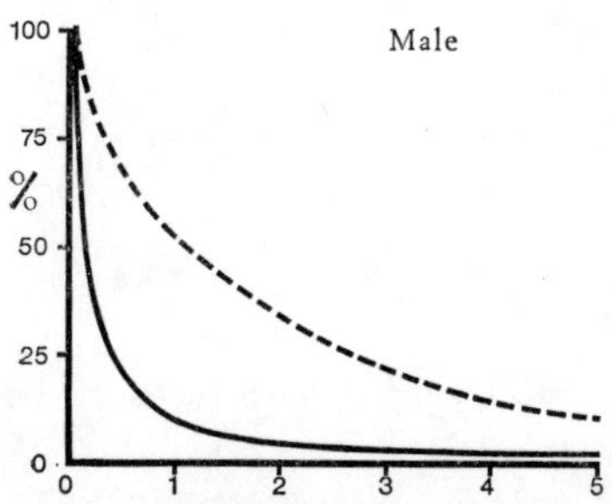

All cases ———
Radical treatment - - - -

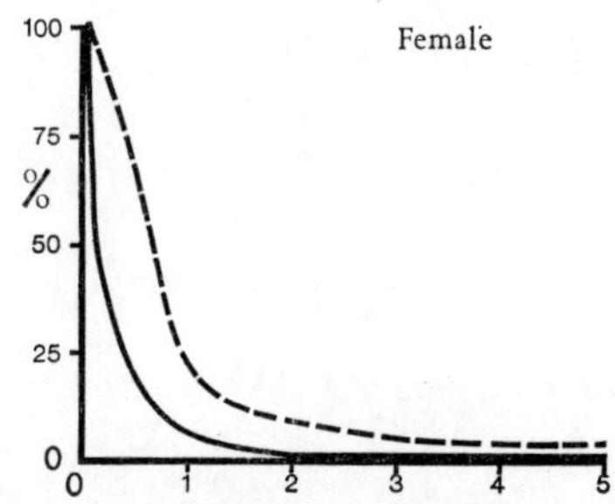

PANCREAS **ICD (8th) 157, 156·2**

INCIDENCE RATE (per 100,000)

Male —— *Female* - - - -

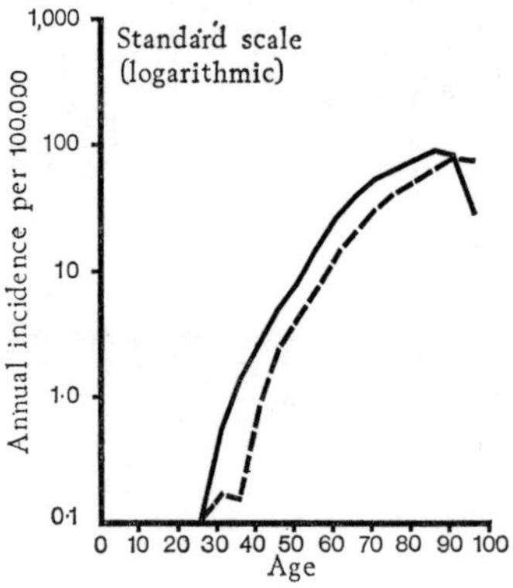

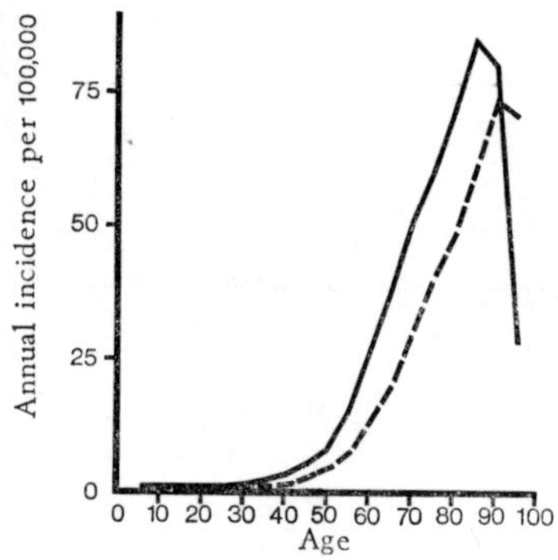

INCIDENCE RATES (per 100,000) by Age

Total cases 1219 *males*; 963 *females* (of which age not stated for 0 *males* and 1 *female*)

Age	M	F	Age	M	F	Age	M	F
0–4	0·0	0·0	*35–39*	1·6	0·1	*70–74*	57·2	36·4
5–9	0·0	0·0	*40–44*	3·4	1·5	*75–79*	65·1	44·1
10–14	0·0	0·0	*45–49*	5·7	3·0	*80–84*	83·4	55·6
15–19	0·0	0·0	*50–54*	9·1	5·0	*85–89*	87·9	72·3
20–24	0·1	0·0	*55–59*	20·6	8·8	*90–94*	30·8	76·6
25–29	0·0	0·1	*60–64*	31·9	17·1	*95+*	0·0	32·2
30–34	0·9	0·2	*65–69*	45·2	23·2	*All ages*	8·6	6·7

SEX AND AGE DISTRIBUTION

	Male	*Female*
Mean age (*years*)	65·3	70·0
95% between ages	41 & 86	46 & 89
Children under 15 (%)	0·0	0·0
Median age (*years*)	65·7	71·0
Proportion by sex (%)	55·9	44·1
Proportion of all cancers by sex (%)	2·8	2·4
Trend over 10 years	++	(+)

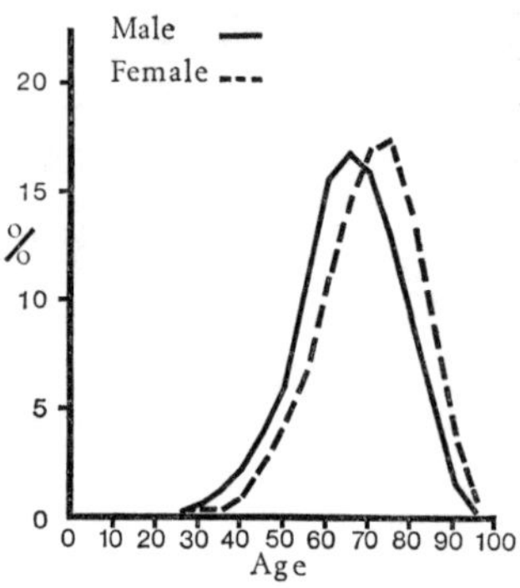

NOTES

Includes: Ampulla of Vater (156·2 in 8th revision, and included in 155·1 in 7th). Details of subdivisions will be found on p. 26.

5-YEAR SURVIVAL RATES BY AGE

Crude—— *Corrected* ----

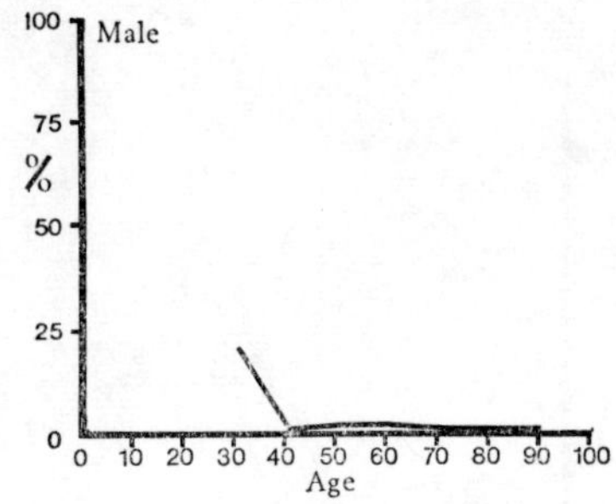

ALL CASES

Total 1018

Male 555
Female 463

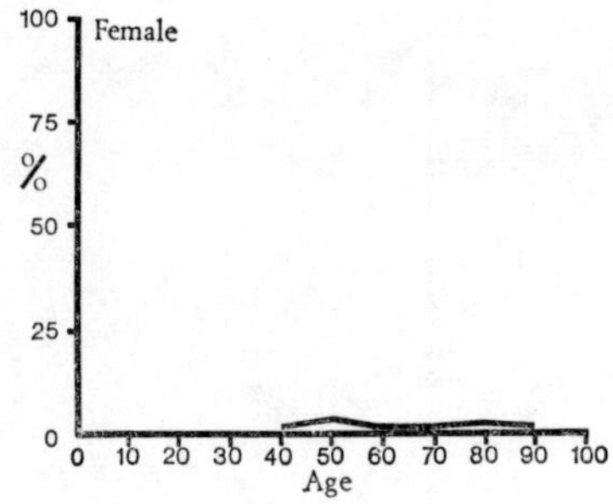

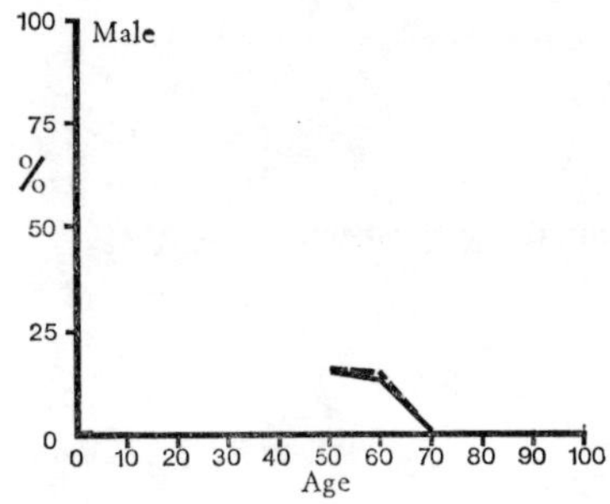

RADICAL TREATMENT

(5·8% of total)
6·5% *male*
5·0% *female*

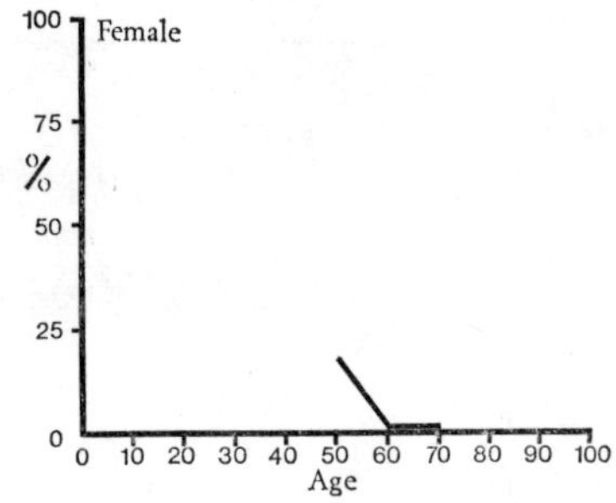

INDICES OF SURVIVAL

	All cases		Radical Treatment	
	Male	*Female*	*Male*	*Female*
FIVE YEAR SURVIVAL RATE (%)				
Crude	0·7	0·4	11·1	4·3
Corrected	*0·9*	*0·5*	*13·2*	*4·7*
Total cases†	555	463	36	23
TEN YEAR SURVIVAL RATE (%)				
Crude	1·5	0·0	12·5	0·0
Corrected	*2·7*	*0·0*	*18·4*	*0·0*
Total cases†	198	260	24	15
SURVIVAL TIME (*months*)				
First quartile (75% S.R.)	0·6	0·6	0·7	0·8
Median (50% S.R.)	**1·6**	**1·5**	**7·7**	**6·5**
Third quartile (25% S.R.)	4·3	4·9	25·3	17·5

† Number of cases on which survival rate is based

ANNUAL SURVIVAL RATES

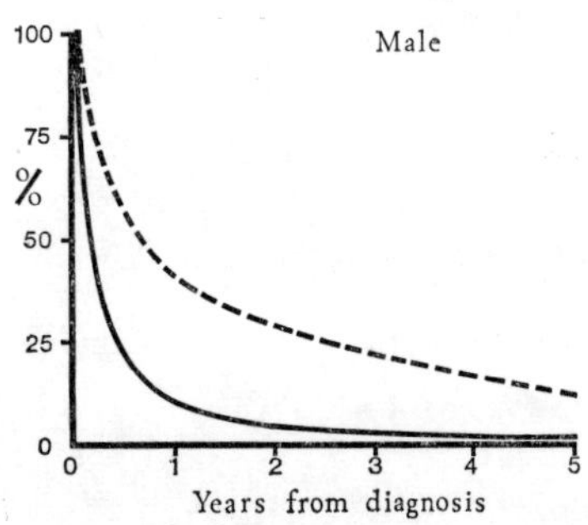

All cases ——
Radical treatment ----

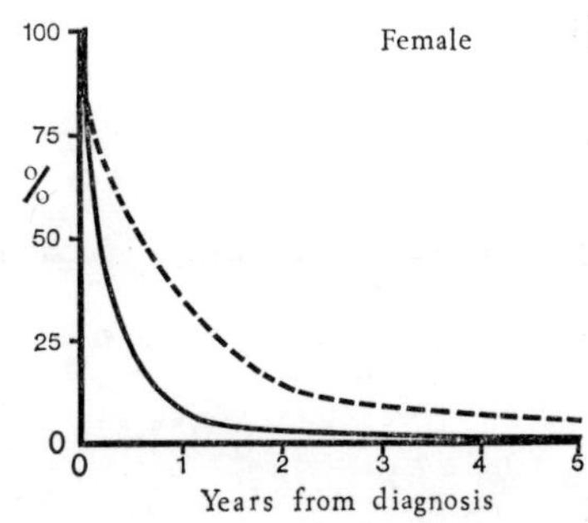

NASAL SINUSES ICD (8th) **160 (part)**

INCIDENCE RATE (per 100,000)

Male —— *Female* ----

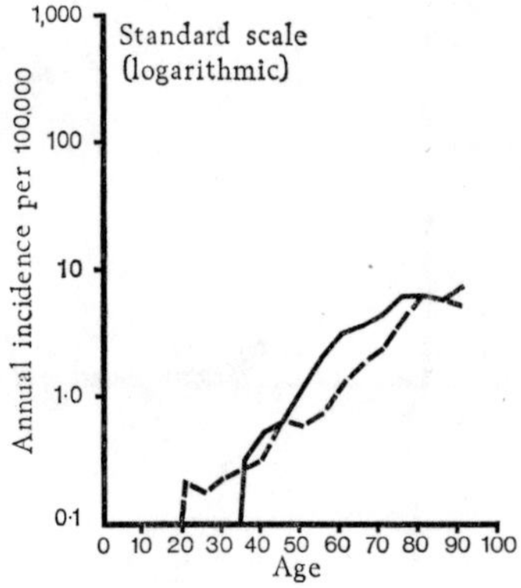

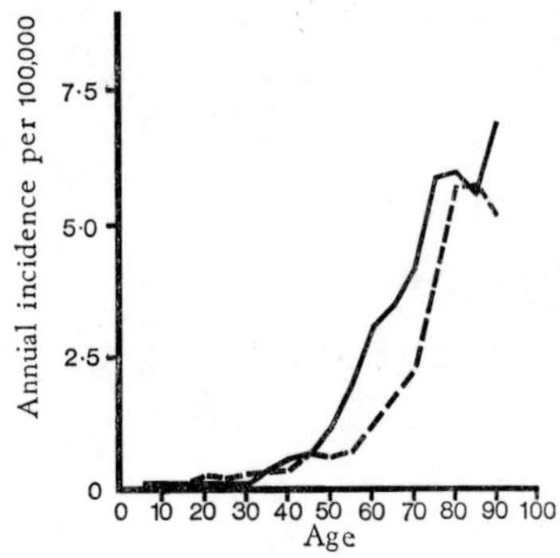

INCIDENCE RATES (per 100,000) by Age

Total cases 128 *males*; 105 *females* (of which age not stated for 0 *males* and 0 *females*)

Age	M	F	Age	M	F	Age	M	F
0–4	0·0	0·0	*35–39*	0·6	0·1	*70–74*	5·4	2·5
5–9	0·0	0·1	*40–44*	0·4	0·5	*75–79*	6·5	5·8
10–14	0·0	0·0	*45–49*	0·8	0·7	*80–84*	4·7	5·5
15–19	0·0	0·1	*50–54*	1·5	0·4	*85–89*	8·0	6·2
20–24	0·0	0·3	*55–59*	2·5	0·9	*90–94*	0·0	0·0
25–29	0·0	0·0	*60–64*	3·6	1·4	*95+*	0·0	0·0
30–34	0·0	0·4	*65–69*	3·1	1·9	*All ages*	0·9	0·7

SEX AND AGE DISTRIBUTION

	Male	*Female*
Mean age (*years*)	62·6	64·2
95% between ages	38 & 85	21 & 87
Children under 15 (%)	0·0	1·0
Median age (*years*)	62·4	68·1
Proportion by sex (%)	55·0	45·0
Proportion of all cancers by sex (%)	0·3	0·3
Trend over 10 years	(–)	(–)

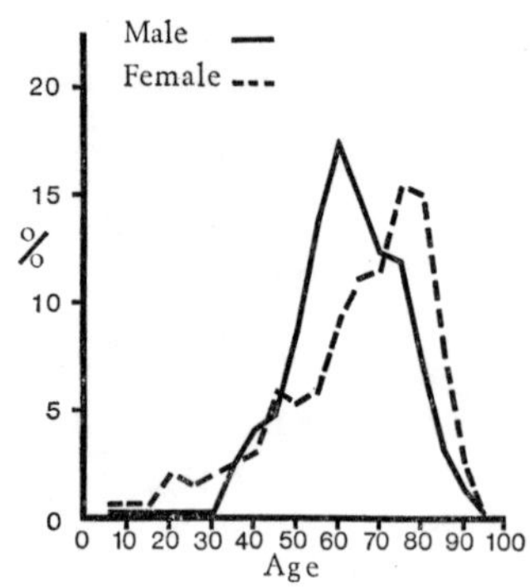

NOTES

Includes: Only nasal cavities and sinuses (160·0, 160·2, 160·8, 160·9 in 8th revision; 160·0, 160·2, 160·7, 160·8, 160·9 in 7th).

Excludes: Eustachian tube and middle ear (160·1 in both 8th and 7th revisions). Further details will be found on p. 34.

5-YEAR SURVIVAL RATES BY AGE

Crude —— *Corrected* ----

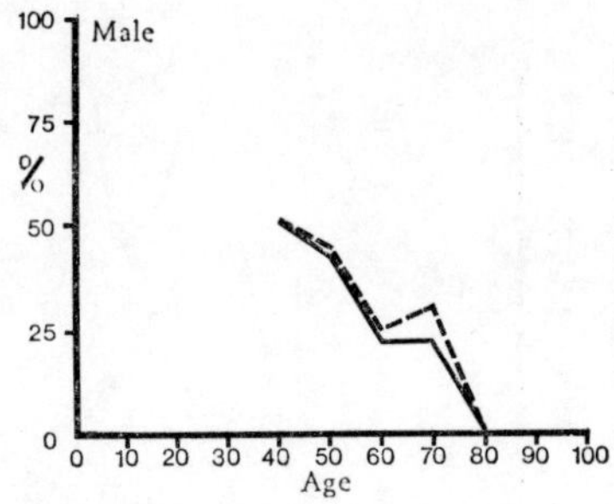

ALL CASES

Total	128
Male	65
Female	63

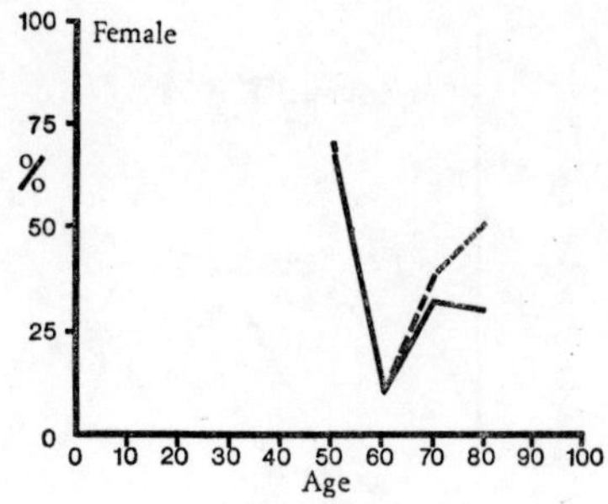

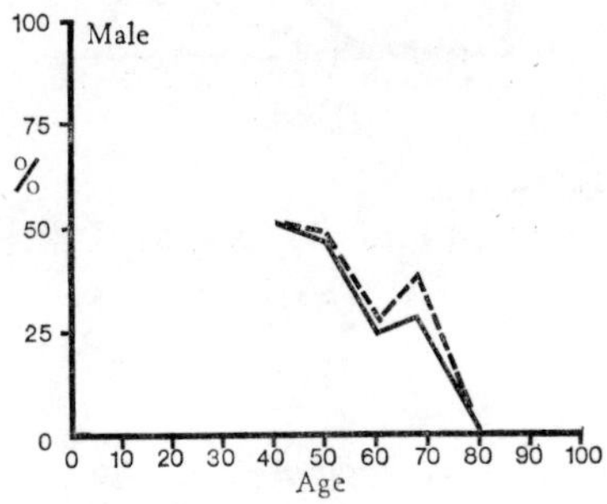

RADICAL TREATMENT

(82·0% of total)
80·0% *male*
84·1% *female*

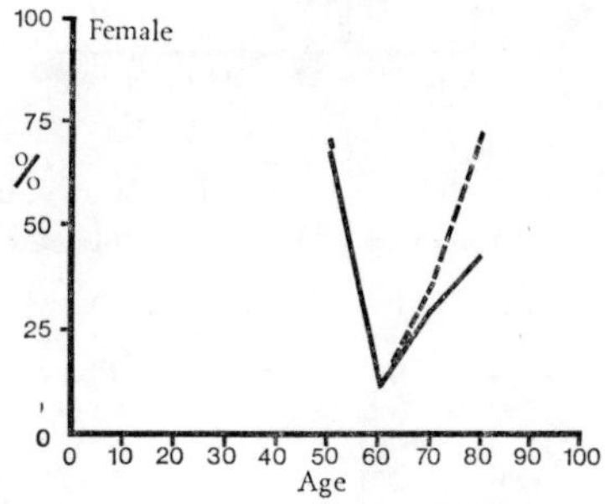

INDICES OF SURVIVAL

	All cases *Male*	All cases *Female*	Radical Treatment *Male*	Radical Treatment *Female*
FIVE YEAR SURVIVAL RATE (%)				
Crude	23·1	31·7	28·8	35·8
Corrected	*29·8*	*38·9*	*35·4*	*41·8*
Total cases†	65	63	52	53
TEN YEAR SURVIVAL RATE (%)				
Crude	20·0	16·9	26·5	22·5
Corrected	*29·5*	*28·9*	*39·8*	*33·8*
Total cases†	75	59	49	40

† Number of cases on which survival rate is based

SURVIVAL TIME (*months*)				
First quartile (75% S.R.)	6·3	6·8	8·7	10·0
Median (50% S.R.)	**15·5**	**22·3**	**31·0**	**29·2**
Third quartile (25% S.R.)	57·0	>60	>60	>60

ANNUAL SURVIVAL RATES

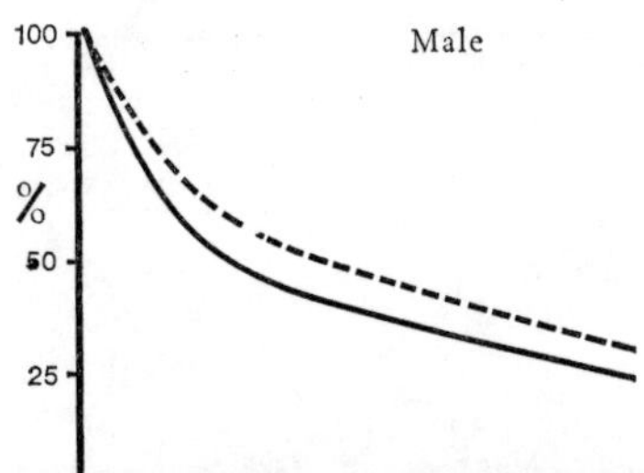

All cases ——
Radical treatment ----

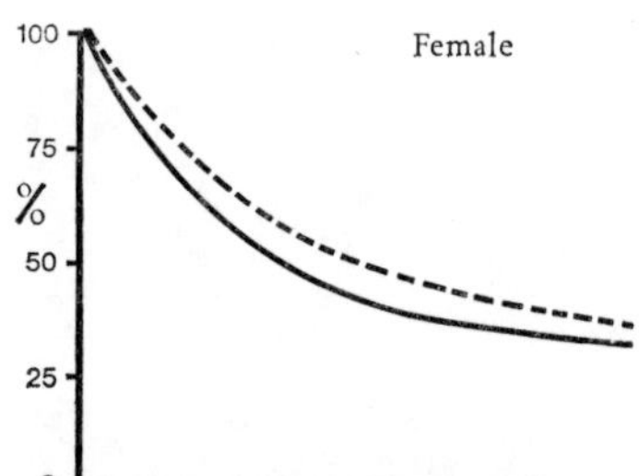

INCIDENCE RATE (per 100,000)

Male —— *Female* - - - -

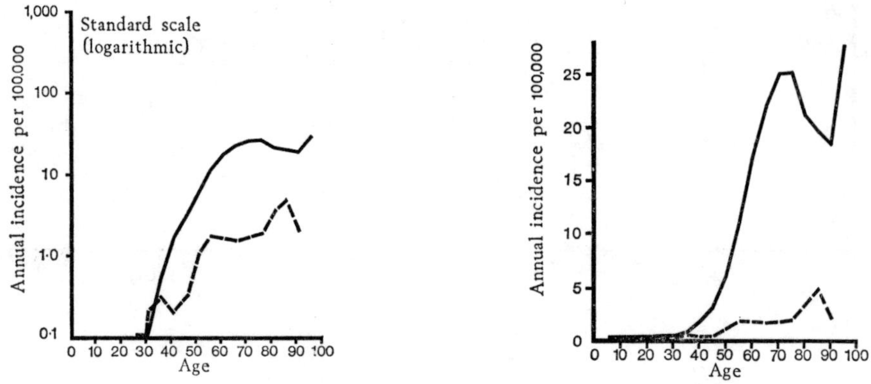

INCIDENCE RATES (per 100,000) by Age

Total cases 643 *males*; 87 *females* (of which age not stated for 1 *male* and 1 *female*)

Age	M	F	Age	M	F	Age	M	F
0–4	0·0	0·0	*35–39*	0·8	0·2	*70–74*	27·2	1·6
5–9	0·0	0·0	*40–44*	2·4	0·2	*75–79*	21·0	2·0
10–14	0·0	0·0	*45–49*	2·8	0·3	*80–84*	20·6	5·5
15–19	0·0	0·0	*50–54*	8·3	1·6	*85–89*	16·0	2·5
20–24	0·0	0·0	*55–59*	13·5	1·4	*90–94*	30·8	0·0
25–29	0·1	0·0	*60–64*	20·0	1·3	*95+*	0·0	0·0
30–34	0·1	0·4	*65–69*	22·2	1·6	*All ages*	4·6	0·6

SEX AND AGE DISTRIBUTION

	Male	*Female*
Mean age (*years*)	62·6	63·0
95% between ages	41 & 83	33 & 85
Children under 15 (%)	0·0	0·0
Median age (*years*)	62·5	62·5
Proportion by sex (%)	88·1	11·9
Proportion of all cancers by sex (%)	1·5	0·2
Trend over 10 years	(−)	(+)

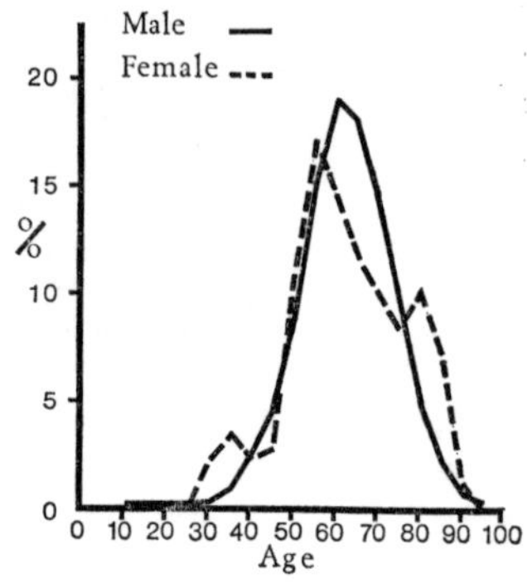

5-YEAR SURVIVAL RATES BY AGE

Crude —— *Corrected* ----

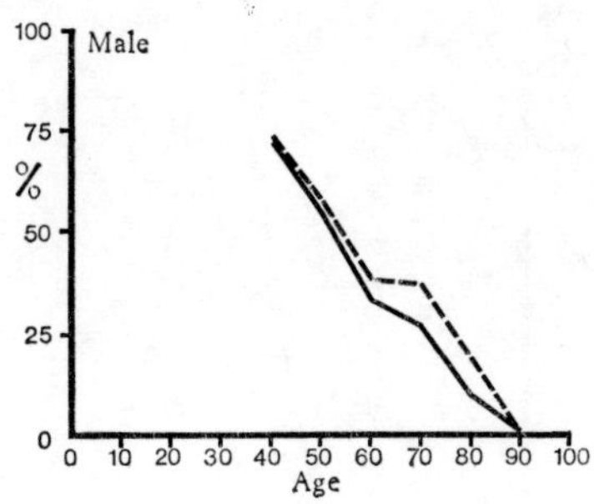

ALL CASES

Total 406
Male 368
Female 38

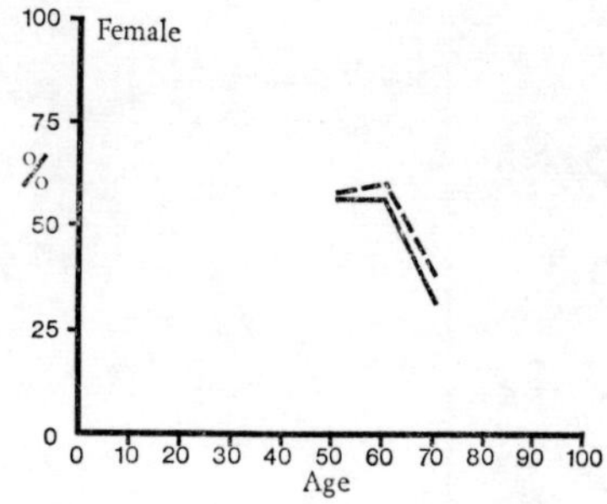

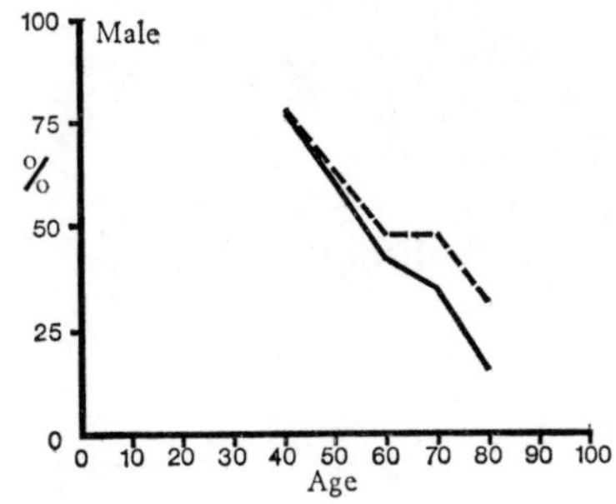

RADICAL TREATMENT

(79·1% of total)
78·5% *male*
84·2% *female*

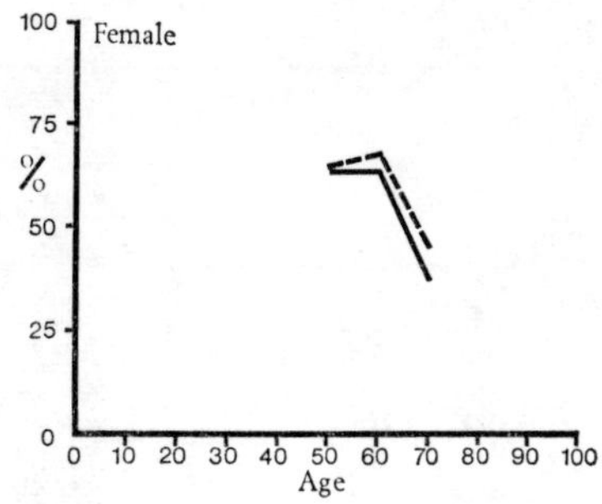

INDICES OF SURVIVAL

	All cases *Male*	All cases *Female*	Radical Treatment *Male*	Radical Treatment *Female*
FIVE YEAR SURVIVAL RATE (%)				
Crude	33·2	39·5	42·2	46·9
Corrected	*42·5*	*46·9*	*52·5*	*53·3*
Total cases†	368	38	289	32
TEN YEAR SURVIVAL RATE (%)				
Crude	23·5	29·6	34·5	53·3
Corrected	*40·9*	*37·8*	*55·4*	*66·4*
Total cases†	294	27	197	15

†Number of cases on which survival rate is based

	All cases *Male*	All cases *Female*	Radical Treatment *Male*	Radical Treatment *Female*
SURVIVAL TIME (*months*)				
First quartile (75% S.R.)	7·2	7·3	11·8	16·8
Median (50% S.R.)	**22·0**	**34·0**	**39·1**	**44·0**
Third quartile (25% S.R.)	>60	>60	>60	>60

ANNUAL SURVIVAL RATES

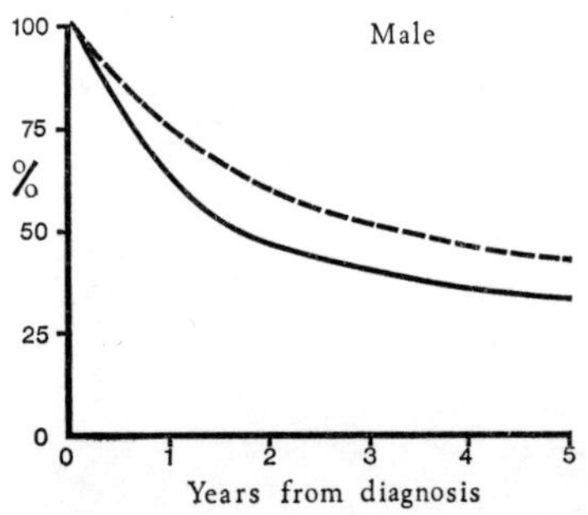

All cases ——
Radical treatment ----

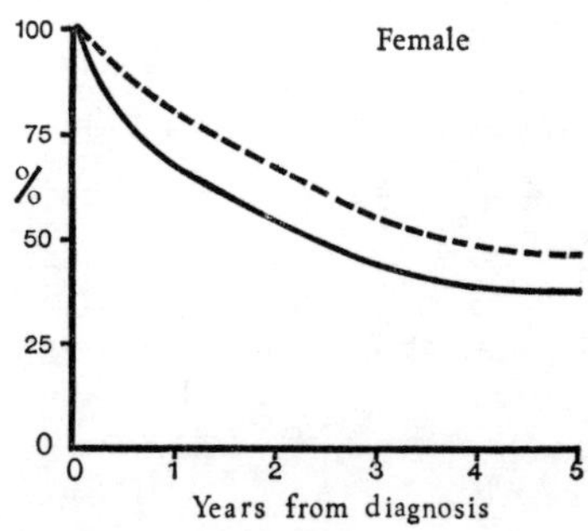

TRACHEA, BRONCHUS AND LUNG

ICD (8th) **162**

INCIDENCE RATE (per 100,000)

Male —— *Female* ----

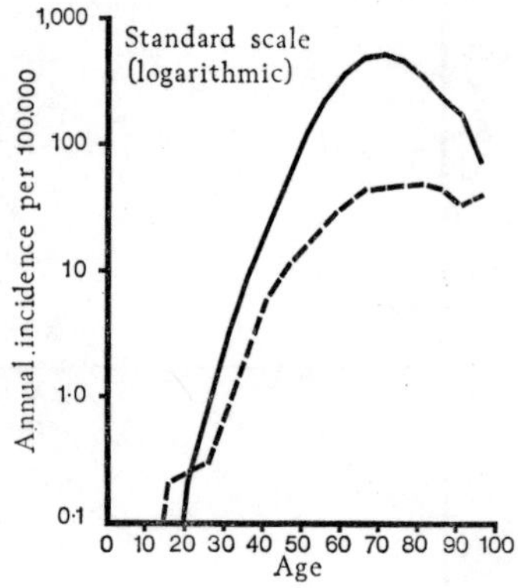

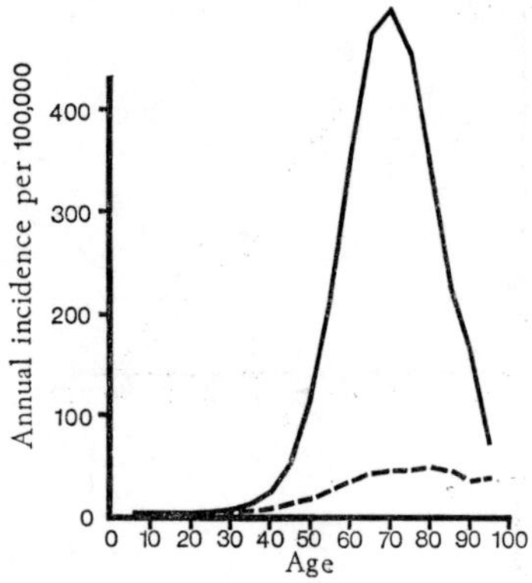

INCIDENCE RATES (per 100,000) by Age

Total cases 12788 *males*; 1710 *females* (of which age not stated for 10 *males* and 2 *females*)

Age	M	F	Age	M	F	Age	M	F
0–4	0·0	0·0	*35–39*	12·4	3·0	*70–74*	491·0	41·8
5–9	0·0	0·0	*40–44*	29·1	8·0	*75–79*	387·3	46·7
10–14	0·1	0·0	*45–49*	67·4	11·8	*80–84*	238·8	46·2
15–19	0·0	0·2	*50–54*	159·2	17·4	*85–89*	181·2	33·6
20–24	0·4	0·2	*55–59*	275·5	29·1	*90–94*	61·5	27·4
25–29	1·1	0·3	*60–64*	453·9	35·9	*95+*	135·5	96·5
30–34	4·7	1·3	*65–69*	497·9	45·1	*All ages*	90·7	11·8

SEX AND AGE DISTRIBUTION

	Male	*Female*
Mean age (*years*)	62·3	63·1
95% between ages	42 & 80	39 & 85
Children under 15 (%)	0·0	0·0
Median age (*years*)	62·4	63·5
Proportion by sex (%)	88·2	11·8
Proportion of all cancers by sex (%)	29·7	4·2
Trend over 10 years	+	++

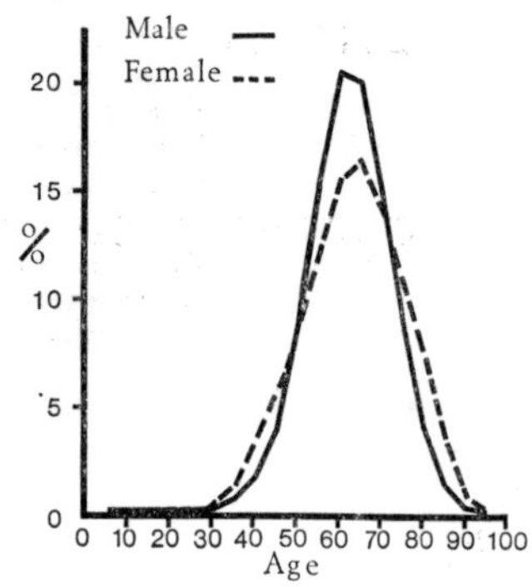

NOTES

Excludes: Pleura (163·0 in 8th revision; 162·2 in 7th). Further details will be found on p. 34.

5-YEAR SURVIVAL RATES BY AGE

Crude —— *Corrected* ----

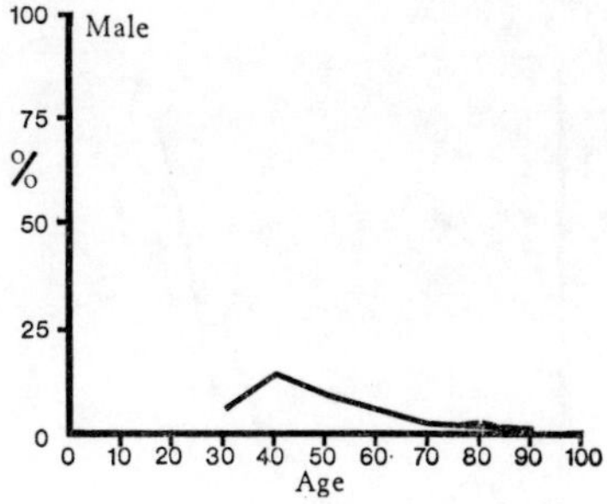

ALL CASES

Total 6987

Male 6236

Female 751

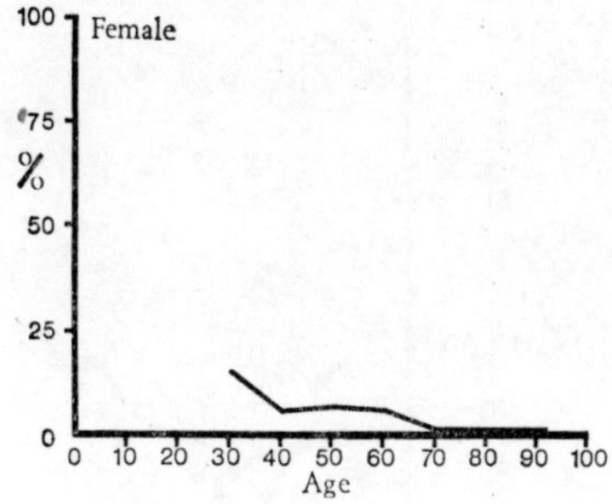

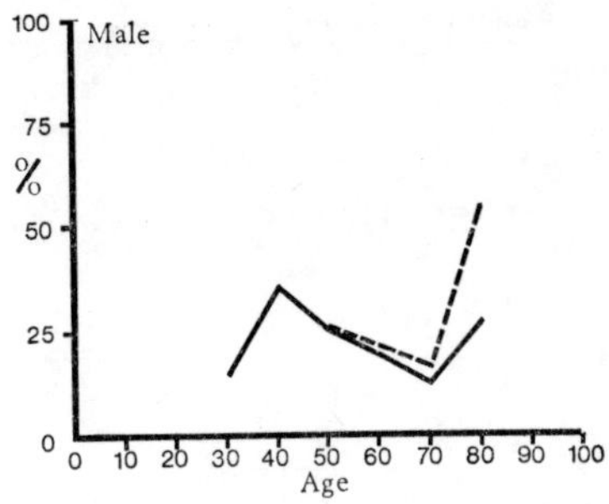

RADICAL TREATMENT

(20·8% of total)

21·6% *male*

14·8% *female*

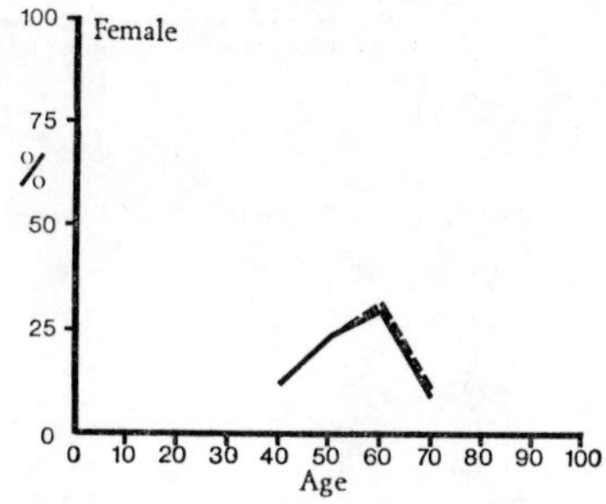

INDICES OF SURVIVAL

	All cases *Male*	All cases *Female*	Radical Treatment *Male*	Radical Treatment *Female*
FIVE YEAR SURVIVAL RATE (%)				
Crude	4·8	3·5	20·5	21·2
Corrected	*5·8*	*4·0*	*23·2*	*22·4*
Total cases†	6236	751	1344	111
TEN YEAR SURVIVAL RATE (%)				
Crude	3·3	2·7	13·8	14·5
Corrected	*4·7*	*3·5*	*18·2*	*17·4*
Total cases†	3400	401	785	69

†Number of cases in which survival rate is based

SURVIVAL TIME (*months*)				
First quartile (75% S.R.)	1·0	0·9	4·0	3·9
Median (50% S.R.)	**3·3**	**12·6**	**11·1**	**10·0**
Third quartile (25% S.R.)	8·5	6·4	37·8	36·3

ANNUAL SURVIVAL RATES

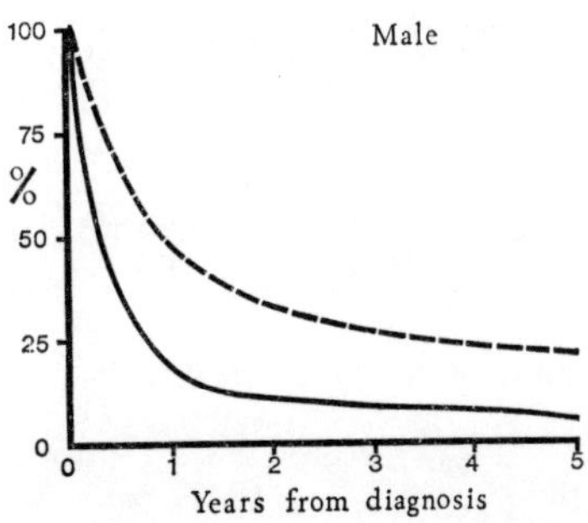

All cases ————

Radical treatment ----

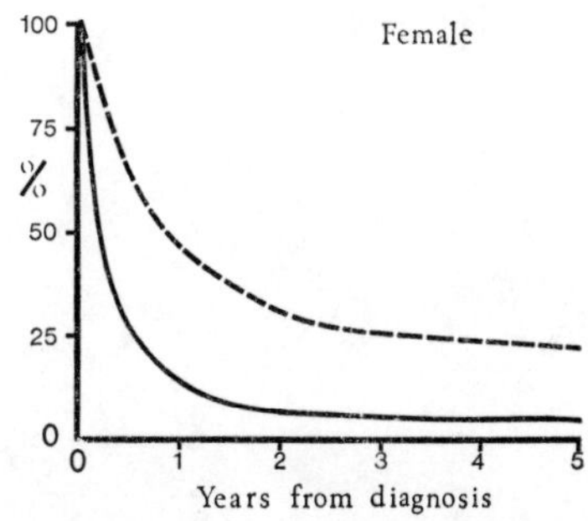

INCIDENCE RATE (per 100,000)

Male —— *Female* ----

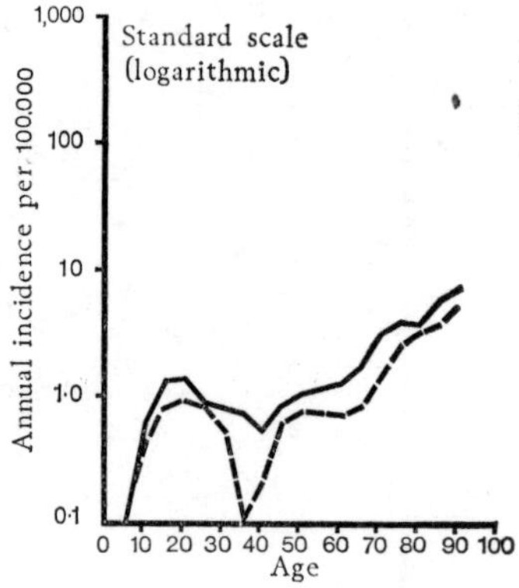

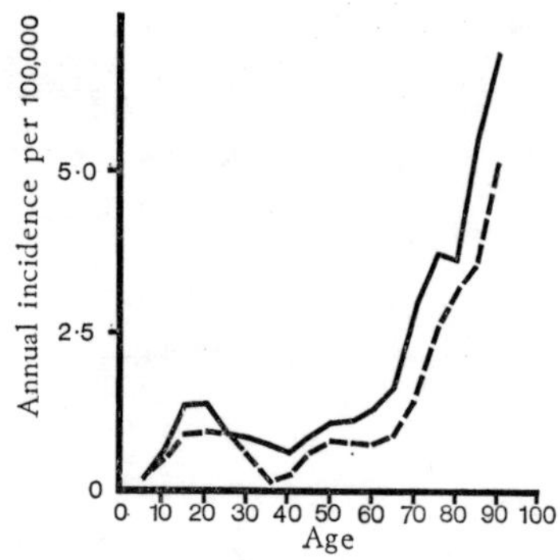

INCIDENCE RATES (per 100,000) by Age

Total cases 142 *males*; 102 *females* (of which age not stated for 0 *males* and 0 *females*)

Age	M	F	Age	M	F	Age	M	F
0–4	0·2	0·1	*35–39*	0·6	0·1	*70–74*	4·1	1·6
5–9	0·1	0·1	*40–44*	0·5	0·3	*75–79*	3·0	3·5
10–14	1·0	0·7	*45–49*	1·1	0·8	*80–84*	4·7	2·5
15–19	1·6	1·0	*50–54*	0·9	0·6	*85–89*	8·0	6·2
20–24	1·0	0·8	*55–59*	1·2	0·8	*90–94*	0·0	0·0
25–29	0·7	0·9	*60–64*	1·3	0·5	*95+*	0·0	0·0
30–34	0·8	0·1	*65–69*	2·0	1·1	*All ages*	1·0	0·7

SEX AND AGE DISTRIBUTION

	Male	*Female*
Mean age (*years*)	44·6	49·4
95% between ages	10 & 84	10 & 87
Children under 15 (%)	10·6	9·8
Median age (*years*)	46·4	52·5
Proportion by sex (%)	58·2	41·8
Proportion of all cancers by sex (%)	0·3	0·3
Trend over 10 years	(–)	(–)

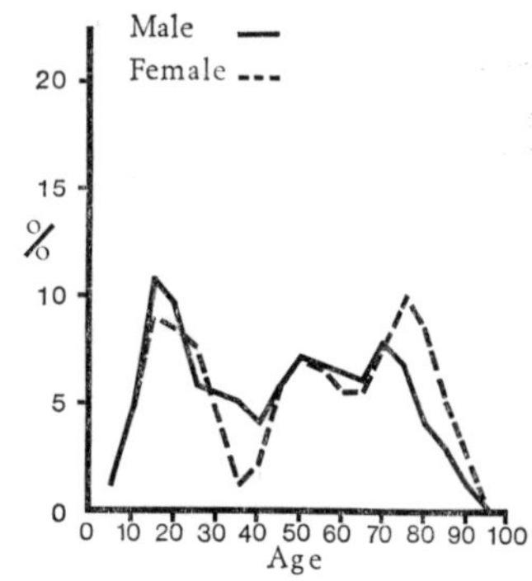

5-YEAR SURVIVAL RATES BY AGE

Crude —— *Corrected* - - - -

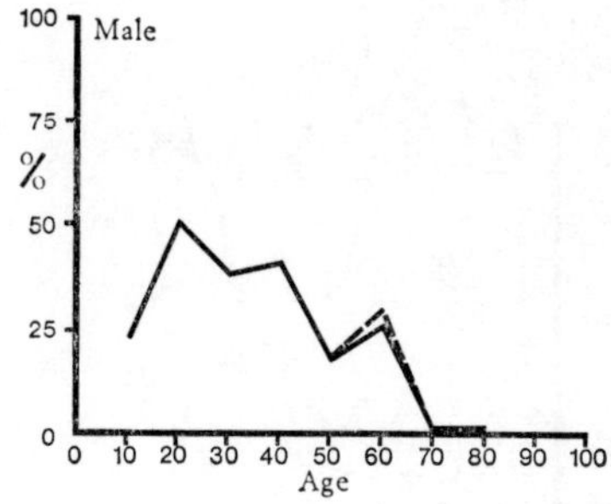

ALL CASES

Total 161
Male 83
Female 78

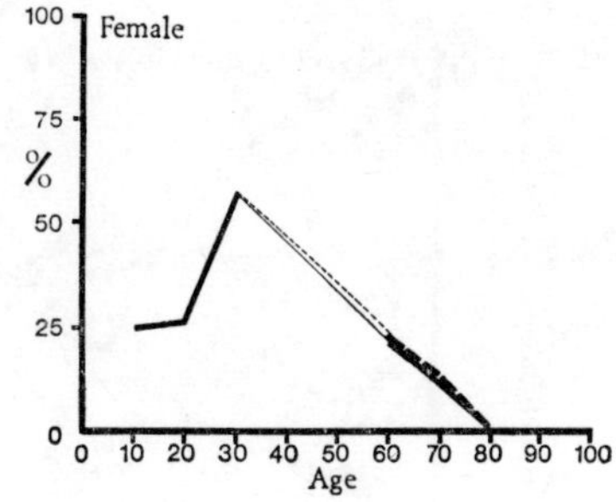

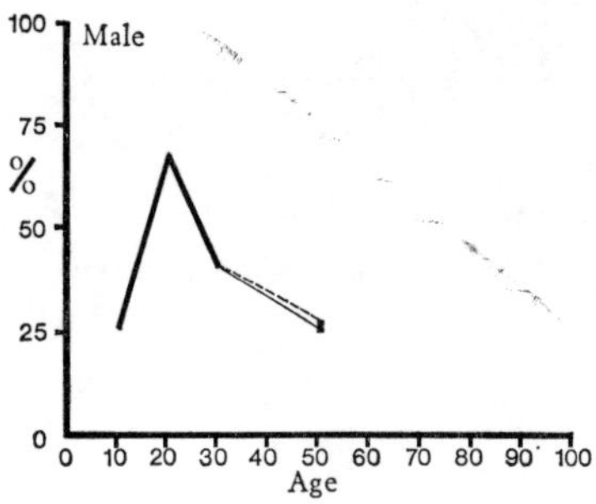

RADICAL TREATMENT

(55·9% of total)
48·2% *male*
64·1% *female*

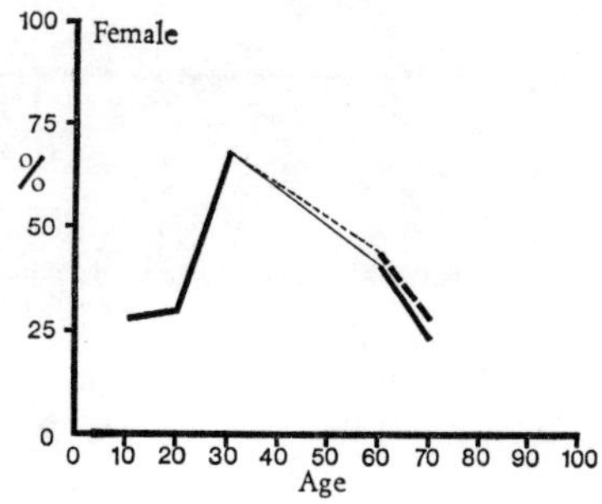

INDICES OF SURVIVAL

	All cases *Male*	All cases *Female*	Radical Treatment *Male*	Radical Treatment *Female*
FIVE YEAR SURVIVAL RATE (%)				
Crude	18·1	23·1	32·5	34·0
Corrected	*21·3*	*25·7*	*35·1*	*36·4*
Total cases†	83	78	40	50
TEN YEAR SURVIVAL RATE (%)				
Crude	14·7	29·4	26·8	44·2
Corrected	*18·3*	*35·7*	*29·5*	*50·2*
Total cases†	75	68	41	43
SURVIVAL TIME (*months*)				
First quartile (75% S.R.)	2·4	4·4	7·8	10·8
Median (50% S.R.)	**8·3**	**14·7**	**16·0**	**23·0**
Third quartile (25% S.R.)	23·8	46·8	>60	>60

† Number of cases on which survival rate is based

ANNUAL SURVIVAL RATES

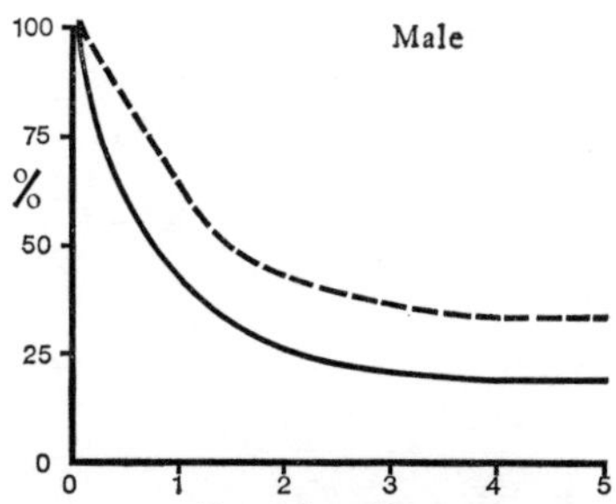

All cases ——
Radical treatment - - - -

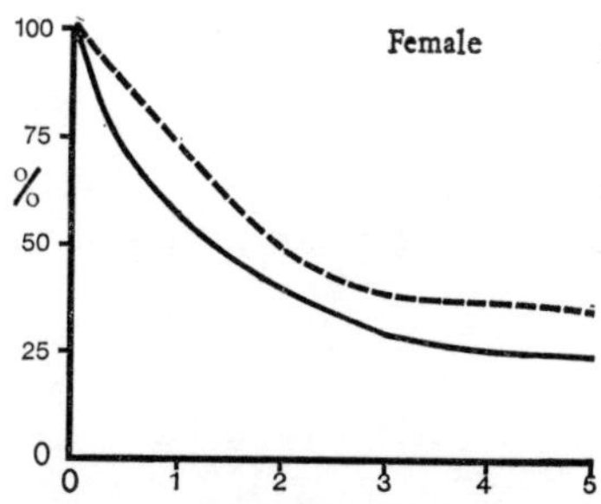

CONNECTIVE TISSUE, ETC. ICD (8th) **158, 171**

INCIDENCE RATE (per 100,000)

Male —— *Female* ----

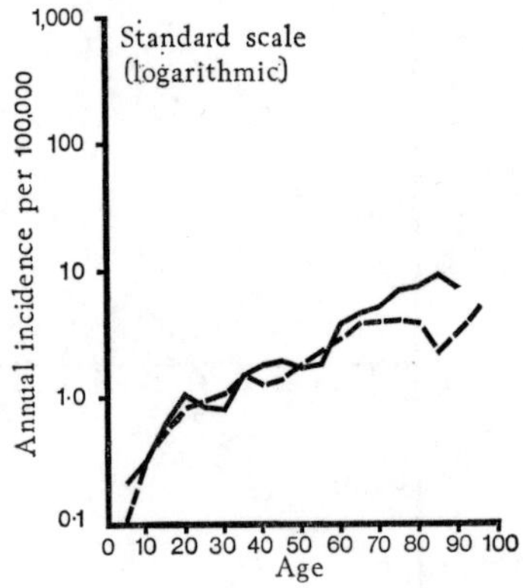

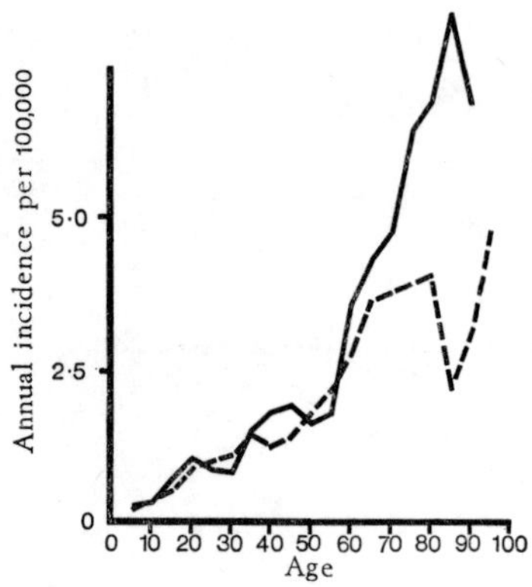

INCIDENCE RATES (per 100,000) by Age

Total cases 223 *males*; 209 *females* (of which age not stated for 0 *males* and 0 *females*)

Age	M	F	Age	M	F	Age	M	F
0–4	0·3	0·2	*35–39*	1·9	1·4	*70–74*	6·6	3·3
5–9	0·1	0·1	*40–44*	1·6	1·0	*75–79*	6·0	4·6
10–14	0·4	0·4	*45–49*	2·1	1·6	*80–84*	8·4	2·0
15–19	0·9	0·5	*50–54*	1·0	1·9	*85–89*	8·0	2·5
20–24	1·1	1·2	*55–59*	2·5	2·3	*90–94*	0·0	5·5
25–29	0·5	0·7	*60–64*	4·9	3·2	*95+*	0·0	0·0
30–34	1·0	1·4	*65–69*	3·4	4·0	*All ages*	1·6	1·4

SEX AND AGE DISTRIBUTION

	Male	*Female*
Mean age (*years*)	51·6	52·6
95% between ages	12 & 84	12 & 82
Children under 15 (%)	3·9	3·9
Median age (*years*)	55·1	55·9
Proportion by sex (%)	51·6	48·4
Proportion of all cancers by sex (%)	0·5	0·5
Trend over 10 years	(−)	(−)

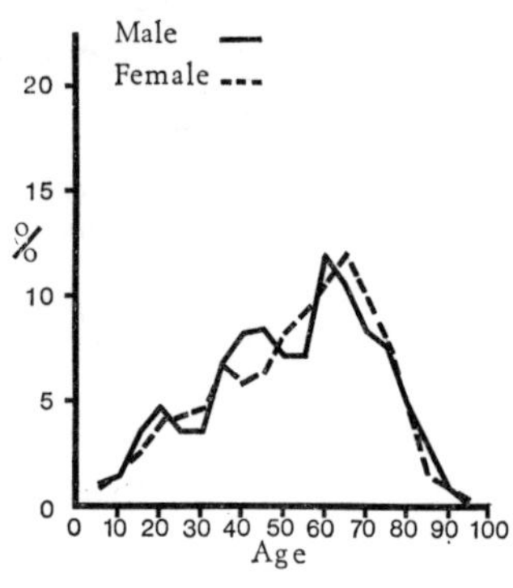

NOTES

Includes: Tumours of peritoneum and retroperitoneum, other than reticuloses.

5-YEAR SURVIVAL RATES BY AGE

Crude —— *Corrected* ----

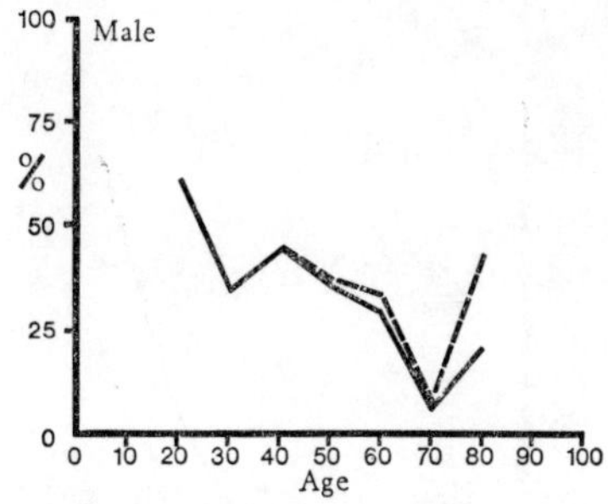

ALL CASES

Total 238
Male 120
Female 118

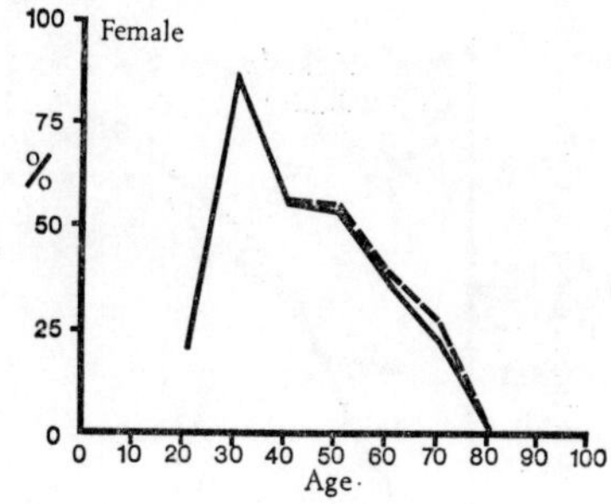

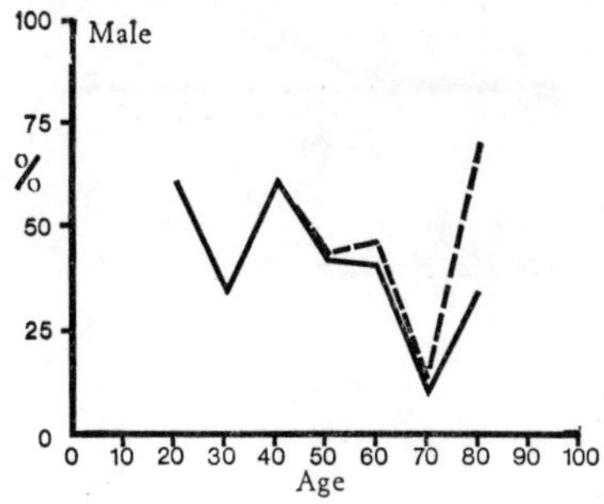

RADICAL TREATMENT

(68·9% of total)
70·0% *male*
67·8% *female*

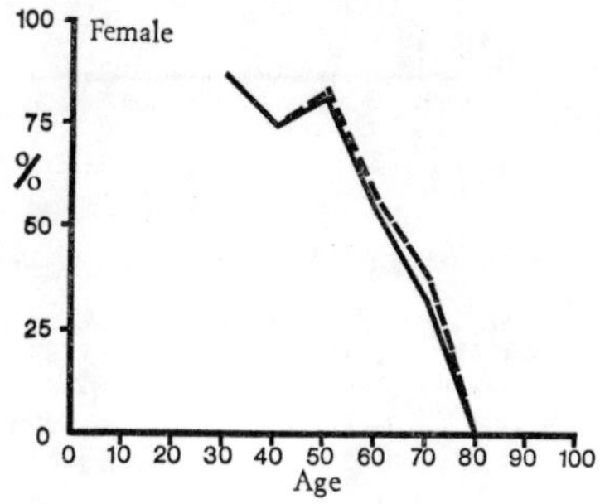

INDICES OF SURVIVAL

	All cases		Radical Treatment	
	Male	*Female*	*Male*	*Female*
FIVE YEAR SURVIVAL RATE (%)				
Crude	30·8	38·1	39·3	55·0
Corrected	*35·3*	*42·2*	*44·5*	*60·3*
Total cases†	120	118	84	80
TEN YEAR SURVIVAL RATE (%)				
Crude	23·5	30·4	37·7	42·9
Corrected	*32·0*	*39·5*	*51·9*	*53·5*
Total cases†	85	79	53	49

† Number of cases on which survival rate is based

SURVIVAL TIME (*months*)				
First quartile (75% S.R.)	4·4	4·3	9·8	17·4
Median (50% S.R.)	**23·0**	**26·0**	**50·0**	**>60**
Third quartile (25% S.R.)	>60	>60	>60	>60

ANNUAL SURVIVAL RATES

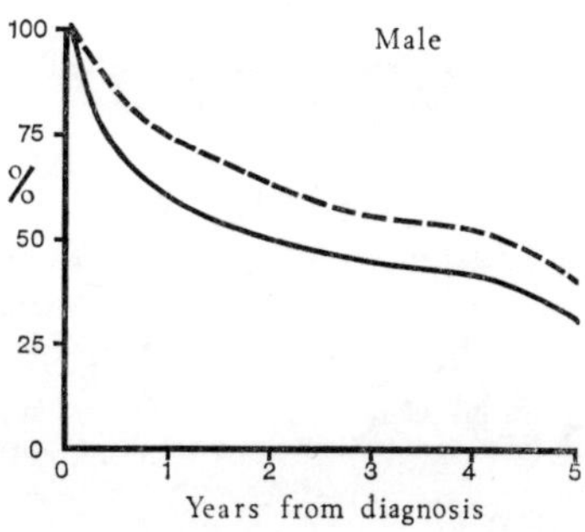

All cases ——
Radical treatment ----

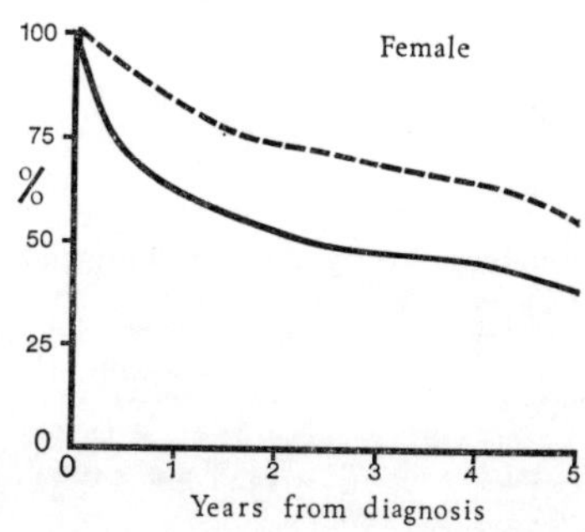

SKIN, FACE AND HEAD **(All histological groups)**

ICD (8th) **172.0–172.4, 173.0–173.4 (part)**

INCIDENCE RATE (per 100,000)

Male —— *Female* ----

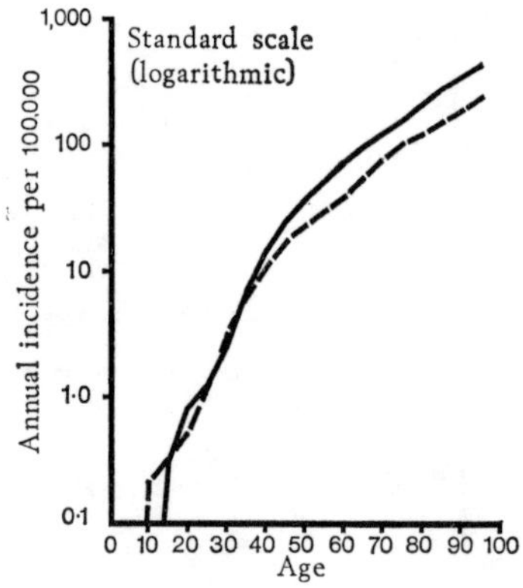

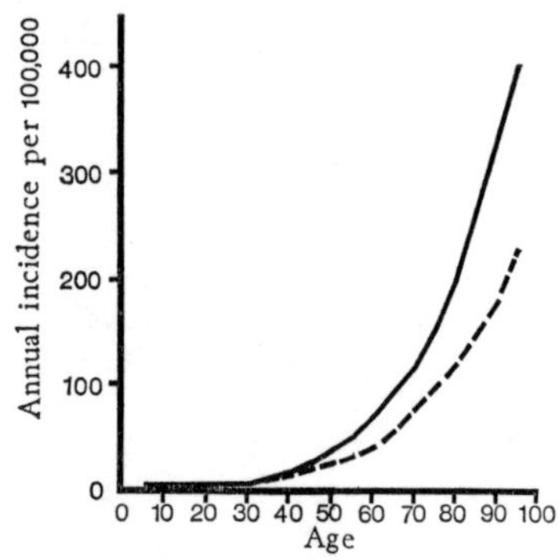

INCIDENCE RATES (per 100,000) by Age

Total cases 3715 *males*; 2989 *females* (of which age not stated for 35 *males* and 25 *females*)

Age	M	F	Age	M	F	Age	M	F
0–4	0·0	0·0	*35–39*	9·7	6·9	*70–74*	135·9	87·5
5–9	0·0	0·1	*40–44*	18·5	13·6	*75–79*	172·6	106·6
10–14	0·0	0·3	*45–49*	27·9	19·3	*80–84*	242·6	135·5
15–19	0·5	0·2	*50–54*	42·9	25·5	*85–89*	327·7	167·0
20–24	1·2	0·9	*55–59*	54·7	31·3	*90–94*	353·6	213·5
25–29	1·2	1·2	*60–64*	85·7	43·6	*95+*	813·0	289·6
30–34	3·6	4·7	*65–69*	98·8	64·4	*All ages*	26·3	20·7

SEX AND AGE DISTRIBUTION

	Male	*Female*
Mean age (*years*)	63·0	65·4
95% between ages	36 & 87	35 & 89
Children under 15 (%)	0·0	0·1
Median age (*years*)	63·0	67·1
Proportion by sex (%)	55·4	44·6
Proportion of all cancers by sex (%)	8·6	7·4
Trend over 10 years	(–)	(–)

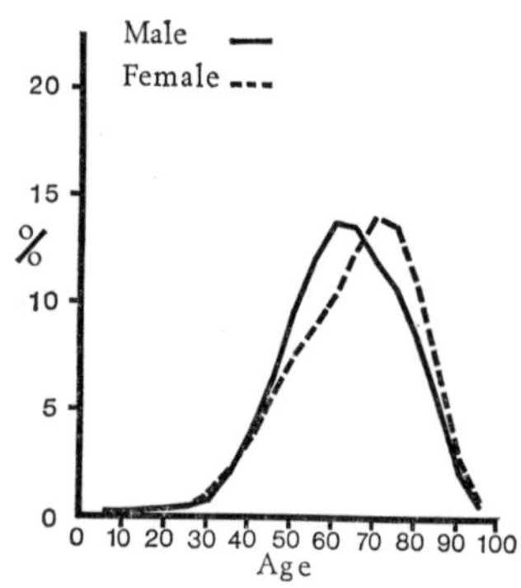

NOTES

The presentation by site groupings which is used here differs from that of the ICD which divides first by histological type into malignant melanoma of skin or into other malignant neoplasm of skin, and thence into localisation by site of lesion, by means of a fourth digit classificatory scheme. Presentation of the same material by each of four histological descriptions, allowing direct comparability with the ICD scheme, will be found on pp. 44-53.

Important. Only cases of melanoma or of squamous-cell carcinoma are followed up routinely. The remainder, chiefly basal-cell carcinoma (rodent ulcers), are not followed up. The data presented on the Fate page opposite refer therefore only to cases of melanoma or squamous-cell carcinoma.

ICD (7th) 190.0–190.4, 191.0–191.4 (part)

SKIN, FACE AND HEAD (Squamous and melanoma only)

5-YEAR SURVIVAL RATES BY AGE

Crude —— *Corrected* ----

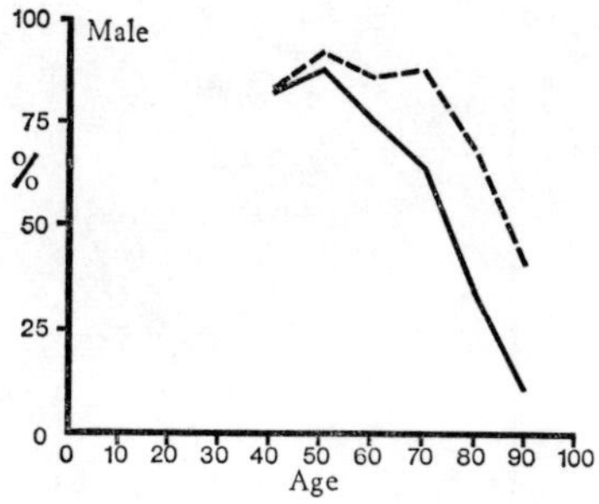

ALL CASES

Total 645
Male 437
Female 208

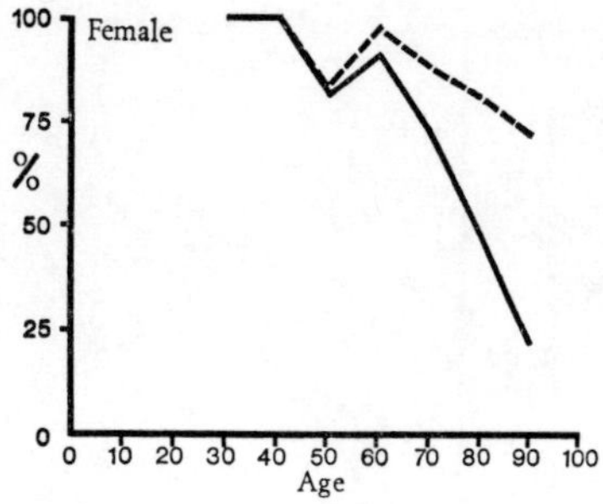

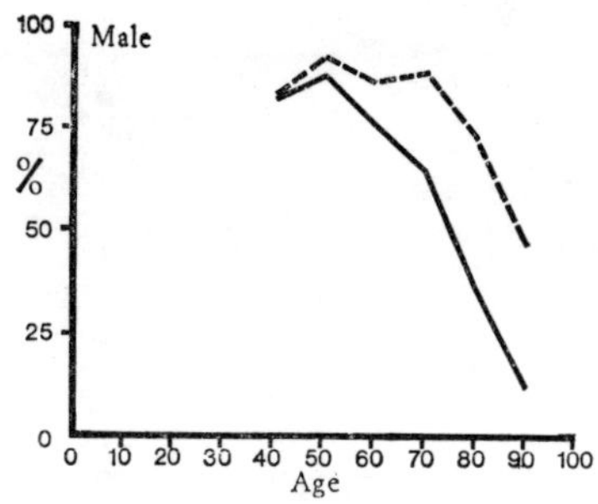

RADICAL TREATMENT

(94·7% of total)
95·2% *male*
93·8% *female*

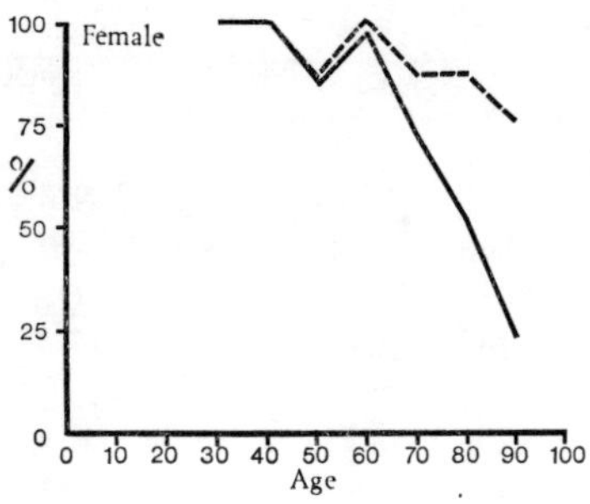

INDICES OF SURVIVAL

	All cases		Radical Treatment	
	Male	*Female*	*Male*	*Female*
FIVE YEAR SURVIVAL RATE (%)				
Crude	57·0	63·5	58·9	66·2
Corrected	*82·0*	*84·5*	*83·5*	*87·6*
Total cases†	437	208	416	195
TEN YEAR SURVIVAL RATE (%)				
Crude	39·5	51·3	40·9	54·9
Corrected	*77·0*	*86·8*	*78·3*	*91·3*
Total cases†	349	230	335	215

†Number of cases on which survival rate is based

SURVIVAL TIME (*months*)				
First quartile (75% S.R.)	25·1	37·5	26·4	43·0
Median (50% S.R.)	**>60**	**>60**	**>60**	**>60**
Third quartile (25% S.R.)	>60	>60	>60	>60

ANNUAL SURVIVAL RATES

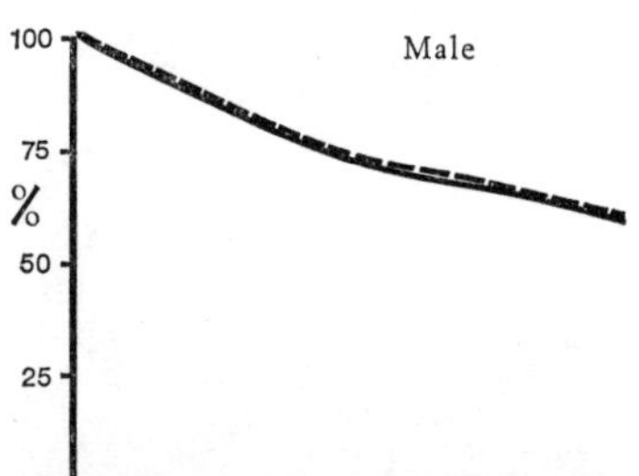

All cases ——
Radical treatment ----

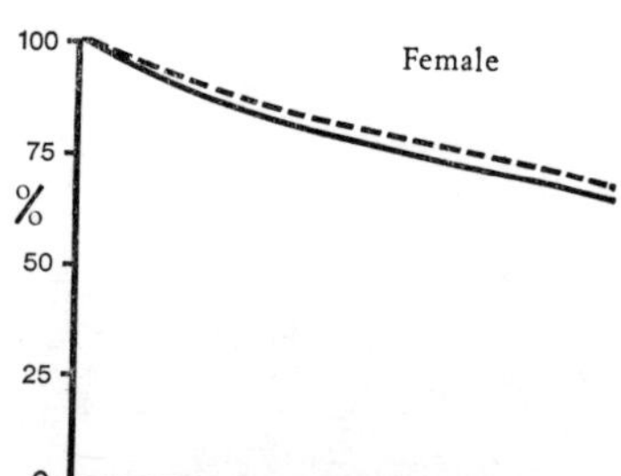

SKIN, TRUNK AND LIMBS **ICD (8th) 172.6–172.9, 173.6–173.9**
(All histological groups)

INCIDENCE RATE (per 100,000)

Male —— *Female* ----

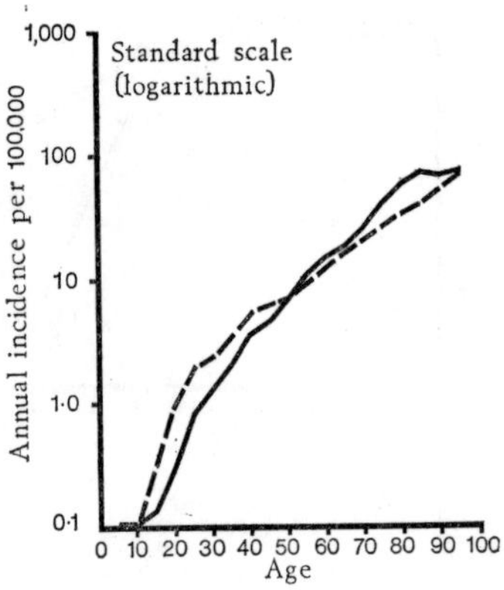

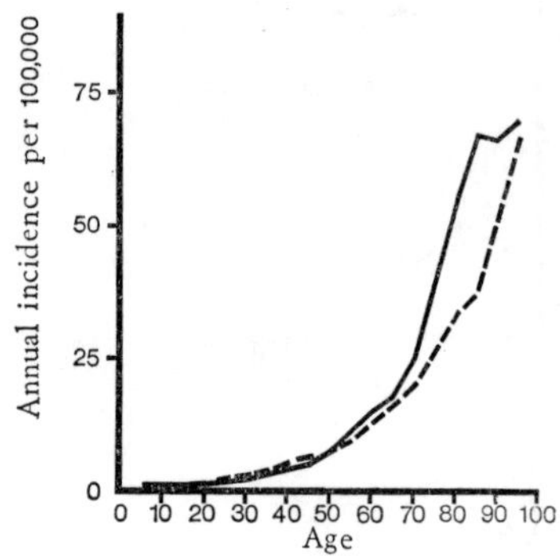

INCIDENCE RATES (per 100,000) by Age

Total cases 829 *males*; 936 *females* (of which age not stated for 2 *males* and 3 *females*)

Age	M	F	Age	M	F	Age	M	F
0–4	0·1	0·0	*35–39*	2·4	4·1	*70–74*	32·9	21·6
5–9	0·1	0·1	*40–44*	4·3	5·7	*75–79*	48·5	31·7
10–14	0·1	0·2	*45–49*	4·3	6·1	*80–84*	65·6	33·8
15–19	0·2	0·5	*50–54*	8·7	6·8	*85–89*	69·3	49·8
20–24	0·5	1·6	*55–59*	12·4	10·7	*90–94*	46·1	49·3
25–29	1·1	2·0	*60–64*	16·7	13·7	*95+*	271·0	160·9
30–34	1·6	2·4	*65–69*	18·4	17·9	*All ages*	5·9	6·5

SEX AND AGE DISTRIBUTION

	Male	*Female*
Mean age (*years*)	62·9	62·0
95% between ages	30 & 87	25 & 89
Children under 15 (%)	0·3	0·3
Median age (*years*)	63·6	64·1
Proportion by sex (%)	47·0	53·0
Proportion of all cancers by sex (%)	1·9	2·3
Trend over 10 years	(+)	(+)

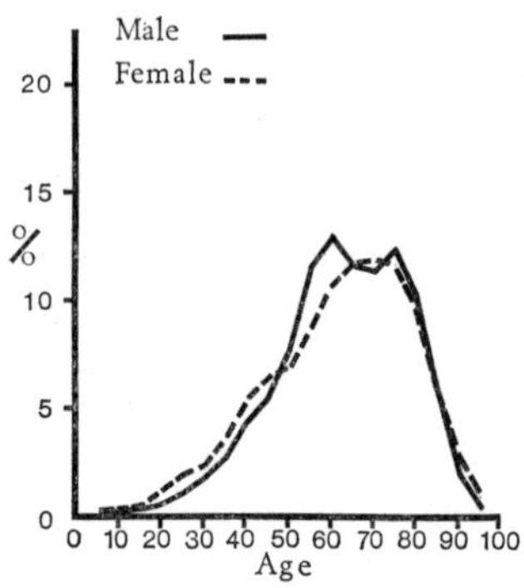

NOTES

The presentation by site groupings which is used here differs from that of the ICD which divides first by histological type into malignant melanoma of skin or into other malignant neoplasm of skin, and thence into localisation by site of lesion, by means of a fourth digit classificatory scheme. Presentation of the same material by each of four histological descriptions, allowing direct comparability with the ICD scheme, will be found on pp. 44-53.

Important. Only cases of melanoma or of squamous-cell carcinoma are followed up routinely. The remainder, chiefly basal-cell carcinoma (rodent ulcers), are not followed up. The data presented on the Fate page opposite refer therefore only to cases of melanoma or squamous-cell carcinoma.

ICD (7th) 190.5–190.9, 191.5–191.9 (part)

SKIN, TRUNK AND LIMBS (Squamous and melanoma only)

5-YEAR SURVIVAL RATES BY AGE

Crude —— *Corrected* ----

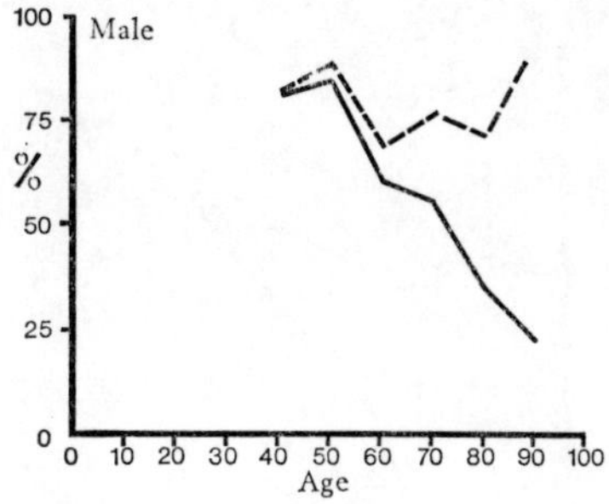

ALL CASES

Total 592
Male 296
Female 296

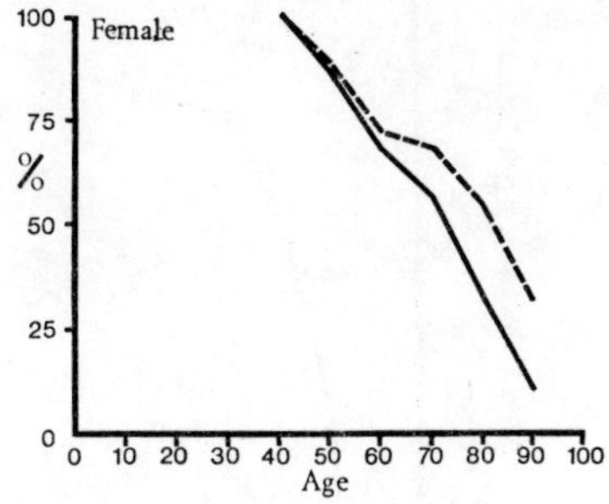

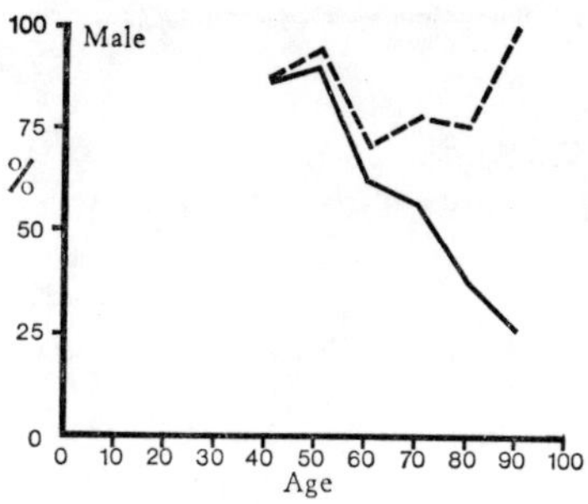

RADICAL TREATMENT

(89·5% of total)
90·2% *male*
88·9% *female*

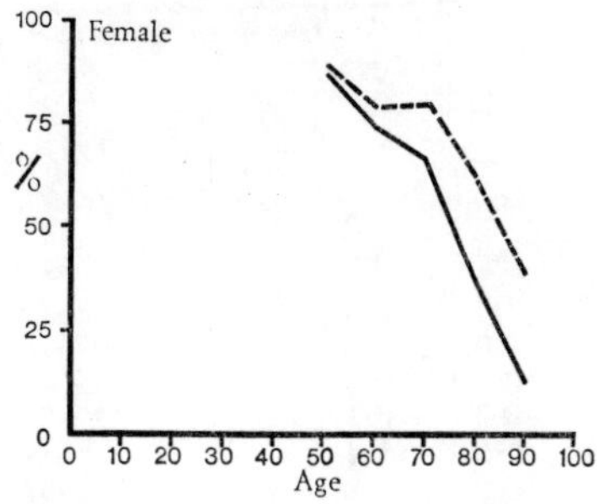

INDICES OF SURVIVAL

	All cases *Male*	All cases *Female*	Radical Treatment *Male*	Radical Treatment *Female*
FIVE YEAR SURVIVAL RATE (%)				
Crude	51·7	51·0	55·8	55·5
Corrected	*67·8*	*61·5*	*72·7*	*65·5*
Total cases†	296	296	267	263
TEN YEAR SURVIVAL RATE (%)				
Crude	27·7	35·0	29·7	37·4
Corrected	*51·7*	*53·9*	*53·9*	*56·5*
Total cases†	220	160	202	147

†Number of cases on which survival rate is based

	All cases *Male*	All cases *Female*	Radical Treatment *Male*	Radical Treatment *Female*
SURVIVAL TIME (*months*)				
First quartile (75% S.R.)	21·6	16·0	28·7	25·0
Median (50% S.R.)	**>60**	**>60**	**>60**	**>60**
Third quartile (25% S.R.)	>60	>60	>60	>60

ANNUAL SURVIVAL RATES

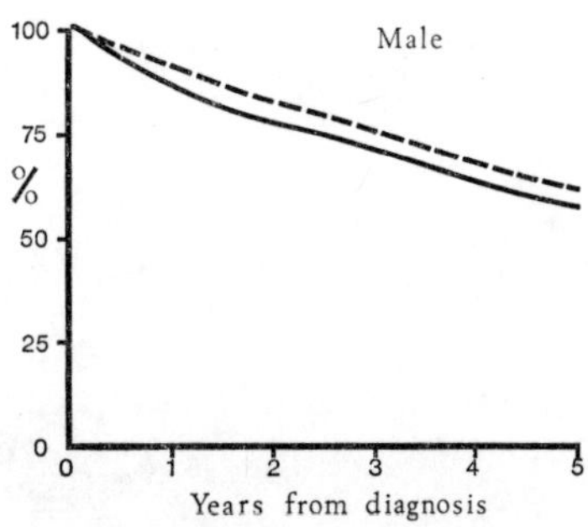

All cases ——
Radical treatment ----

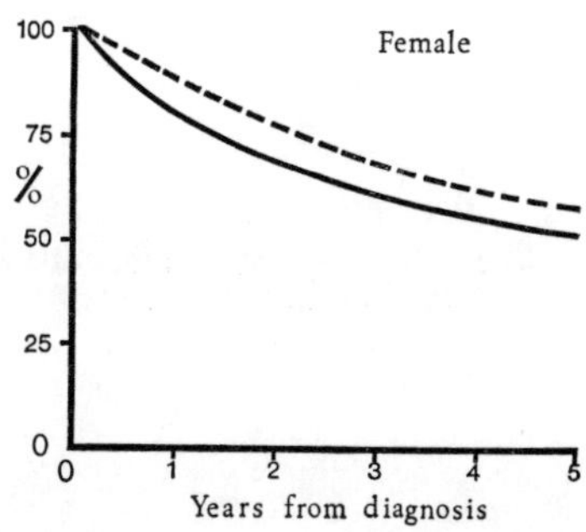

INCIDENCE RATE (per 100,000)

Male —— *Female* ----

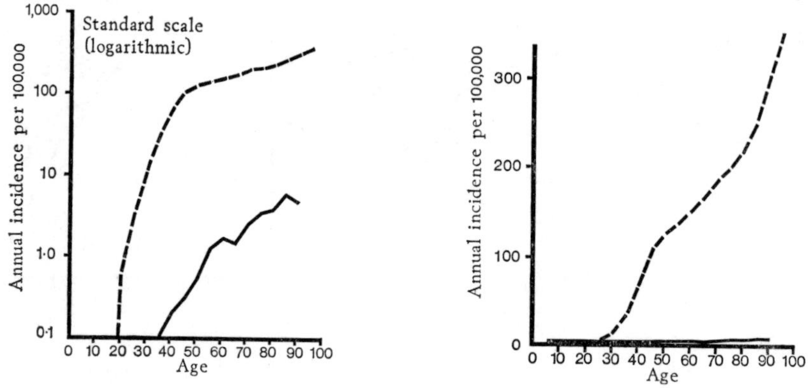

INCIDENCE RATES (per 100,000) by Age

Total cases 70 *males*; 9976 *females* (of which age not stated for 0 *males* and 10 *females*)

Age	M	F	Age	M	F	Age	M	F
0–4	0·0	0·0	*35–39*	0·2	43·1	*70–74*	3·8	191·9
5–9	0·0	0·0	*40–44*	0·3	89·4	*75–79*	2·5	208·3
10–14	0·0	0·0	*45–49*	0·3	120·2	*80–84*	5·6	236·3
15–19	0·0	0·1	*50–54*	0·7	128·9	*85–89*	5·3	295·3
20–24	0·0	1·4	*55–59*	1·8	144·8	*90–94*	0·0	339·4
25–29	0·0	5·2	*60–64*	1·4	154·8	*95+*	0·0	450·5
30–34	0·0	18·0	*65–69*	1·3	179·5	*All ages*	0·5	69·1

SEX AND AGE DISTRIBUTION

	Male	*Female*
Mean age (*years*)	63·9	59·6
95% between ages	39 & 86	35 & 86
Children under 15 (%)	0·0	0·0
Median age (*years*)	62·8	59·0
Proportion by sex (%)	0·7	99·3
Proportion of all cancers by sex (%)	0·2	24·6
Trend over 10 years	(−)	(−)

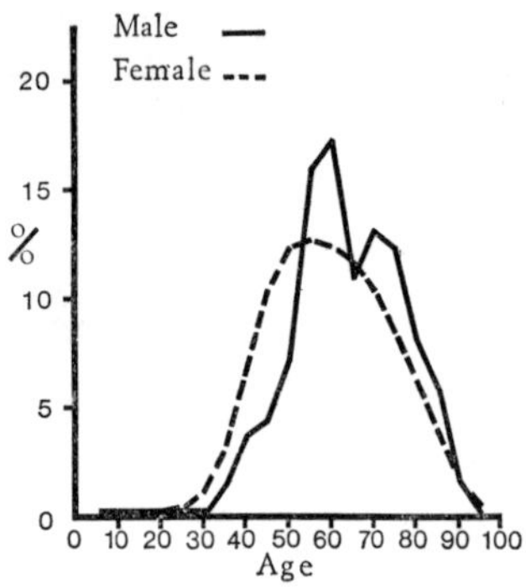

NOTES

Includes: All malignant tumours of breast. No attempt has been made to include subdivisions by any system of clinical staging (e.g. TNM).

5-YEAR SURVIVAL RATES BY AGE

Crude —— *Corrected* ----

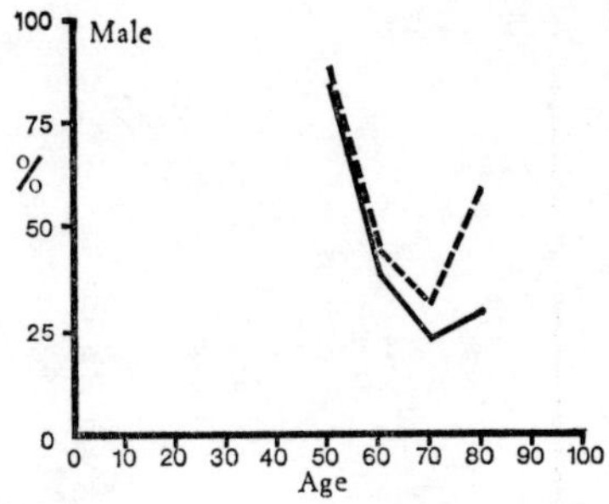

ALL CASES

Total 5805
Male 49
Female 5756

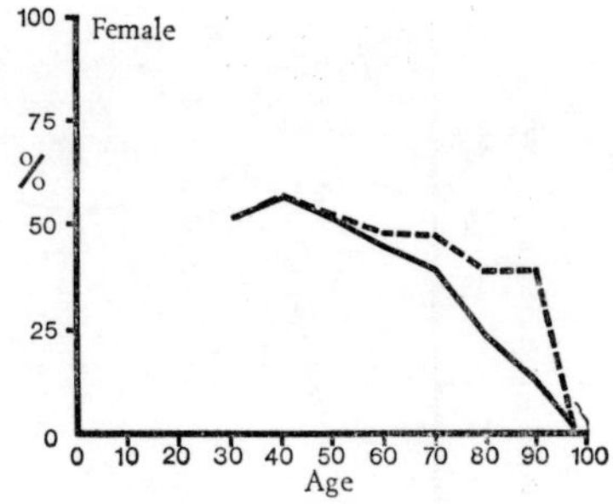

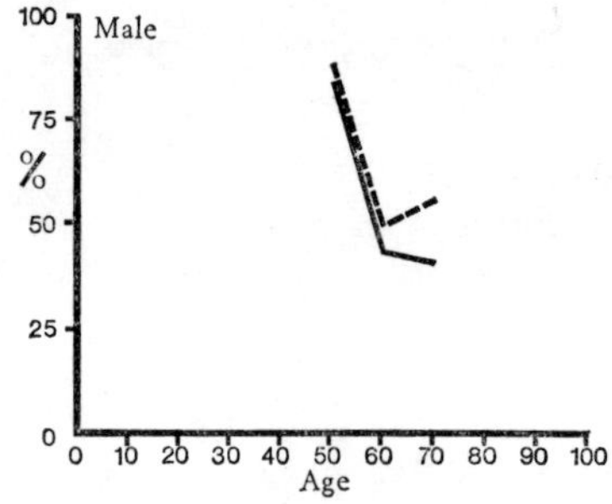

RADICAL TREATMENT

(78·9% of total)
75·5% *male*
78·9% *female*

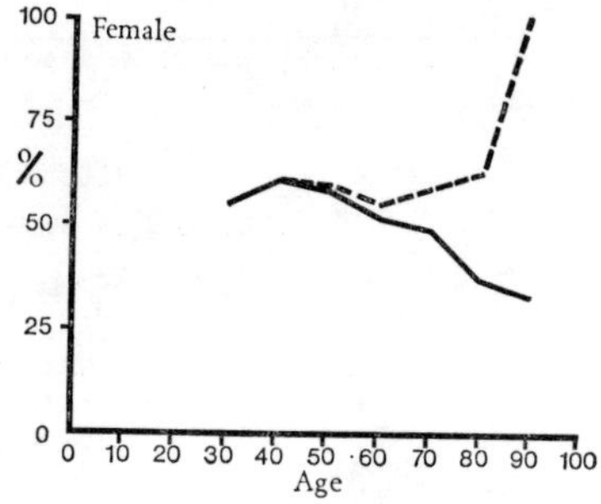

INDICES OF SURVIVAL

	All cases		Radical Treatment	
	Male	*Female*	*Male*	*Female*
FIVE YEAR SURVIVAL RATE (%)				
Crude	44·7	42·6	59·5	52·2
Corrected	*58·2*	*49·0*	*71·2*	*57·8*
Total cases†	49	5756	37	4544
TEN YEAR SURVIVAL RATE (%)				
Crude	21·9	28·8	26·5	34·5
Corrected	*31·6*	*38·2*	*42·1*	*43·6*
Total cases†	41	4283	34	3495
SURVIVAL TIME (*months*)				
First quartile (75% S.R.)	16·3	15·7	41·0	25·9
Median (50% S.R.)	**45·5**	**44·7**	**>60**	**>60**
Third quartile (25% S.R.)	>60	>60	>60	>60

† Number of cases on which survival rate is based

ANNUAL SURVIVAL RATES

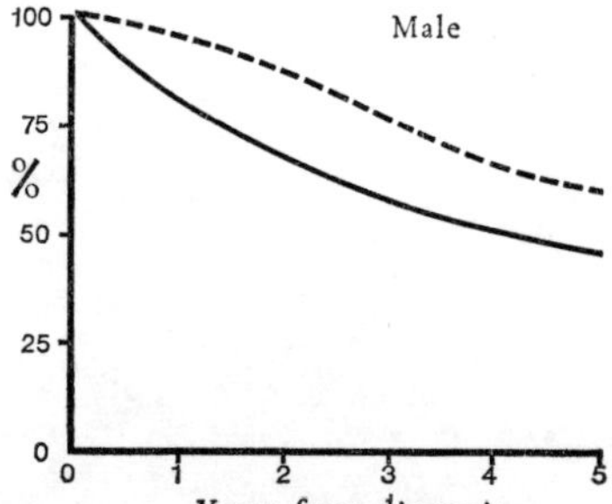

All cases ——
Radical treatment ----

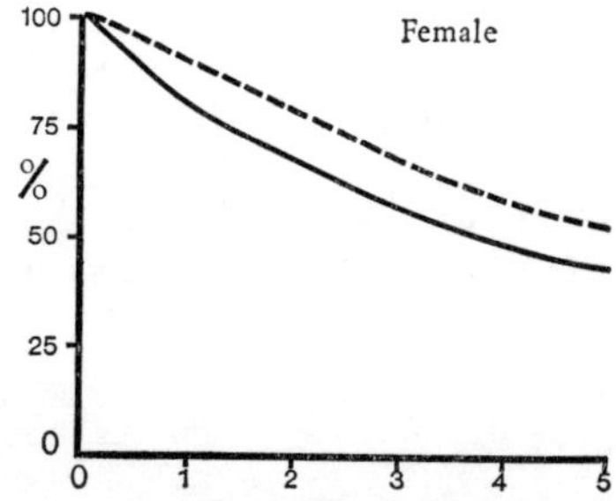

INCIDENCE RATE (per 100,000)

Female ----

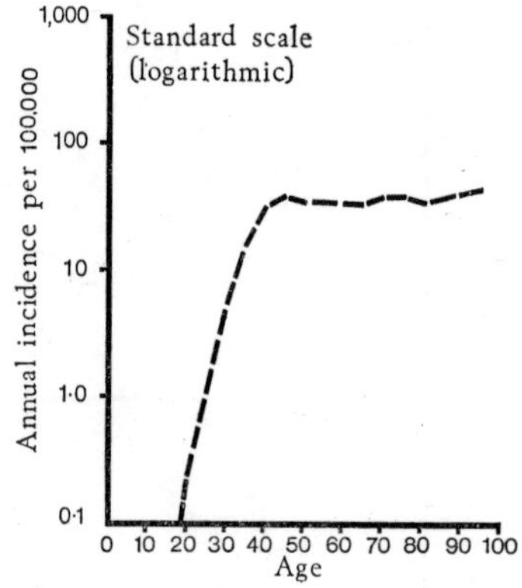

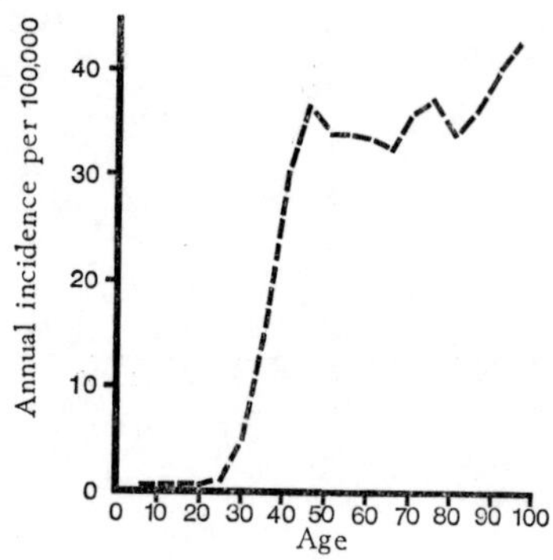

INCIDENCE RATES (per 100,000) by Age

Total cases 2514 *females* (of which age not stated for 4 *females*)

Age	F	Age	F	Age	F
0–4	0·0	*35–39*	21·7	*70–74*	38·9
5–9	0·0	*40–44*	37·9	*75–79*	33·7
10–14	0·0	*45–49*	34·6	*80–84*	33·3
15–19	0·1	*50–54*	32·4	*85–89*	42·4
20–24	0·3	*55–59*	34·8	*90–94*	27·4
25–29	1·9	*60–64*	31·4	*95+*	128·7
30–34	8·1	*65–69*	33·3	*All ages*	17·4

SEX AND AGE DISTRIBUTION

	Female
Mean age (*years*)	55·0
95% between ages	33 & 84
Children under 15 (%)	0·0
Median age (*years*)	53·5
Proportion by sex (%)	100
Proportion of all cancers by sex (%)	6·2
Trend over 10 years	(–)

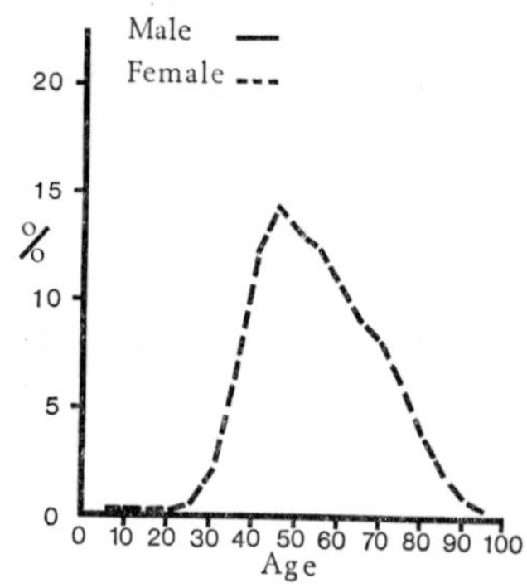

NOTES

Includes: Only cases of invasive carcinoma. Further details will be found on p. 60.

Excludes: Cases of carcinoma-in-situ (Stage 0), which are to be found on p. 88.

5-YEAR SURVIVAL RATES BY AGE

Crude —— *Corrected* ----

ALL CASES

Total 1430
Female 1430

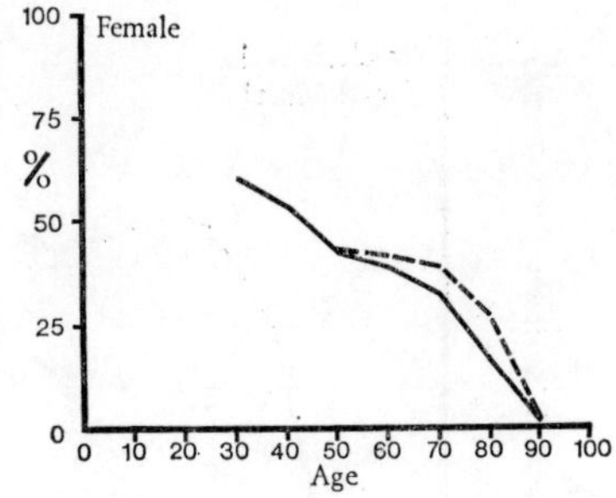

RADICAL TREATMENT

(81·6% of total)
81·6% *female*

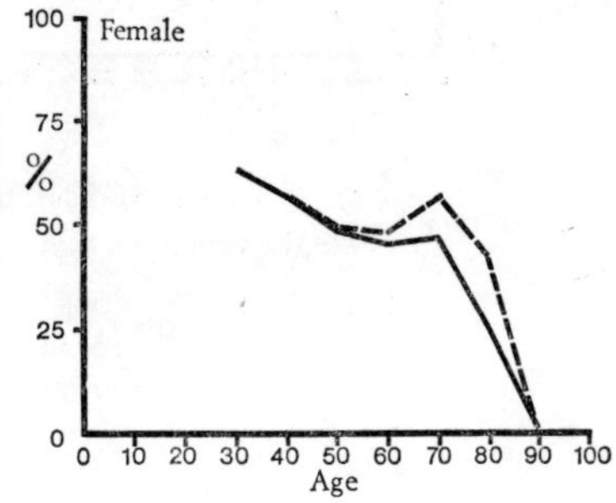

INDICES OF SURVIVAL

	All cases *Female*	Radical Treatment *Female*
FIVE YEAR SURVIVAL RATE (%)		
Crude	39·7	48·1
Corrected	*43·5*	*51·7*
Total cases†	1430	1167
TEN YEAR SURVIVAL RATE (%)		
Crude	31·0	37·8
Corrected	*38·4*	*45·7*
Total cases†	1299	1044
SURVIVAL TIME (*months*)		
First quartile (75% S.R.)	8·2	14·3
Median (50% S.R.)	**29·7**	**52·5**
Third quartile (25% S.R.)	>60	>60

† Number of cases on which survival rate is based

ANNUAL SURVIVAL RATES

All cases ————

Radical treatment - - - -

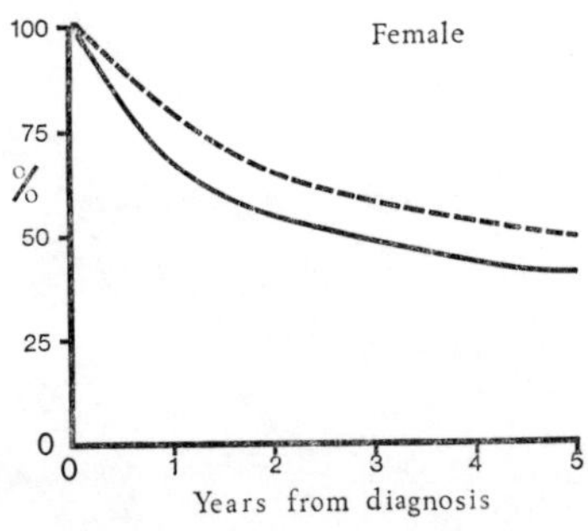

ENDOMETRIUM ICD (8th) **182.0**

INCIDENCE RATE (per 100,000)

Female - - - -

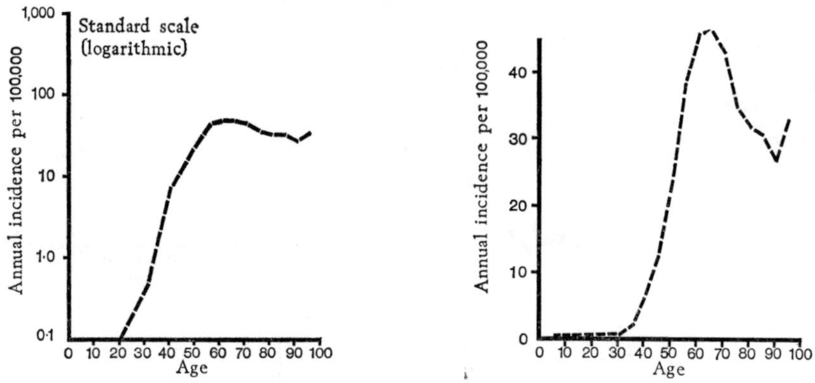

INCIDENCE RATES (per 100,000) by Age

Total cases 1986 *females* (of which age not stated for 2 *females*)

Age	F	Age	F	Age	F
0–4	0·0	*35–39*	2·9	*70–74*	37·5
5–9	0·0	*40–44*	10·0	*75–79*	30·0
10–14	0·0	*45–49*	14·4	*80–84*	34·3
15–19	0·1	*50–54*	31·6	*85–89*	23·7
20–24	0·1	*55–59*	44·5	*90–94*	38·3
25–29	0·3	*60–64*	45·5	*95+*	0·0
30–34	0·4	*65–69*	46·8	*All ages*	13·8

SEX AND AGE DISTRIBUTION

	Female
Mean age (*years*)	60·9
95% between ages	41 & 83
Children under 15 (%)	0·0
Median age (*years*)	60·4
Proportion by sex (%)	100
Proportion of all cancers by sex (%)	4·9
Trend over 10 years	(–)

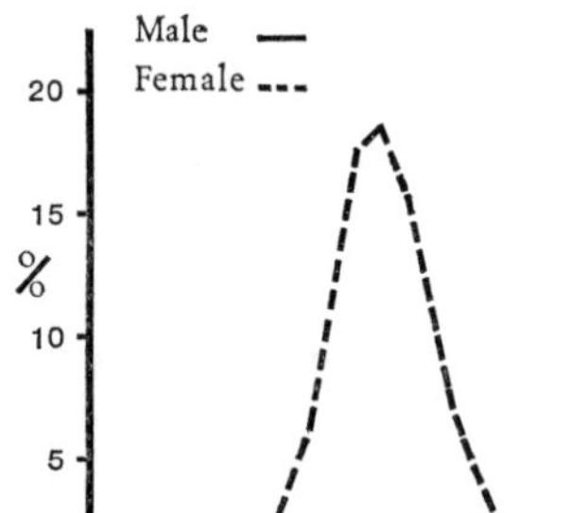

NOTES

Excludes: Sarcoma of uterus, which is classified with OTHER UTERUS.

5-YEAR SURVIVAL RATES BY AGE

Crude —— *Corrected* ----

ALL CASES

Total 1004
Female 1004

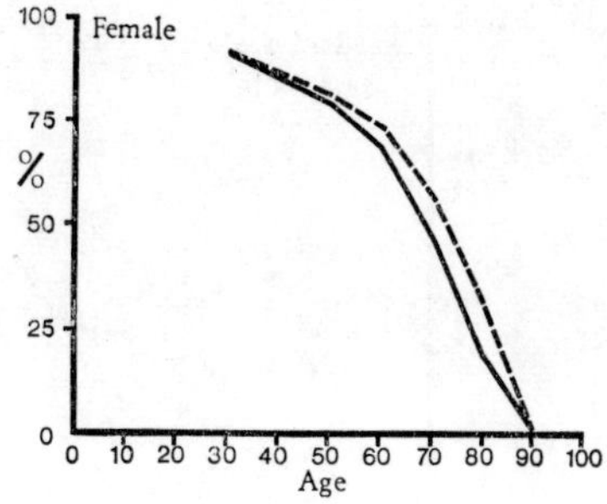

RADICAL TREATMENT

(87·4% of total)
87·4% *female*

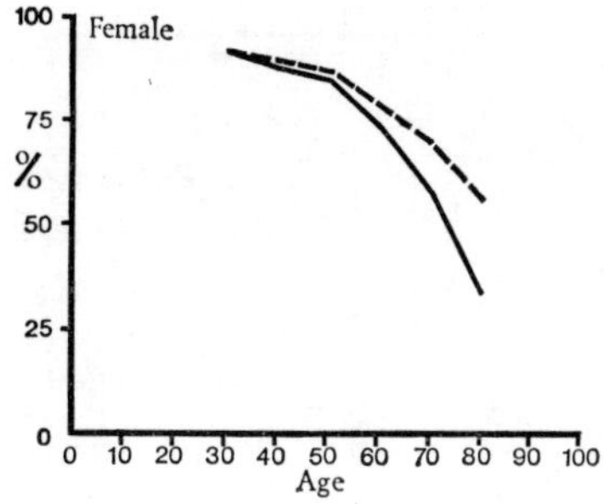

INDICES OF SURVIVAL

	All cases *Female*	Radical Treatment *Female*
FIVE YEAR SURVIVAL RATE (%)		
Crude	62·2	70·6
Corrected	*69·6*	*77·5*
Total cases†	1004	877
TEN YEAR SURVIVAL RATE (%)		
Crude	50·0	56·6
Corrected	*64·6*	*71·9*
Total cases†	820	721
SURVIVAL TIME (*months*)		
First quartile (75% S.R.)	22·1	42·0
Median (50% S.R.)	**>60**	**>60**
Third quartile (25% S.R.)	>60	>60

† Number of cases on which survival rate is based

ANNUAL SURVIVAL RATES

All cases ——
Radical treatment ----

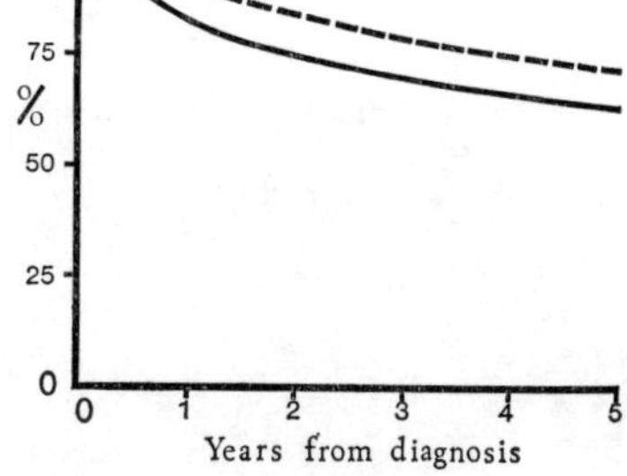

OTHER UTERUS ICD (8th) **181, 182.9**

INCIDENCE RATE (per 100,000)

Female ----

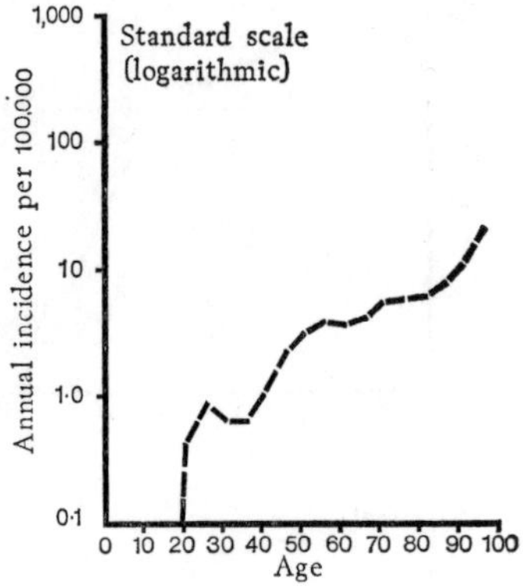

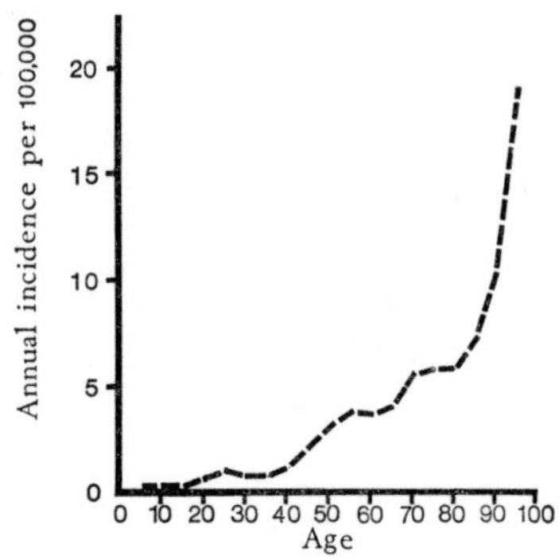

INCIDENCE RATES (per 100,000) by Age

Total cases 256 *females* (of which age not stated for 1 *female*)

Age	F	Age	F	Age	F
0–4	0·0	*35–39*	0·9	*70–74*	5·8
5–9	0·0	*40–44*	1·2	*75–79*	5·5
10–14	0·0	*45–49*	2·6	*80–84*	6·0
15–19	0·0	*50–54*	3·2	*85–89*	10·0
20–24	0·8	*55–59*	3·9	*90–94*	10·9
25–29	0·9	*60–64*	3·0	*95+*	64·4
30–34	0·3	*65–69*	5·9	*All ages*	1·8

SEX AND AGE DISTRIBUTION

	Female
Mean age (*years*)	59·8
95% between ages	25 & 89
Children under 15 (%)	0·0
Median age (*years*)	59·6
Proportion by sex (%)	100
Proportion of all cancers by sex (%)	0·6
Trend over 10 years	(–)

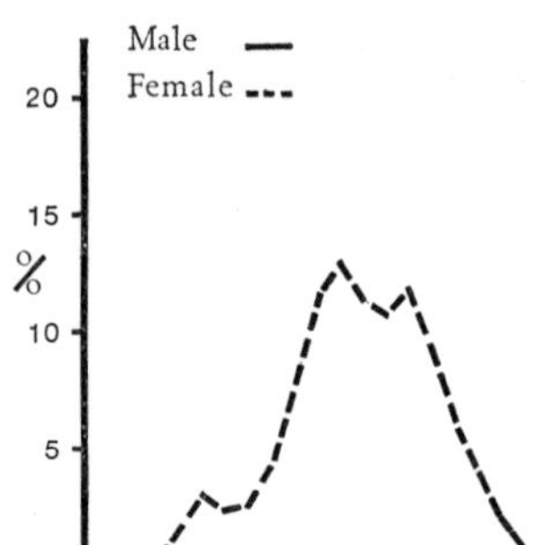

NOTES

Includes: Sarcoma of uterus (60%); uterus, not further specified (25%); mesodermal mixed tumours (carcinosarcoma) (10%); chorionepithelioma (5%). (The figures in parenthesis give the proportionate composition of the group).

5-YEAR SURVIVAL RATES BY AGE

Crude —— *Corrected* - - - -

ALL CASES

Total 152
Female 152

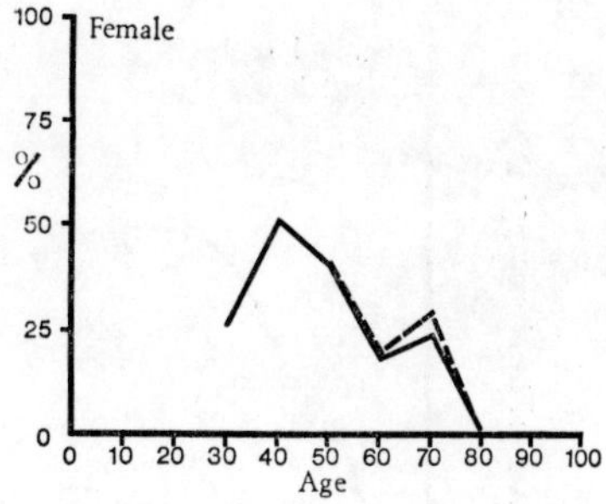

RADICAL TREATMENT

(63·8 % of total)
63·8 % *female*

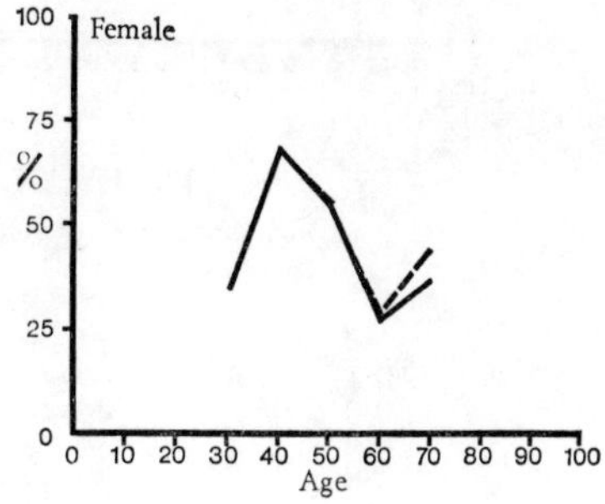

INDICES OF SURVIVAL

	All cases *Female*	Radical Treatment *Female*
FIVE YEAR SURVIVAL RATE (%)		
Crude	27·0	41·2
Corrected	*30·5*	*44·6*
Total cases†	152	97
TEN YEAR SURVIVAL RATE (%)		
Crude	29·9	36·5
Corrected	*38·2*	*44·9*
Total cases†	87	63

† Number of cases on which survival rate is based

SURVIVAL TIME (*months*)		
First quartile (75 % S.R.)	2·0	9·0
Median (50 % S.R.)	**9·4**	**21·5**
Third quartile (25 % S.R.)	>60	>60

ANNUAL SURVIVAL RATES

All cases ——
Radical treatment - - - -

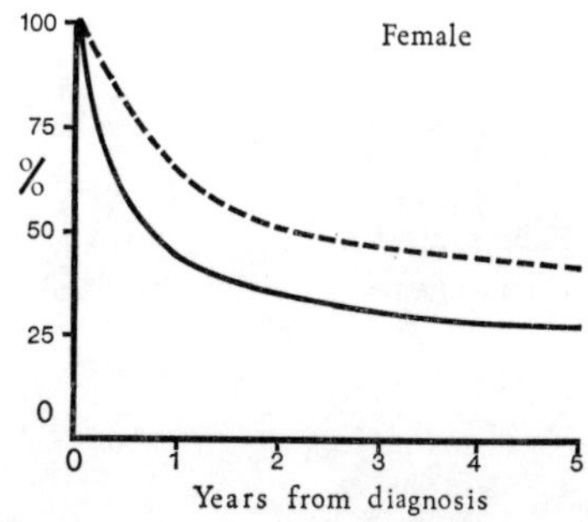

INCIDENCE RATE (per 100,000)

Female ----

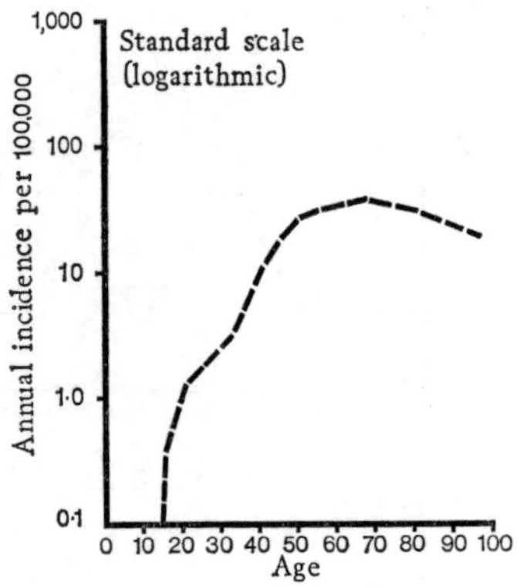

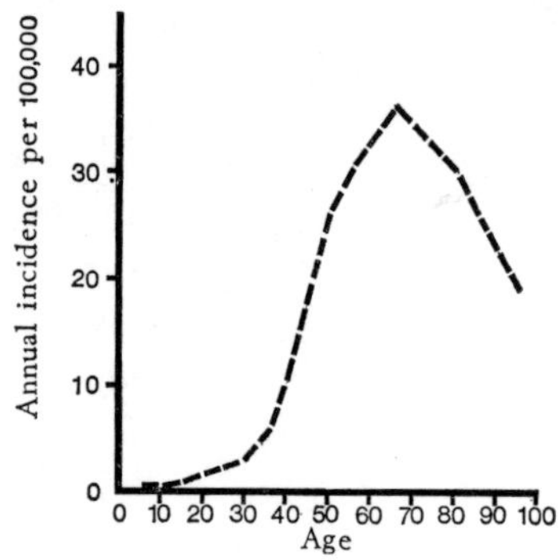

INCIDENCE RATES (per 100,000) by Age

Total cases 1898 *females* (of which age not stated for 2 *females*)

Age	F	Age	F	Age	F
0–4	0·0	*35–39*	6·6	*70–74*	32·7
5–9	0·1	*40–44*	14·7	*75–79*	30·8
10–14	0·0	*45–49*	22·3	*80–84*	27·3
15–19	0·9	*50–54*	30·8	*85–89*	22·4
20–24	1·6	*55–59*	29·8	*90–94*	21·9
25–29	1·9	*60–64*	36·6	*95+*	0·0
30–34	3·2	*65–69*	35·1	*All ages*	13·1

SEX AND AGE DISTRIBUTION

	Female
Mean age (*years*)	57·9
95% between ages	31 & 83
Children under 15 (%)	0·1
Median age (*years*)	57·9
Proportion by sex (%)	100
Proportion of all cancers by sex (%)	4·7
Trend over 10 years	(–)

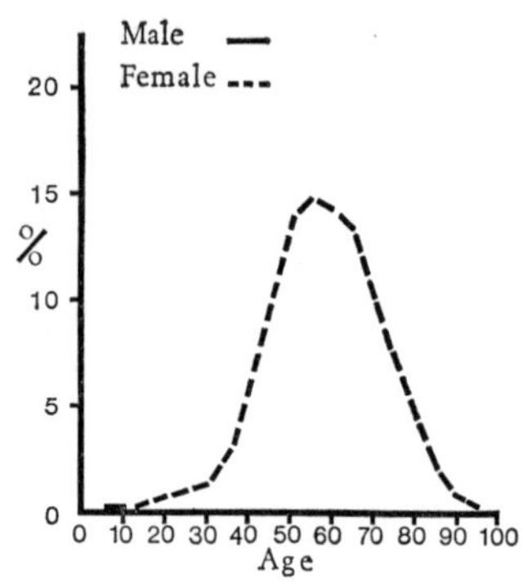

NOTES

Includes: Fallopian tube.

Excludes: Broad ligament, which is classified with OTHER FEMALE GENITALIA.

5-YEAR SURVIVAL RATES BY AGE

Crude —— *Corrected* ----

ALL CASES

Total 1154
Female 1154

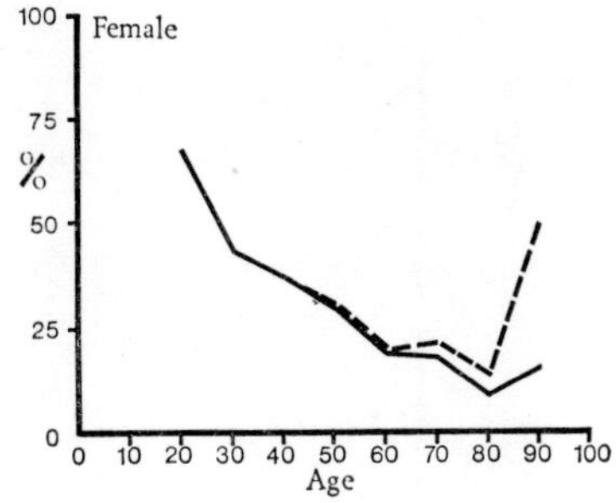

RADICAL TREATMENT

(51·8% of total)
51·8% *female*

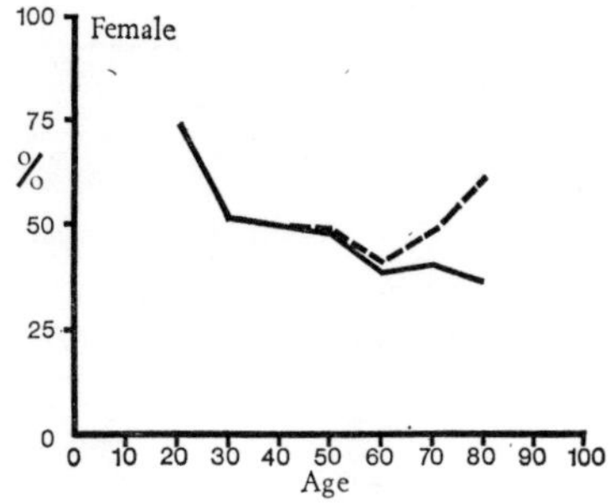

INDICES OF SURVIVAL

	All cases *Female*	Radical Treatment *Female*
FIVE YEAR SURVIVAL RATE (%)		
Crude	23·2	43·6
Corrected	*25·6*	*46·8*
Total cases†	1154	598
TEN YEAR SURVIVAL RATE (%)		
Crude	21·8	36·7
Corrected	*26·9*	*43·6*
Total cases†	760	439

† Number of cases on which survival rate is based

SURVIVAL TIME (*months*)		
First quartile (75% S.R.)	2·7	11·6
Median (50% S.R.)	**9·7**	**38·3**
Third quartile (25% S.R.)	46·9	>60

ANNUAL SURVIVAL RATES

All cases ——

Radical treatment ----

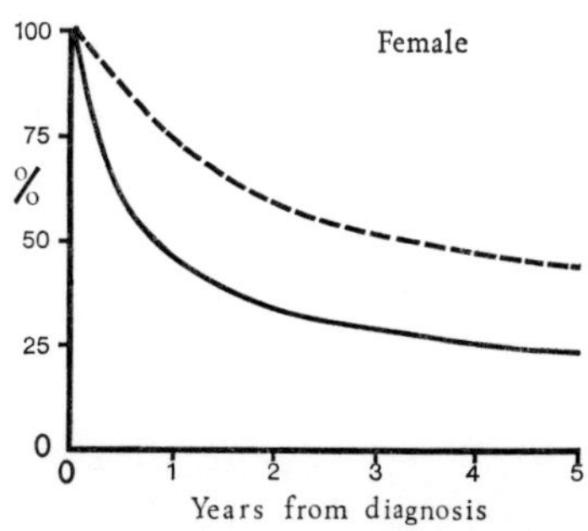

VULVA ICD (8th) **184.1**

INCIDENCE RATE (per 100,000)

Female ----

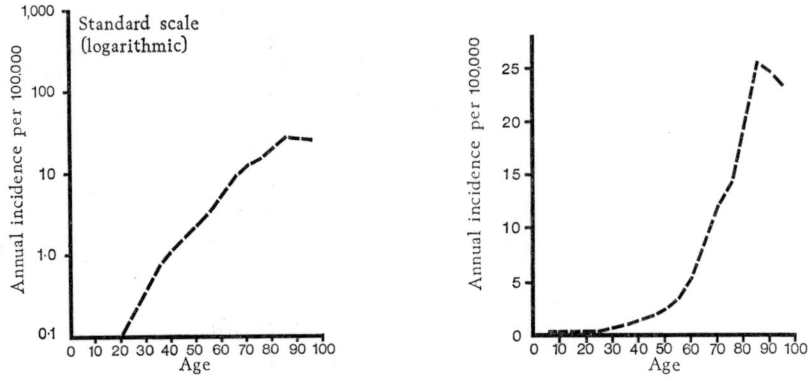

INCIDENCE RATES (per 100,000) by Age

Total cases 420 *females* (of which age not stated for 1 *female*)

Age	F	Age	F	Age	F
0–4	0·0	*35–39*	0·9	*70–74*	13·0
5–9	0·0	*40–44*	1·4	*75–79*	15·6
10–14	0·0	*45–49*	1·7	*80–84*	25·3
15–19	0·0	*50–54*	2·6	*85–89*	24·9
20–24	0·1	*55–59*	3·8	*90–94*	21·9
25–29	0·3	*60–64*	6·7	*95+*	32·2
30–34	0·5	*65–69*	10·9	*All ages*	2·9

SEX AND AGE DISTRIBUTION

	Female
Mean age (*years*)	67·2
95% between ages	36 & 89
Children under 15 (%)	0·0
Median age (*years*)	68·8
Proportion by sex (%)	100
Proportion of all cancers by sex (%)	1·0
Trend over 10 years	(−)

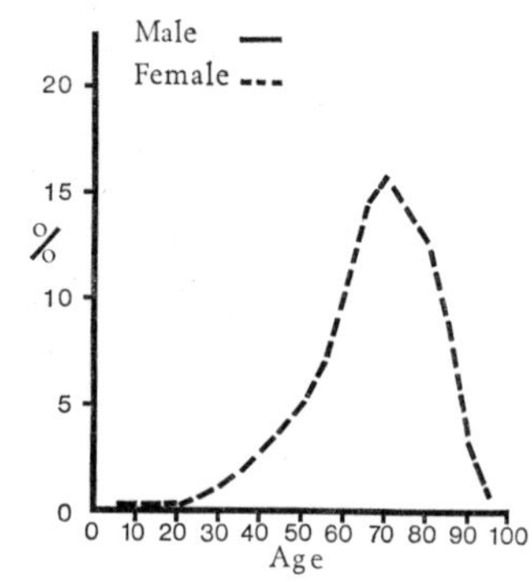

5-YEAR SURVIVAL RATES BY AGE

Crude —— *Corrected* ----

ALL CASES

Total 234
Female 234

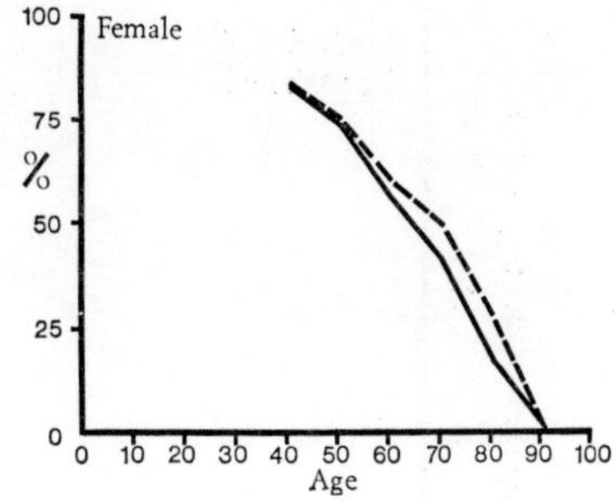

RADICAL TREATMENT

(85·9% of total)
85·9% *female*

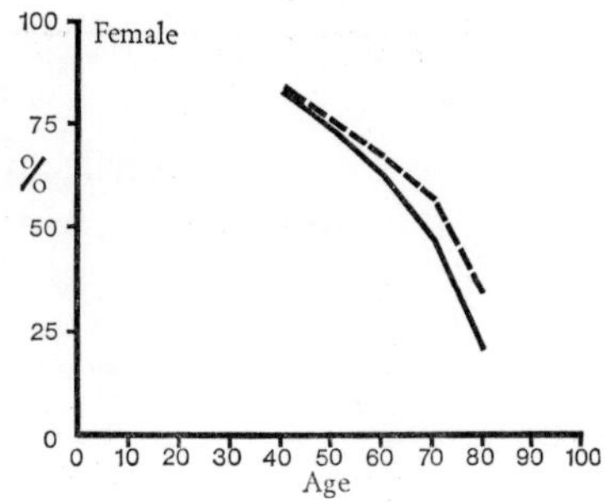

INDICES OF SURVIVAL

	All Cases *Female*	Radical Treatment *Female*
FIVE YEAR SURVIVAL RATE (%)		
Crude	40·6	47·3
Corrected	*52·2*	*59·1*
Total cases†	234	201
TEN YEAR SURVIVAL RATE (%)		
Crude	29·2	32·3
Corrected	*47·9*	*51·7*
Total cases†	178	158

† Number of cases on which survival rate is based

SURVIVAL TIME (*months*)		
First quartile (75% S.R.)	6·9	10·7
Median (50% S.R.)	**29·7**	**51·5**
Third quartile (25% S.R.)	>60	>60

ANNUAL SURVIVAL RATES

All cases ——

Radical treatment ----

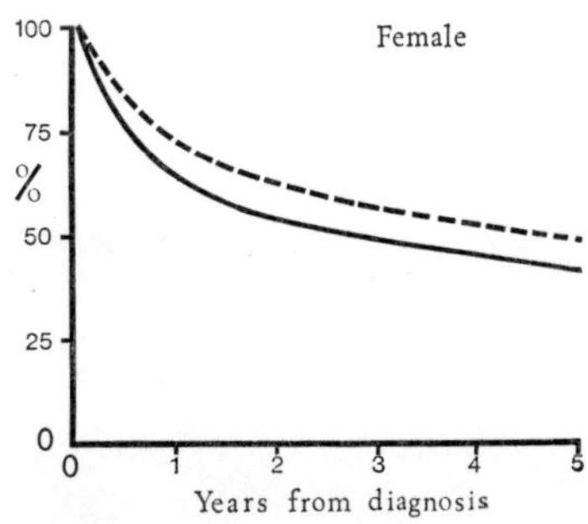

OTHER FEMALE GENITALIA

ICD (8th) **184 (rem.)**

INCIDENCE RATE (per 100,000)

Female ----

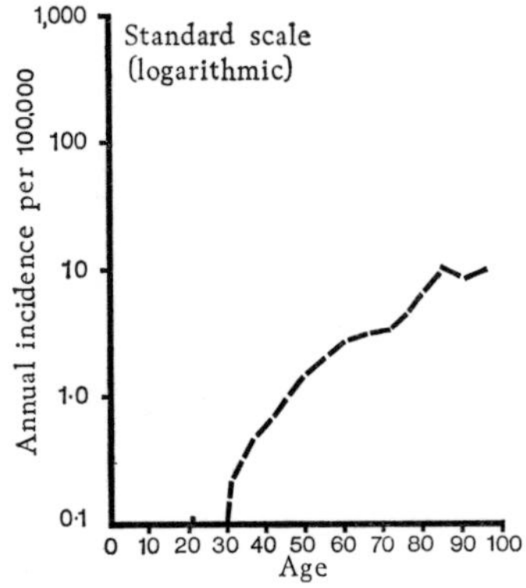

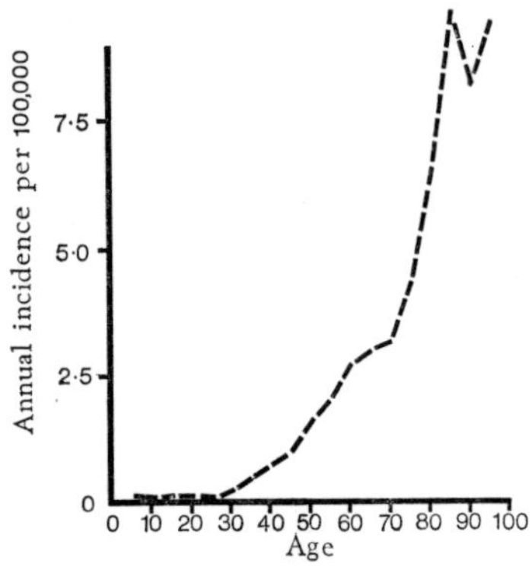

INCIDENCE RATES (per 100,000) by Age

Total cases 169 *females* (of which age not stated for 0 *females*)

Age	F	Age	F	Age	F
0–4	0·1	*35–39*	0·5	*70–74*	4·1
5–9	0·0	*40–44*	0·8	*75–79*	4·3
10–14	0·0	*45–49*	1·1	*80–84*	10·4
15–19	0·1	*50–54*	2·0	*85–89*	7·5
20–24	0·0	*55–59*	2·0	*90–94*	10·9
25–29	0·0	*60–64*	3·4	*95+*	0·0
30–34	0·3	*65–69*	2·3	*All ages*	1·2

SEX AND AGE DISTRIBUTION

	Female
Mean age (*years*)	63·7
95% between ages	34 & 88
Children under 15 (%)	0·6
Median age (*years*)	63·8
Proportion by sex (%)	100
Proportion of all cancers by sex (%)	0·4
Trend over 10 years	(+)

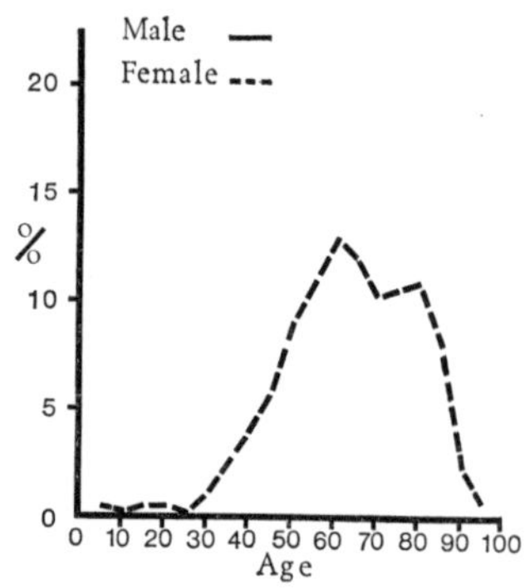

NOTES

Includes: Vagina (65%); "carcinoma uteri et ovarii", etc. (25%); broad ligament (1%); female genitalia, not further specified (9%). (The figures in parenthesis give the proportionate composition of the group).

5-YEAR SURVIVAL RATES BY AGE

Crude —— *Corrected* ----

ALL CASES

Total 82
Female 82

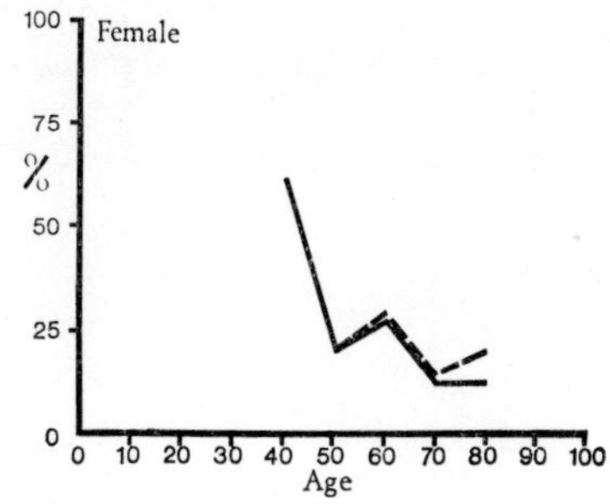

RADICAL TREATMENT

(68·3% of total)
68·3% *female*

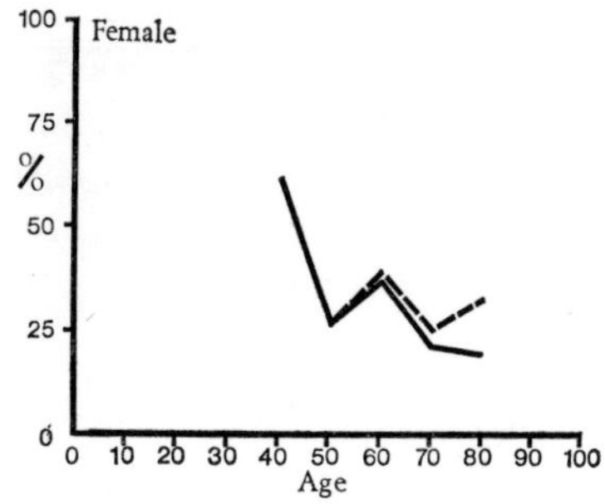

INDICES OF SURVIVAL

	All cases *Female*	Radical Treatment *Female*
FIVE YEAR SURVIVAL RATE (%)		
Crude	19·5	28·6
Corrected	*23·9*	*34·0*
Total cases†	82	56
TEN YEAR SURVIVAL RATE (%)		
Crude	7·3	14·2
Corrected	*10·9*	*19·9*
Total cases†	55	28
SURVIVAL TIME (*months*)		
First quartile (75% S.R.)	4·6	10·8
Median (50% S.R.)	**14·0**	**24·0**
Third quartile (25% S.R.)	44·8	>60

† Number of cases on which survival rate is based

ANNUAL SURVIVAL RATES

All cases ——————

Radical treatment - - - -

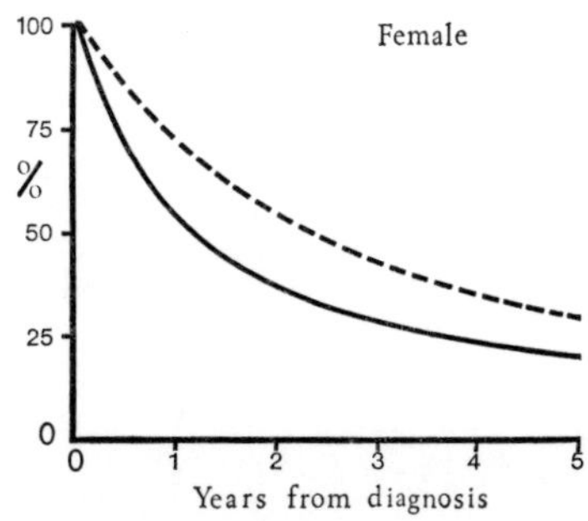

PROSTATE ICD (8th) **185**

INCIDENCE RATE (per 100,000)

Male ——

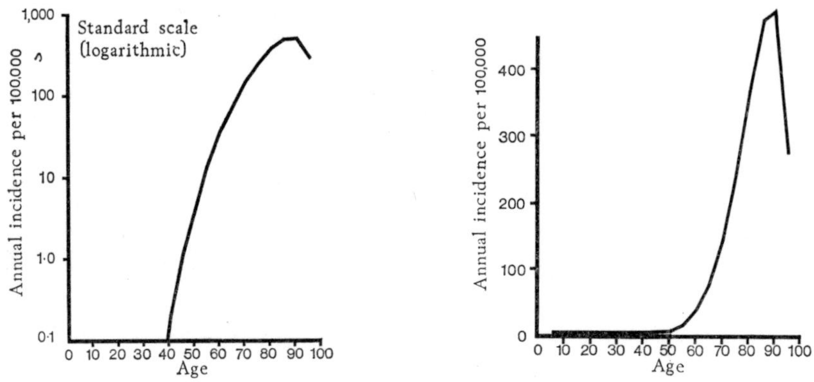

INCIDENCE RATES (per 100,000) by Age

Total cases 3038 *males* (of which age not stated for 8 *males*)

Age	M	Age	M	Age	M
0–4	0·0	*35–39*	0·0	*70–74*	196·6
5–9	0·0	*40–44*	0·5	*75–79*	317·3
10–14	0·0	*45–49*	1·8	*80–84*	455·2
15–19	0·0	*50–54*	6·2	*85–89*	519·5
20–24	0·0	*55–59*	21·3	*90–94*	292·1
25–29	0·0	*60–64*	55·1	*95+*	135·5
30–34	0·0	*65–69*	103·5	*All ages*	21·5

SEX AND AGE DISTRIBUTION

	Male
Mean age (years)	72·9
95% between ages	54 & 89
Children under 15 (%)	0·0
Median age (*years*)	73·6
Proportion by sex (%)	100
Proportion of all cancers by sex (%)	7·0
Trend over 10 years	(−)

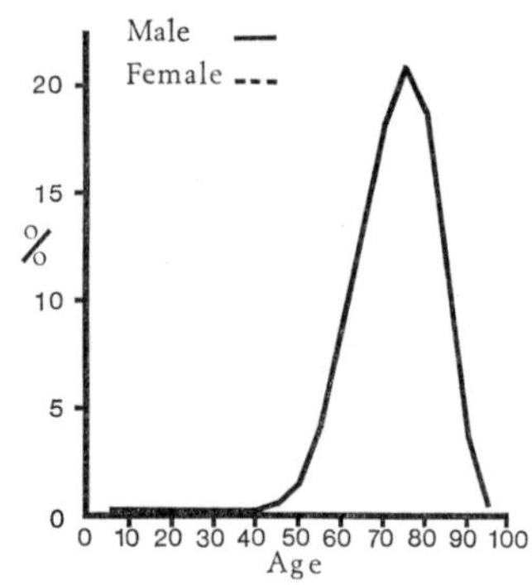

NOTES

Interpretations of what constitutes radical treatment at this site have not always shown consistency, particularly over the period of time used in the calculation of survival rates. It is evident for instance from the sharp discrepancy between the numbers of cases on which the survival rate for radical treatment are based at 5 years and at 10 years. It has not proved practicable to reassess the ascription of the treatment policy of earlier cases for better comparison with the more recent, but it is unlikely that such inconsistencies are of any importance in the later figures.

5-YEAR SURVIVAL RATES BY AGE

Crude —— *Corrected* ----

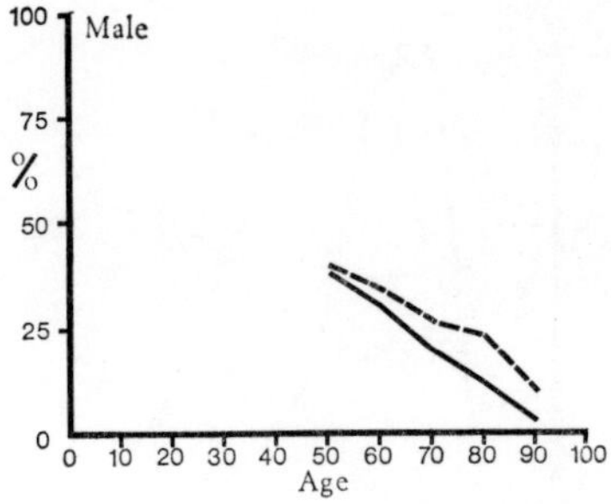

ALL CASES

Total 1715
Male 1715

RADICAL TREATMENT

(0·9% of total)
0·9% *male*

INDICES OF SURVIVAL

	All cases *Male*	Radical Treatment *Male*
FIVE YEAR SURVIVAL RATE (%)		
Crude	17·0	46·7
Corrected	*27·1*	*70·5*
Total cases†	1715	15
TEN YEAR SURVIVAL RATE (%)		
Crude	8·1	22·0
Corrected	*21·1*	*54·3*
Total cases†	952	59

† Number of cases on which survival rate is based

SURVIVAL TIME (*months*)		
First quartile (75% S.R.)	2·0	22·8
Median (50% S.R.)	**14·9**	**54·5**
Third quartile (25% S.R.)	41·4	>60

ANNUAL SURVIVAL RATES

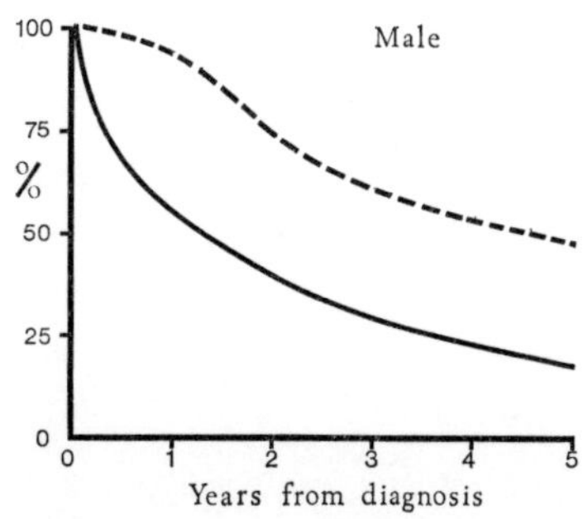

All cases ————
Radical treatment ----

INCIDENCE RATE (per 100,000)

Male ——

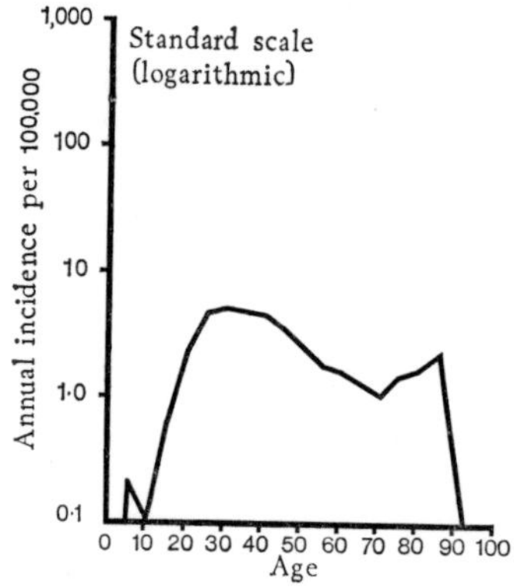

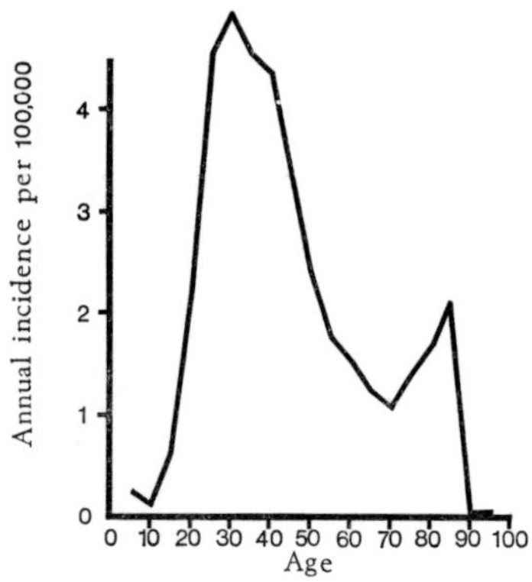

INCIDENCE RATES (per 100,000) by Age

Total cases 321 *males* (of which age not stated for 2 *males*)

Age	M	Age	M	Age	M
0–4	0·4	*35–39*	4·7	*70–74*	1·6
5–9	0·0	*40–44*	3·9	*75–79*	1·0
10–14	0·2	*45–49*	2·7	*80–84*	2·8
15–19	1·1	*50–54*	2·0	*85–89*	0·0
20–24	3·5	*55–59*	1·4	*90–94*	0·0
25–29	5·5	*60–64*	1·6	*95+*	0·0
30–34	4·4	*65–69*	0·7	*All ages*	2·3

SEX AND AGE DISTRIBUTION

	Male
Mean age (*years*)	37·6
95% between ages	15 & 72
Children under 15 (%)	2·2
Median age (*years*)	36·2
Proportion by sex (%)	100
Proportion of all cancers by sex (%)	0·7
Trend over 10 years	(–)

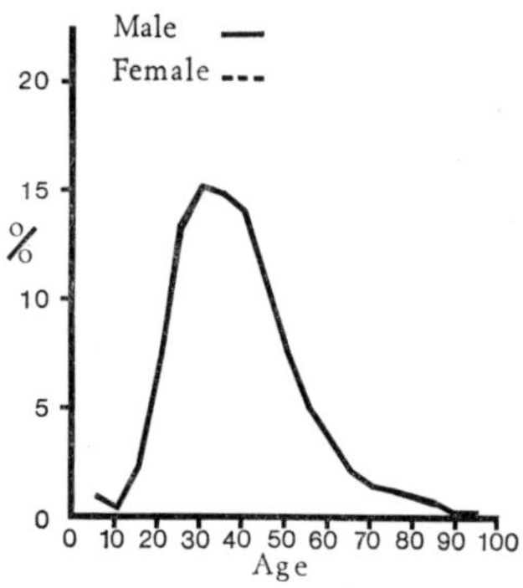

5-YEAR SURVIVAL RATES BY AGE

Crude —— *Corrected* ----

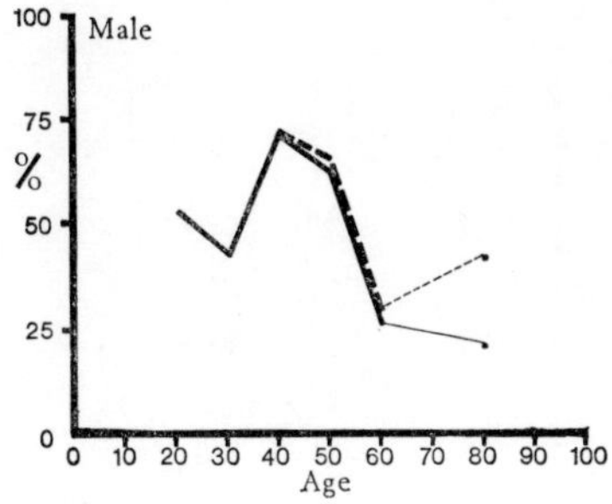

ALL CASES

Total 178
Male 178

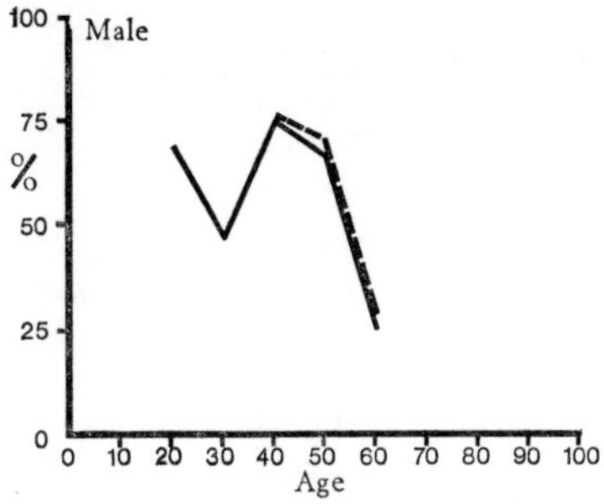

RADICAL TREATMENT

(87·6% of total)
87·6% *male*

INDICES OF SURVIVAL

	All cases *Male*	Radical Treatment *Male*
FIVE YEAR SURVIVAL RATE (%)		
Crude	51·1	57·1
Corrected	*53·1*	*59·0*
Total cases†	178	156
TEN YEAR SURVIVAL RATE (%)		
Crude	52·9	59·8
Corrected	*60·3*	*66·7*
Total cases†	140	122
† Number of cases on which survival rate is based		
SURVIVAL TIME (*months*)		
First quartile (75% S.R.)	10·4	12·6
Median (50% S.R.)	**>60**	**>60**
Third quartile (25% S.R.)	>60	>60

ANNUAL SURVIVAL RATES

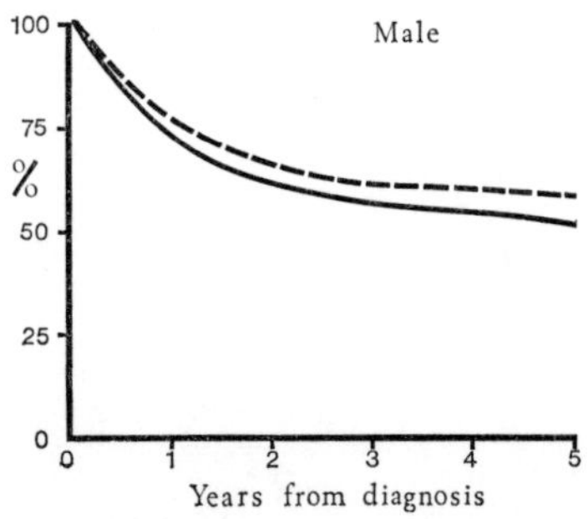

All cases ————

Radical treatment ----

PENIS ICD (8th) **187.0**

INCIDENCE RATE (per 100,000)

Male ——

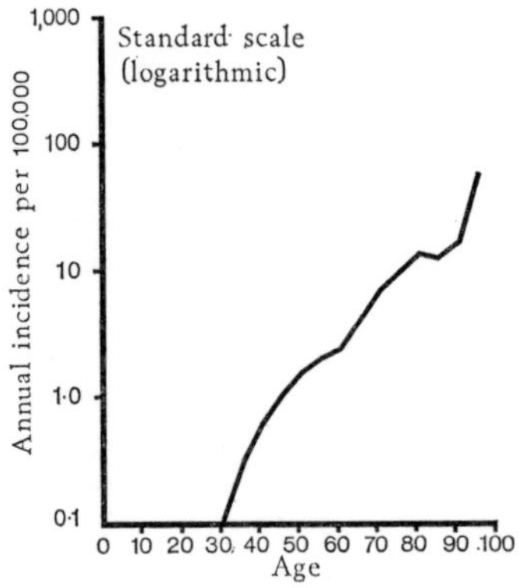

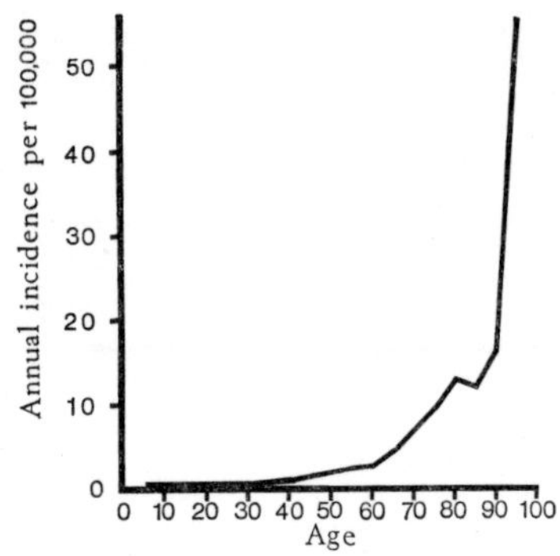

INCIDENCE RATES (per 100,000) by Age

Total cases 174 *males* (of which age not stated for 0 *males*)

Age	M	Age	M	Age	M
0–4	0·0	*35–39*	0·5	*70–74*	7·3
5–9	0·0	*40–44*	0·8	*75–79*	12·0
10–14	0·0	*45–49*	1·3	*80–84*	13·1
15–19	0·0	*50–54*	1·8	*85–89*	8·0
20–24	0·0	*55–59*	2·1	*90–95*	61·5
25–29	0·0	*60–64*	2·5	*95+*	0·0
30–34	0·2	*65–69*	6·0	*All ages*	1·2

SEX AND AGE DISTRIBUTION

	Male
Mean age (*years*)	64·8
95% between ages	37 & 89
Children under 15 (%)	0·0
Median age (*years*)	66·5
Proportion by sex (%)	100
Proportion of all cancers by sex (%)	0·4
Trend over 10 years	(+)

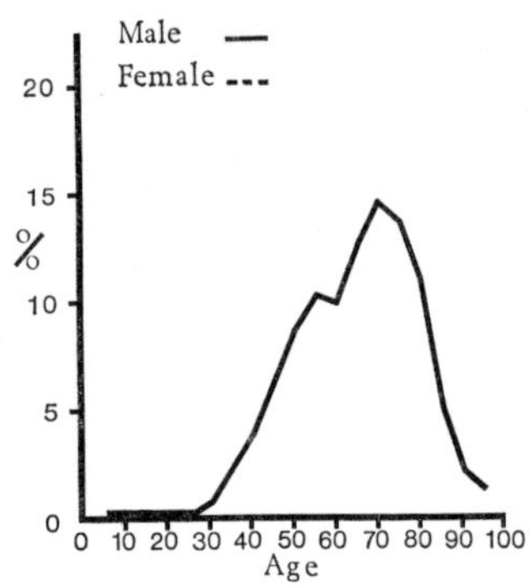

5-YEAR SURVIVAL RATES BY AGE

Crude —— *Corrected* ----

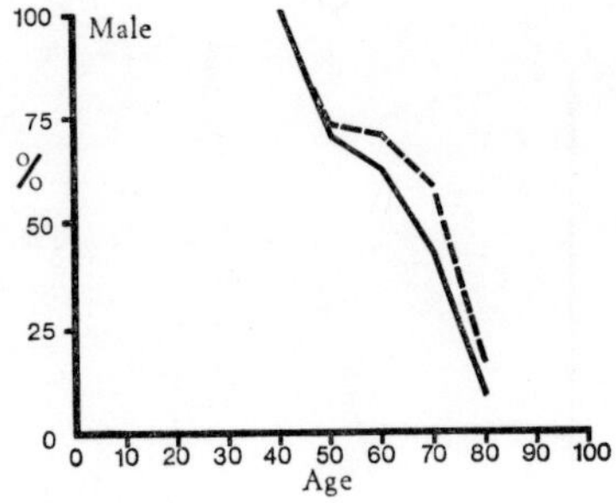

ALL CASES

Total	79
Male	79

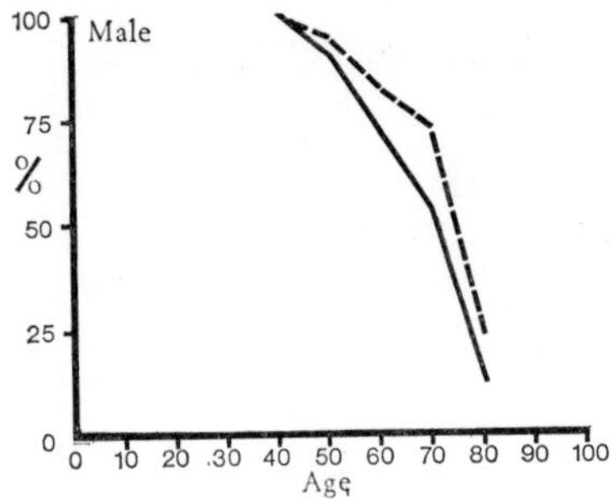

RADICAL TREATMENT

(79·7% of total)
79·7% *male*

INDICES OF SURVIVAL

	All cases *Male*	Radical Treatment *Male*
FIVE YEAR SURVIVAL RATE (%)		
Crude	48·1	58·7
Corrected	*64·5*	*78·5*
Total cases†	79	63
TEN YEAR SURVIVAL RATE (%)		
Crude	37·4	40·9
Corrected	*68·7*	*72·5*
Total cases†	107	93
SURVIVAL TIME (*months*)		
First quartile (75% S.R.)	9·3	25·5
Median (50% S.R.)	**57·5**	**>60**
Third quartile (25% S.R.)	>60	>60

† Number of cases on which survival rate is based

ANNUAL SURVIVAL RATES

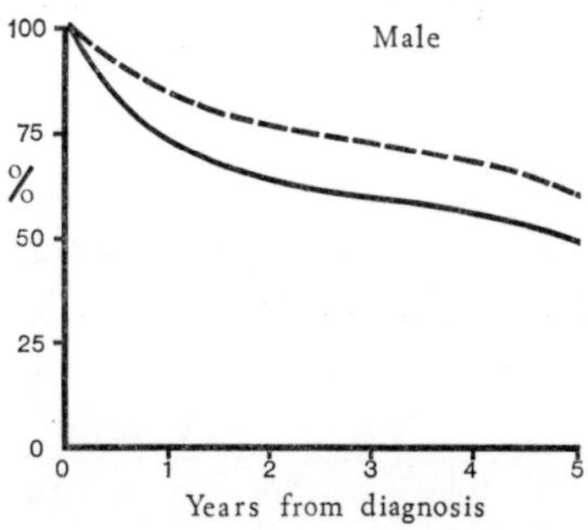

All cases ——

Radical treatment ----

SCROTUM ICD (8th) **172.5, 173.5**

INCIDENCE RATE (per 100,000)

Male ——

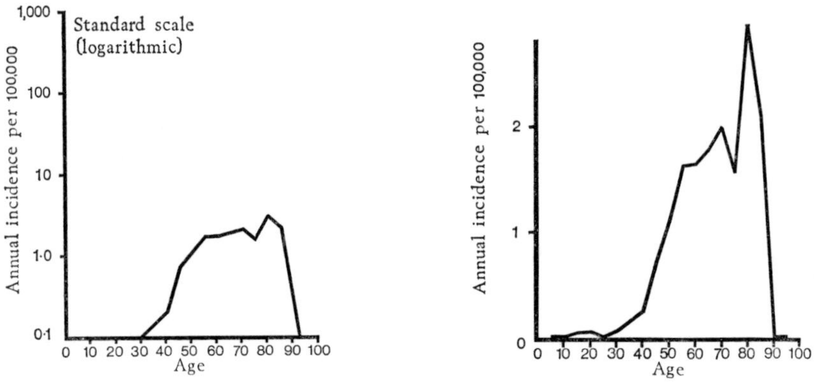

INCIDENCE RATES (per 100,000) by Age

Total cases 77 *males* (of which age not stated for 0 *males*)

Age	M	Age	M	Age	M
0–4	0·0	*35–39*	0·2	*70–74*	0·6
5–9	0·0	*40–44*	0·3	*75–79*	3·0
10–14	0·0	*45–49*	1·1	*80–84*	2·8
15–19	0·1	*50–54*	1·1	*85–89*	0·0
20–24	0·0	*55–59*	2·1	*90–94*	0·0
25–29	0·0	*60–64*	0·9	*95+*	0·0
30–34	0·1	*65–69*	2·9	*All ages*	0·5

SEX AND AGE DISTRIBUTION

	Male
Mean age (*years*)	58·4
95% between ages	35 & 82
Children under 15 (%)	0·0
Median age (*years*)	57·6
Proportion by sex (%)	100
Proportion of all cancers by sex (%)	0·2
Trend over 10 years	(–)

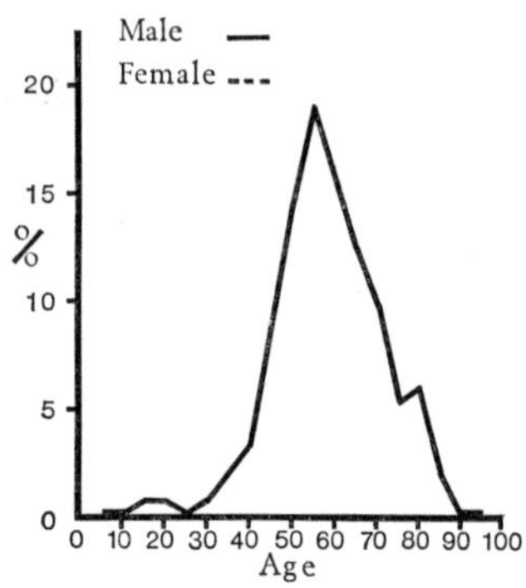

NOTES

The incidence of epitheliomatous tumours of the scrotum represented here is approximately four times greater than it is in the rest of Britain. The Region from which these figures come includes a large part of the light engineering manufactories of the country, and men in such work who also come into close contact with mineral oils in the groin area show an increased incidence of scrotal epitheliomata.

5-YEAR SURVIVAL RATES BY AGE

Crude —— *Corrected* - - - -

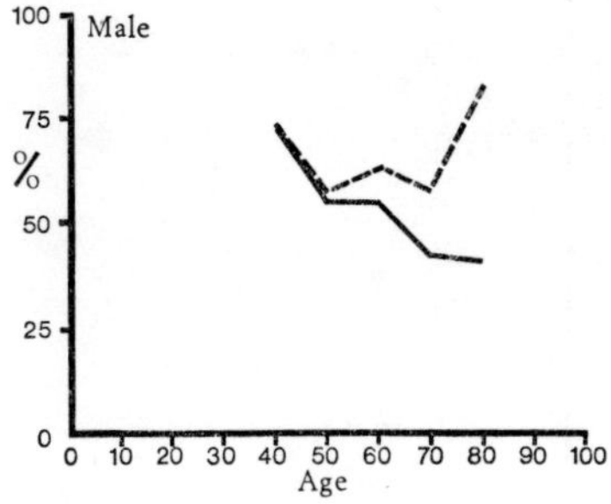

ALL CASES

Total	60
Male	60

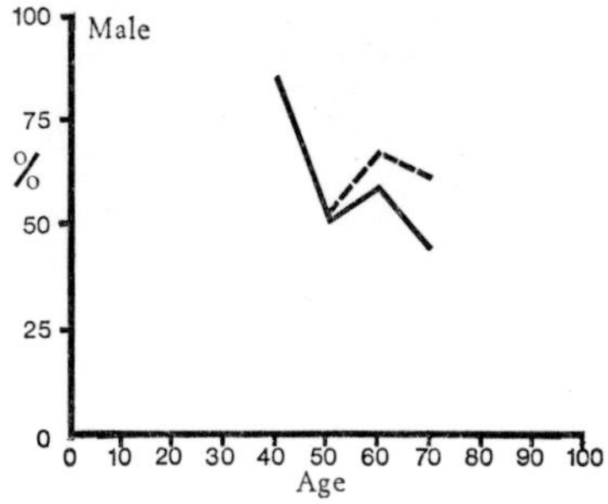

RADICAL TREATMENT

(88·3% of total)
88·3% *male*

INDICES OF SURVIVAL

	All cases *Male*	Radical Treatment *Male*
FIVE YEAR SURVIVAL RATE (%)		
Crude	50·0	54·7
Corrected	*61·8*	*67·0*
Total cases†	60	53
TEN YEAR SURVIVAL RATE (%)		
Crude	31·3	30·0
Corrected	*49·0*	*45·9*
Total cases†	32	30
SURVIVAL TIME (*months*)		
First quartile (75% S.R.)	11·9	21·0
Median (50% S.R.)	**>60**	**>60**
Third quartile (25% S.R.)	>60	>60

† Number of cases on which survival rate is based

ANNUAL SURVIVAL RATES

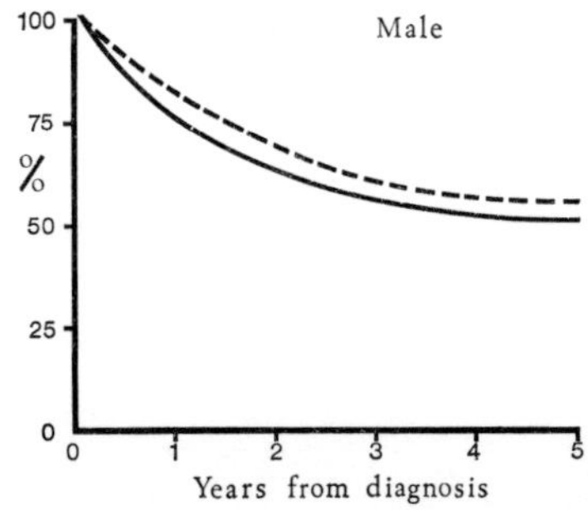

All cases ————

Radical treatment - - - -

BLADDER ICD (8th) **188**

INCIDENCE RATE (per 100,000)

Male ——— *Female* - - - -

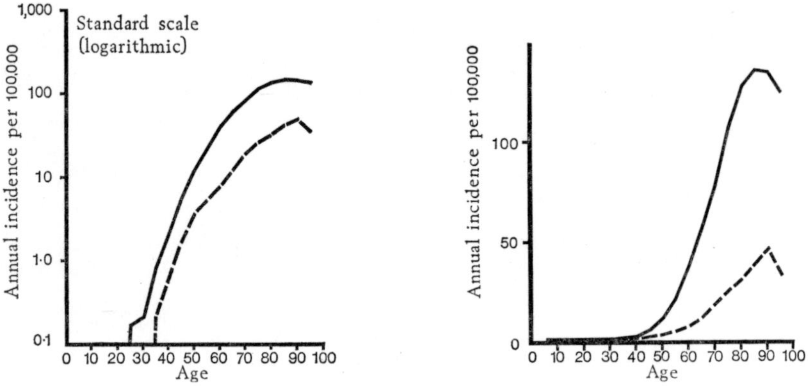

INCIDENCE RATES (per 100,000) by Age

Total cases 1870 *males*; 611 *females* (of which age not stated for 2 *males* and 0 *females*)

Age	M	F	Age	M	F	Age	M	F
0–4	0·0	0·0	*35–39*	1·4	0·4	*70–74*	95·5	23·1
5–9	0·0	0·0	*40–44*	2·6	0·7	*75–79*	122·6	27·9
10–14	0·1	0·0	*45–49*	7·7	2·6	*80–84*	134·9	34·8
15–19	0·1	0·0	*50–54*	15·2	4·2	*85–89*	135·9	48·6
20–24	0·0	0·0	*55–59*	27·7	6·0	*90–94*	123·0	32·8
25–29	0·3	0·0	*60–64*	50·3	8·8	*95+*	135·5	32·2
30–34	0·1	0·0	*65–69*	65·4	14·5	*All ages*	13·3	4·2

SEX AND AGE DISTRIBUTION

	Male	*Female*
Mean age (*years*)	66·6	69·6
95% between ages	45 & 86	46 & 89
Children under 15 (%)	0·1	0·0
Median age (*years*)	66·9	70·9
Proportion by sex (%)	75·4	24·6
Proportion of all cancers by sex (%)	4·3	1·5
Trend over 10 years	(+)	(+)

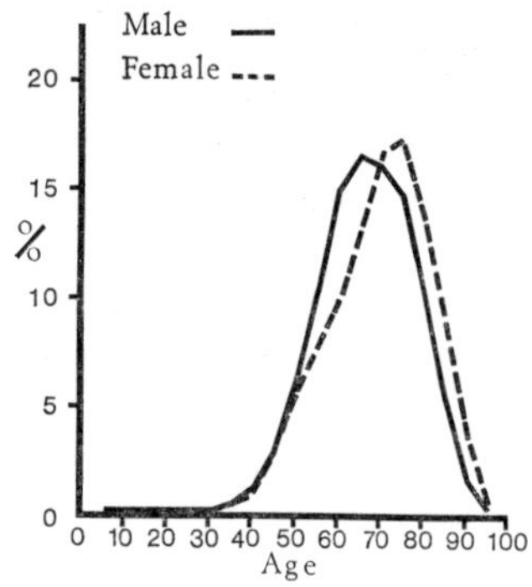

NOTES

Excludes: Papilloma of bladder (see p. 86).

5-YEAR SURVIVAL RATES BY AGE

Crude —— *Corrected* - - - -

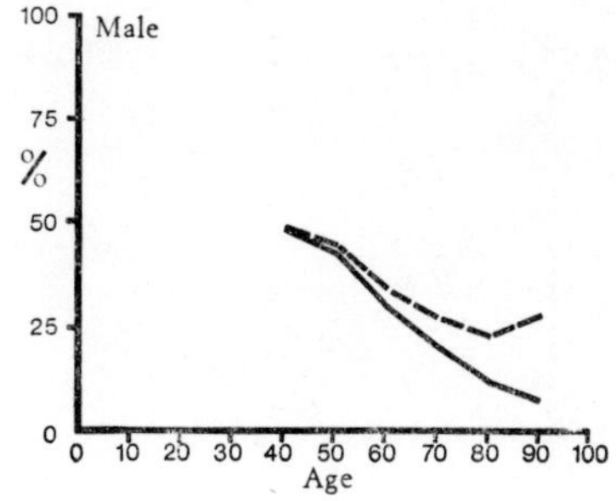

ALL CASES

Total 1326

Male 986
Female 340

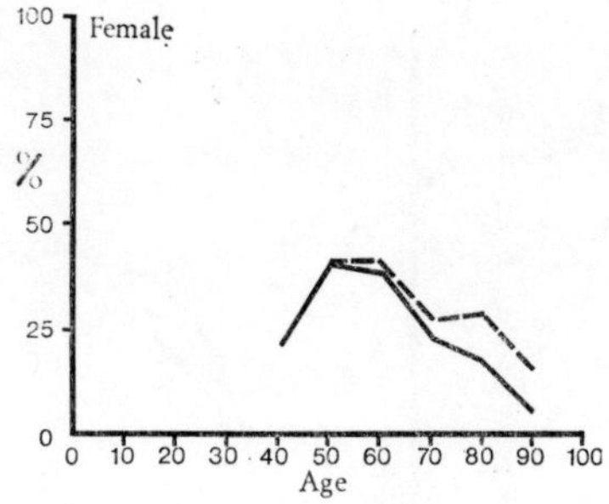

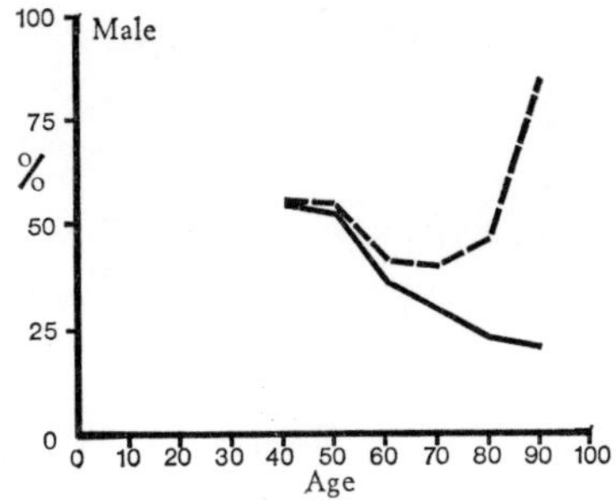

RADICAL TREATMENT

(64·9% of total)
66·9% *male*
58·8% *female*

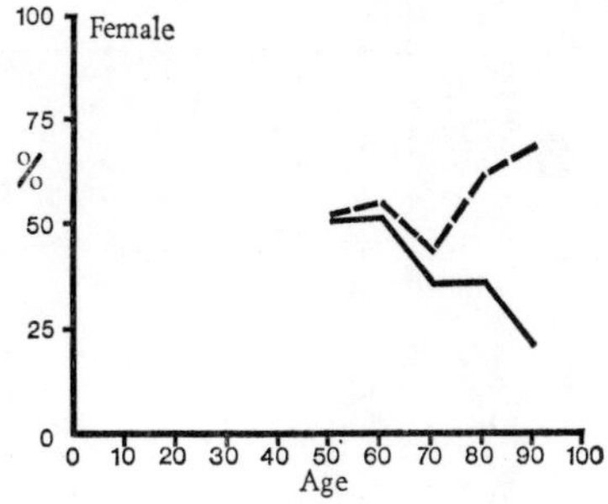

INDICES OF SURVIVAL

	All cases *Male*	All cases *Female*	Radical Treatment *Male*	Radical Treatment *Female*
FIVE YEAR SURVIVAL RATE (%)				
Crude	23·8	25·0	34·7	41·5
Corrected	*32·4*	*32·1*	*44·5*	*50·1*
Total cases†	986	340	660	200
TEN YEAR SURVIVAL RATE (%)				
Crude	17·1	15·2	24·7	25·7
Corrected	*32·1*	*25·1*	*41·2*	*38·8*
Total cases†	794	257	519	148
SURVIVAL TIME (*months*)				
First quartile (75% S.R.)	3·3	2·1	8·8	13·4
Median (50% S.R.)	**12·9**	**13·3**	**28·0**	**43·5**
Third quartile (25% S.R.)	55·2	>60	>60	>60

† Number of cases on which survival rate is based

ANNUAL SURVIVAL RATES

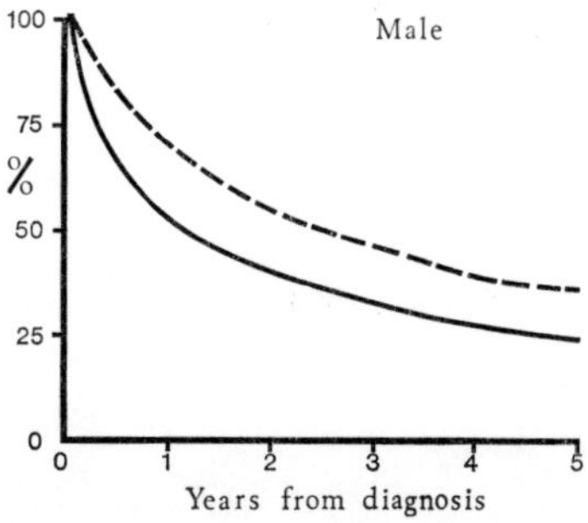

All cases ——

Radical treatment - - - -

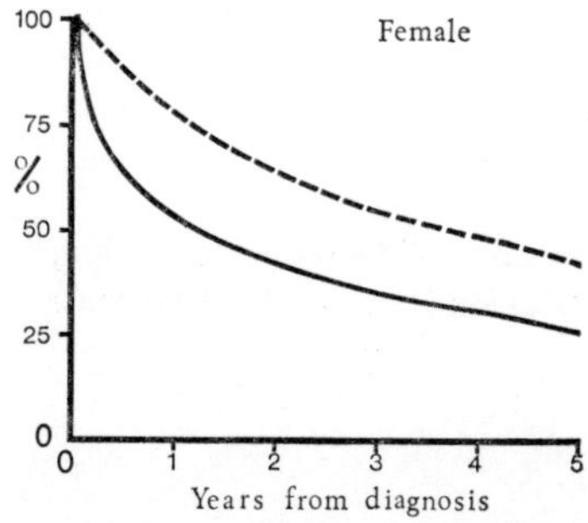

KIDNEY AND OTHER URINARY ORGANS

INCIDENCE RATE (per 100,000)

Male —— *Female* ----

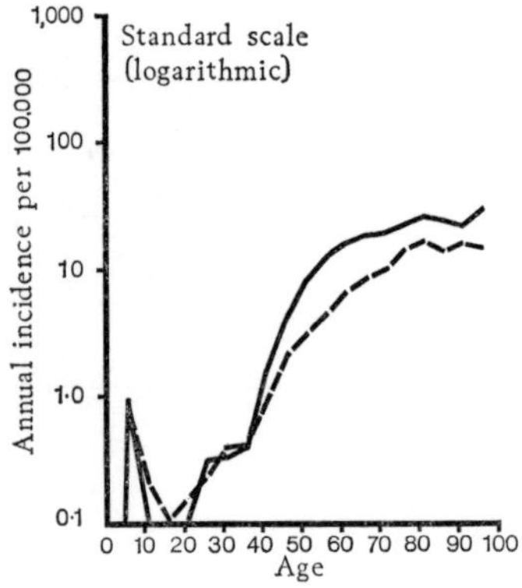

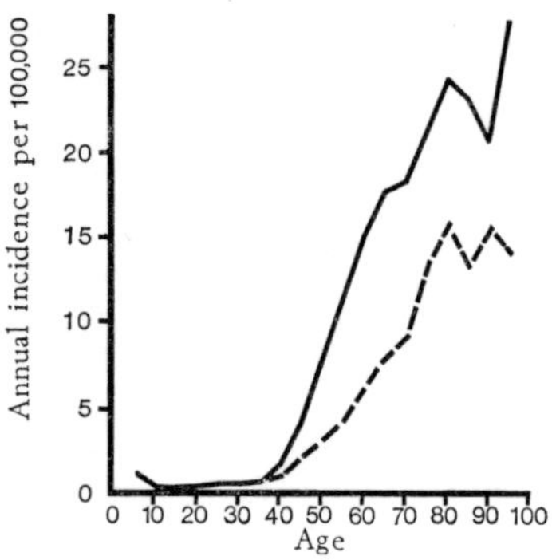

INCIDENCE RATES (per 100,000) by Age

Total cases 657 *males*; 400 *females* (of which age not stated for 0 *males* and 0 *females*)

Age	M	F	Age	M	F	Age	M	F
0–4	1·6	1·3	*35–39*	0·5	0·4	*70–74*	19·3	10·1
5–9	0·2	0·5	*40–44*	2·6	1·2	*75–79*	24·0	17·3
10–14	0·0	0·0	*45–49*	5·1	2·6	*80–84*	24·4	12·4
15–19	0·0	0·2	*50–54*	10·6	3·1	*85–89*	18·6	15·0
20–24	0·3	0·1	*55–59*	13·0	5·0	*90–94*	30·8	16·4
25–29	0·3	0·3	*60–64*	17·5	7·4	*95+*	0·0	0·0
30–34	0·3	0·4	*65–60*	17·5	8·2	*All ages*	4·7	2·8

SEX AND AGE DISTRIBUTION

	Male	*Female*
Mean age (*years*)	59·3	62·1
95% between ages	4 & 84	4 & 87
Children under 15 (%)	3·2	4·8
Median age (*years*)	60·2	65·0
Proportion by sex (%)	62·2	37·8
Proportion of all cancers by sex (%)	1·5	1·0
Trend over 10 years	(+)	(+)

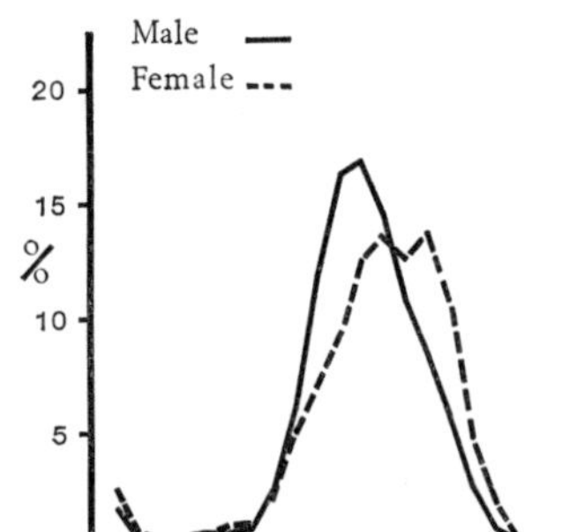

NOTES

Includes: Kidney, ureters, urethra, and other or unspecified urinary organs.

Excludes: Urachus (189·9 in 8th revision, 181·7 in 7th) which is classified with extra-gonadal developmental tumours, (see ENDOCRINE GLANDS, ETC., p. 72).

ICD (7th) **180, 181.7, 181.8** **KIDNEY AND OTHER URINARY ORGANS**

5-YEAR SURVIVAL RATES BY AGE

Crude —— *Corrected* ----

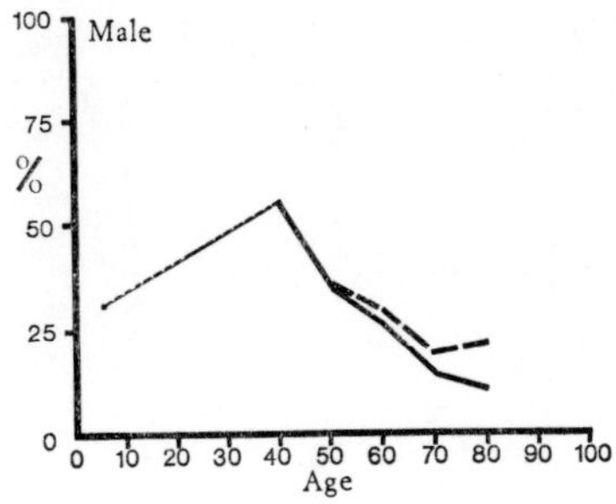

ALL CASES

Total 465
Male 294
Female 171

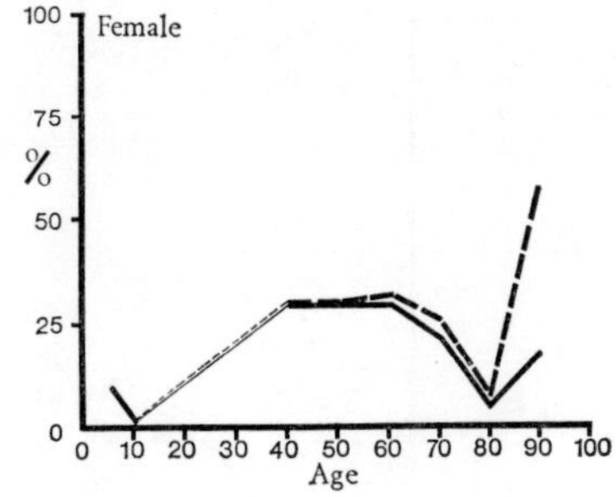

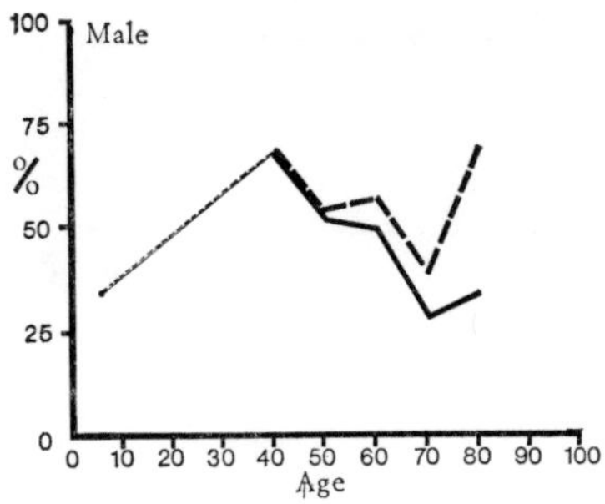

RADICAL TREATMENT

(55·7% of total)
54·1% *male*
58·5% *female*

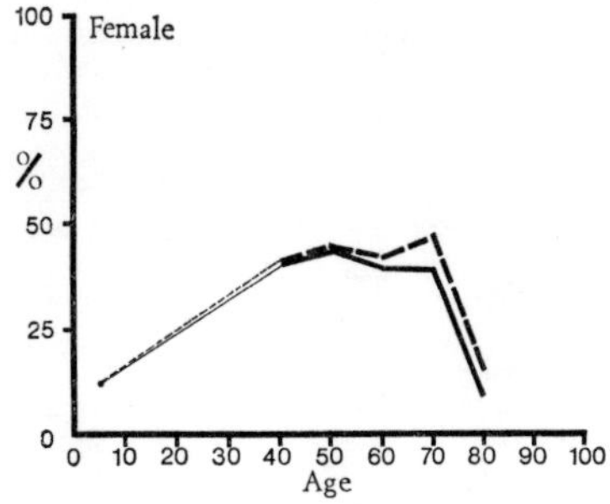

INDICES OF SURVIVAL

	All cases *Male*	All cases *Female*	Radical Treatment *Male*	Radical Treatment *Female*
FIVE YEAR SURVIVAL RATE (%)				
Crude	26·2	19·9	46·5	32·0
Corrected	*31·4*	*23·5*	*53·2*	*36·3*
Total cases†	294	171	159	100
TEN YEAR SURVIVAL RATE (%)				
Crude	17·9	17·4	29·0	30·0
Corrected	*26·9*	*24·2*	*41·1*	*39·1*
Total cases†	190	144	100	80
SURVIVAL TIME (*months*)				
First quartile (75% S.R.)	2·1	2·2	10·8	9·8
Median (50% S.R.)	**8·7**	**10·8**	**47·5**	**26·0**
Third quartile (25% S.R.)	>60	37·8	>60	>60

† Number of cases on which survival rate is based

ANNUAL SURVIVAL RATES

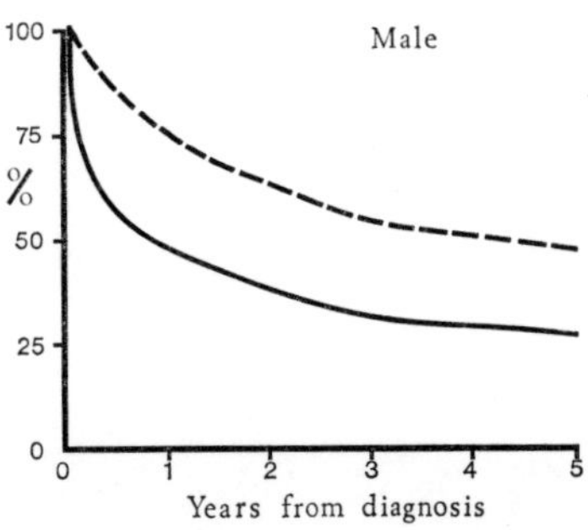

All cases ——
Radical treatment ----

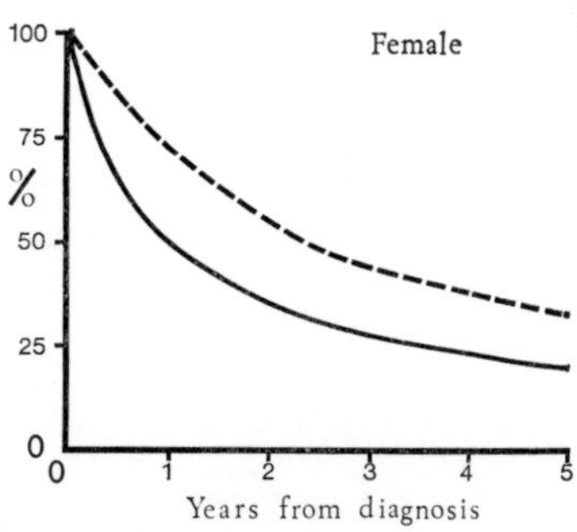

INCIDENCE RATE (per 100,000)

Male —— *Female* ----

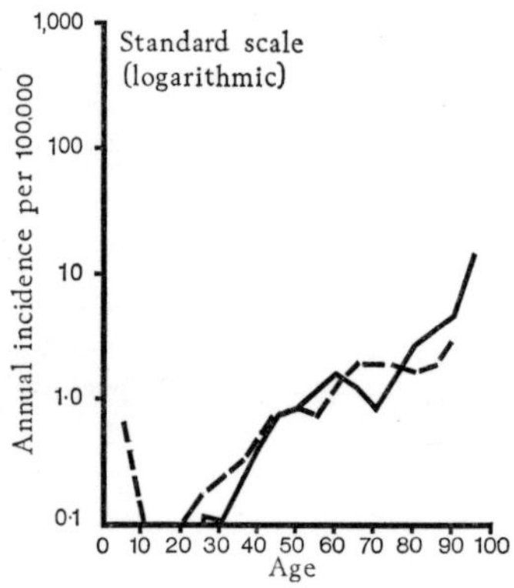

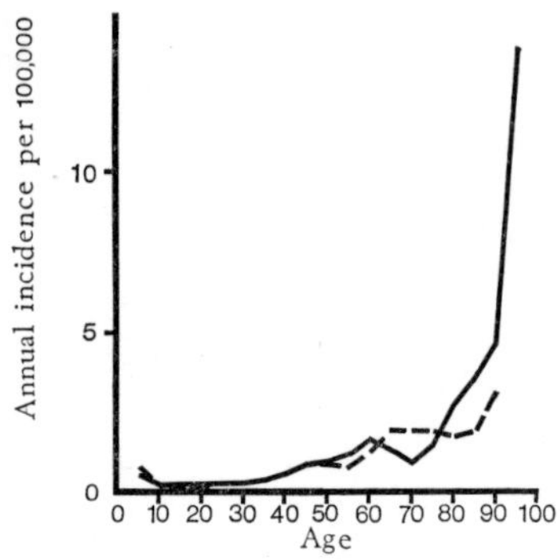

INCIDENCE RATES (per 100,000) by Age

Total cases 76 *males*; 95 *females* (of which age not stated for 1 *male* and 1 *female*)

Age	M	F	Age	M	F	Age	M	F
0–4	0·7	1·0	*35–39*	0·4	0·3	*70–74*	0·9	1·6
5–9	0·0	0·2	*40–44*	0·5	0·7	*75–79*	2·0	2·0
10–14	0·1	0·0	*45–49*	0·9	0·8	*80–84*	3·7	1·0
15–19	0·0	0·0	*50–54*	0·7	0·7	*85–89*	2·7	3·7
20–24	0·1	0·1	*55–59*	1·4	0·7	*90–94*	15·4	0·0
25–29	0·1	0·2	*60–64*	1·6	1·7	*95+*	0·0	0·0
30–34	0·1	0·2	*65–69*	0·7	1·9	*All ages*	0·5	0·7

SEX AND AGE DISTRIBUTION

	Male	*Female*
Mean age (*years*)	51·0	51·7
95% between ages	1 & 86	1 & 86
Children under 15 (%)	12·0	13·8
Median age (*years*)	55·2	58·3
Proportion by sex (%)	44·4	55·6
Proportion of all cancers by sex (%)	0·2	0·2
Trend over 10 years	(−)	(+)

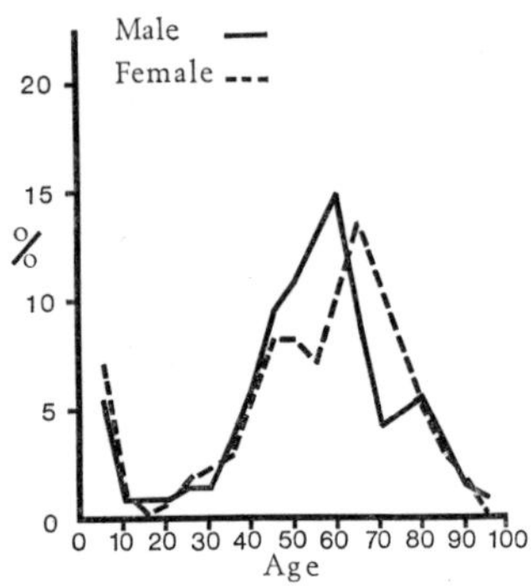

NOTES

Excludes: Eyelid (classified with SKIN); optic nerve (classified with cranial nerves in OTHER NERVOUS TISSUES).

5-YEAR SURVIVAL RATES BY AGE

Crude —— *Corrected* ----

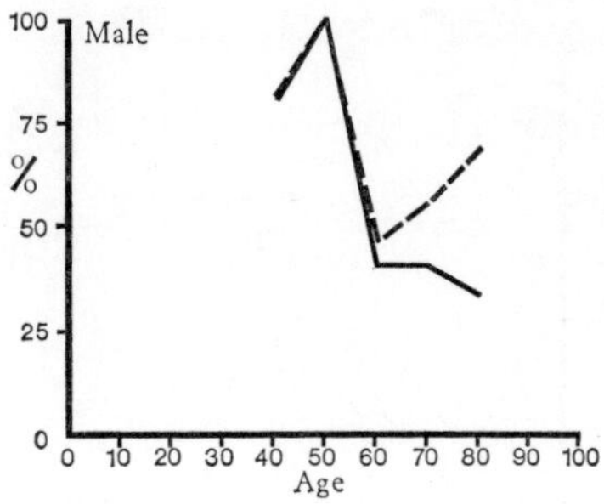

ALL CASES

Total 90
Male 40
Female 50

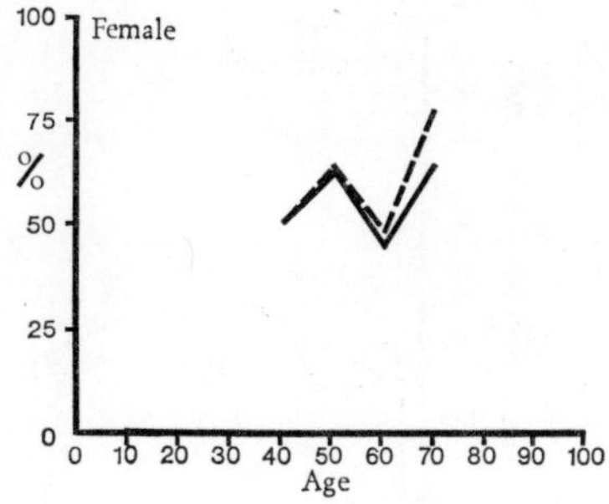

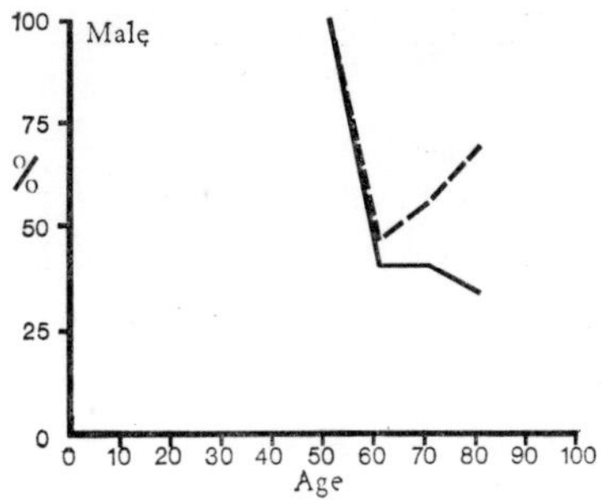

RADICAL TREATMENT

(98·9% of total)
97·5% *male*
100·0% *female*

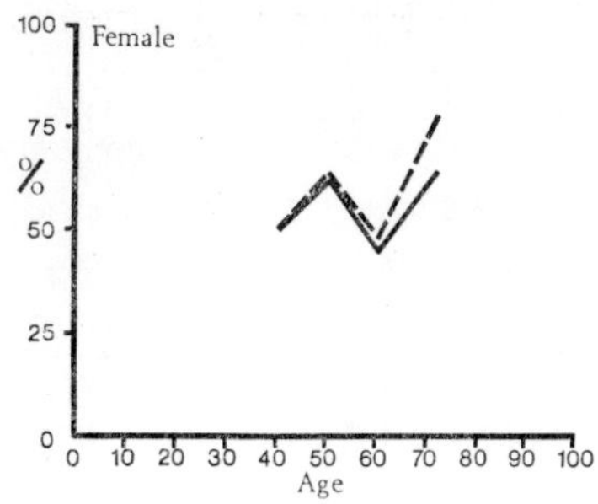

INDICES OF SURVIVAL

	All cases *Male*	All cases *Female*	Radical Treatment *Male*	Radical Treatment *Female*
FIVE YEAR SURVIVAL RATE (%)				
Crude	57·5	58·0	59·0	58·0
Corrected	*70·3*	*64·2*	*72·5*	*64·2*
Total cases†	40	50	39	50
TEN YEAR SURVIVAL RATE (%)				
Crude	25·0	47·1	24·0	50·0
Corrected	*33·9*	*53·1*	*33·4*	*55·9*
Total cases†	28	17	25	16
SURVIVAL TIME (*months*)				
First quartile (75% S.R.)	19·8	29·3	20·5	29·3
Median (50% S.R.)	**>60**	**>60**	**>60**	**>60**
Third quartile (25% S.R.)	>60	>60	>60	>60

† Number of cases on which survival rate is based

ANNUAL SURVIVAL RATES

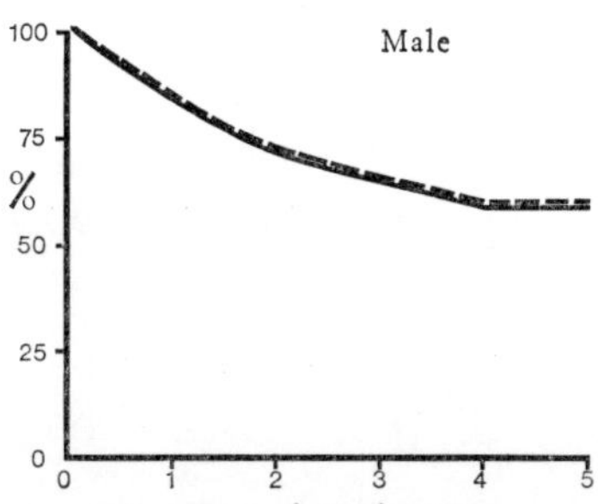

All cases ——
Radical treatment ----

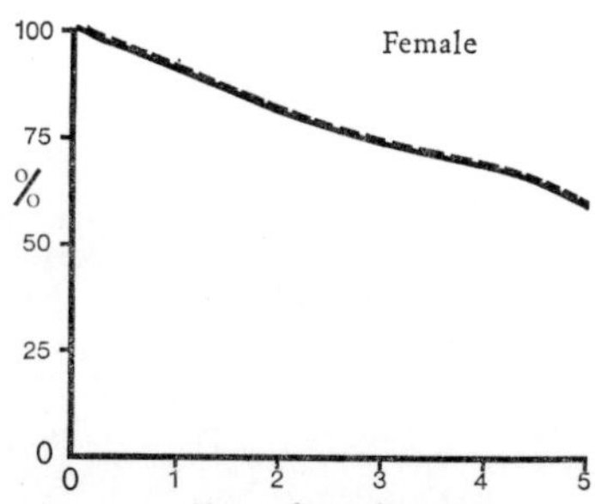

BRAIN

ICD (8th) **191, 192.1, 225.0, .2, .3, .4, .9, 238.1, .3, .4, .5, .9**

INCIDENCE RATE (per 100,000)

Male —— *Female* ----

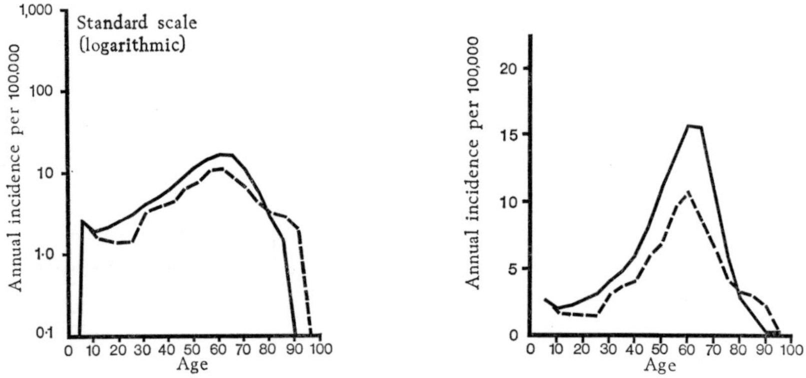

INCIDENCE RATES (per 100,000) by Age

Total cases 854 *males*; 620 *females* (of which age not stated for 1 *male* and 0 *females*)

Age	M	F	Age	M	F	Age	M	F
0–4	2·9	3·2	*35–39*	4·9	2·9	*70–74*	7·6	4·7
5–9	2·0	1·7	*40–44*	6·8	5·0	*75–79*	3·0	3·2
10–14	1·6	1·5	*45–49*	9·1	6·3	*80–84*	1·9	3·0
15–19	2·4	1·3	*50–54*	12·9	7·1	*85–89*	0·0	2·5
20–24	2·3	1·4	*55–59*	14·1	11·9	*90–94*	0·0	0·0
25–29	3·4	1·4	*60–64*	17·5	8·8	*95+*	0·0	0·0
30–34	4·3	4·3	*65–69*	12·5	7·7	*All ages*	6·1	4·3

SEX AND AGE DISTRIBUTION

	Male	*Female*
Mean age (*years*)	46·2	46·7
95% between ages	3 & 72	2 & 77
Children under 15 (%)	8·8	11·2
Median age (*years*)	50·6	51·3
Proportion by sex (%)	57·9	42·1
Proportion of all cancers by sex (%)	2·0	1·5
Trend over 10 years	(+)	(+)

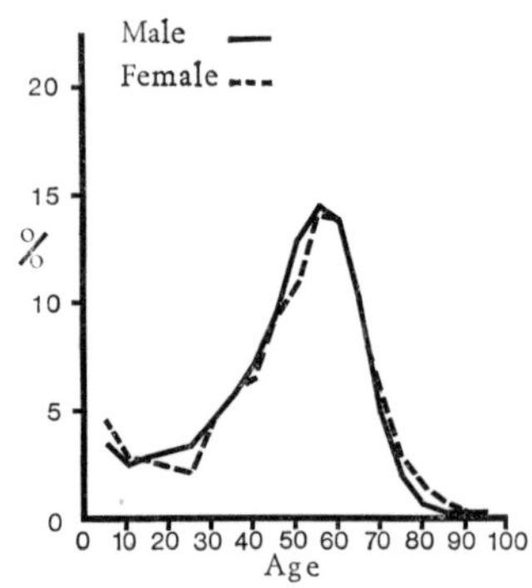

NOTES

Includes: Benign and unspecified tumours of the central nervous system (225 and 238 in 8th revision; 223 and 237 in 7th; but excluding peripheral nervous system).
Cerebral meninges (192·1 in 8th revision; 193·2 in 7th).

Excludes: Cranial nerves, which are classified with OTHER NERVOUS TISSUE.

ICD (7th) **193.0, 193.2**
223 (part)
237 (part)

5-YEAR SURVIVAL RATES BY AGE

Crude —— *Corrected* - - - -

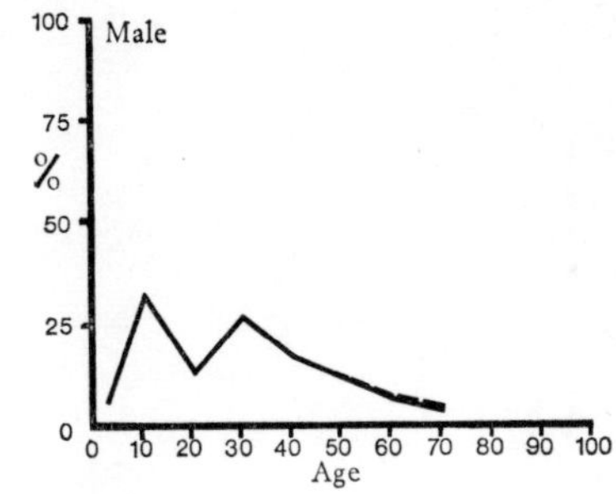

ALL CASES

Total 749
Male 399
Female 350

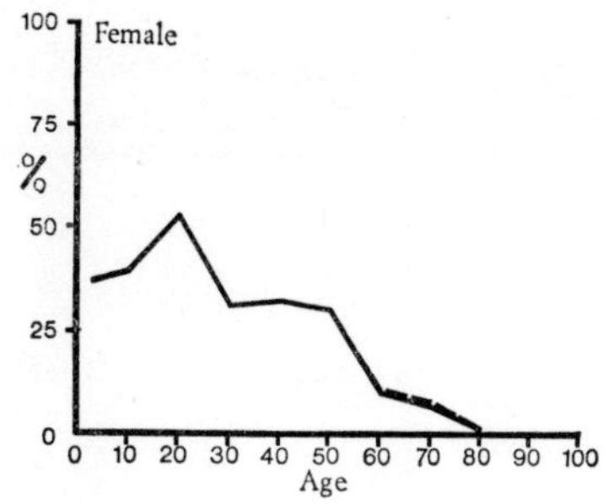

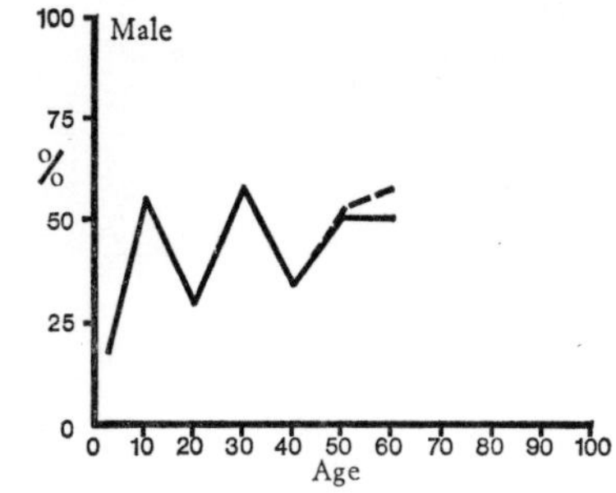

RADICAL TREATMENT

(25·0% of total)
20·3% *male*
30·3% *female*

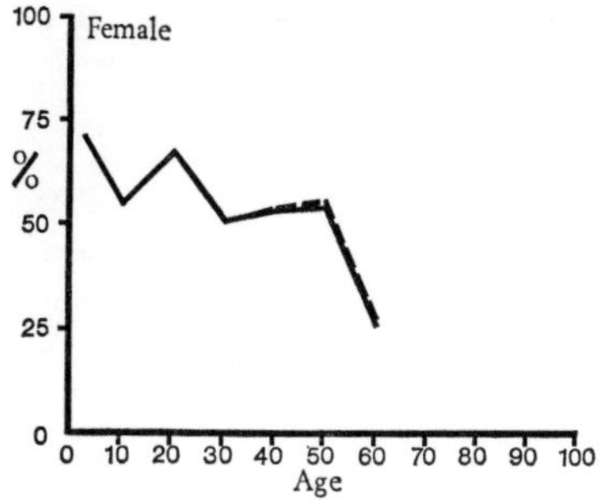

INDICES OF SURVIVAL

	All cases *Male*	All cases *Female*	Radical Treatment *Male*	Radical Treatment *Female*
FIVE YEAR SURVIVAL RATE (%)				
Crude	11·5	24·3	40·7	50·9
Corrected	*12·4*	*25·5*	*42·3*	*52·2*
Total cases†	399	350	81	106
TEN YEAR SURVIVAL RATE (%)				
Crude	13·7	12·9	49·4	50·0
Corrected	*15·7*	*14·2*	*53·4*	*53·0*
Total cases†	328	286	81	62
SURVIVAL TIME (*months*)				
First quartile (75% S.R.)	0·7	0·8	8·0	8·1
Median (50% S.R.)	**2·1**	**3·7**	**36·5**	**>60**
Third quartile (25% S.R.)	11·1	49·4	>60	>60

† Number of cases on which survival rate is based

ANNUAL SURVIVAL RATES

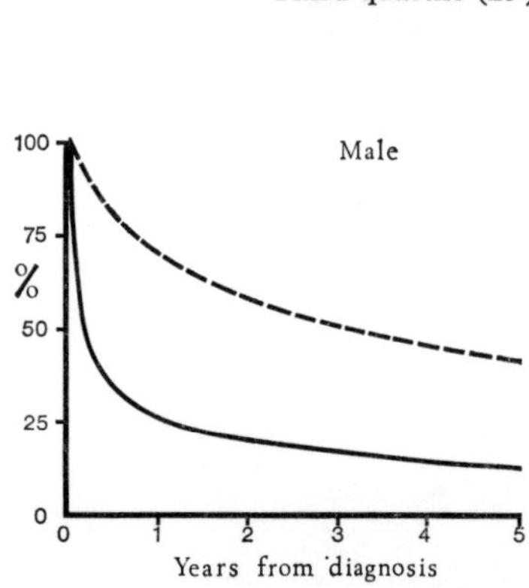

All cases ——
Radical treatment - - - -

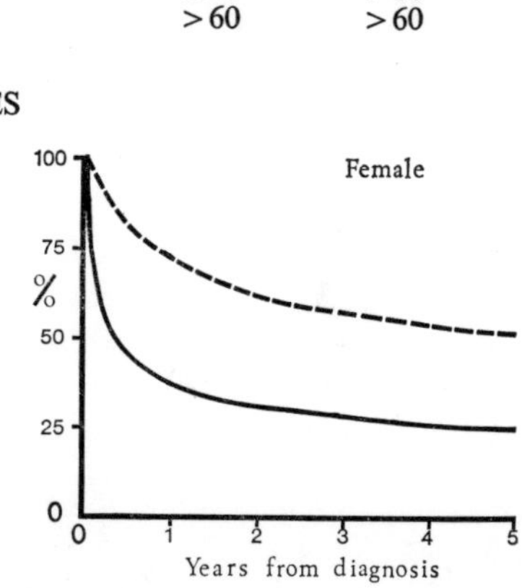

OTHER NERVOUS TISSUE

ICD (8th) **192 (part)**

INCIDENCE RATE (per 100,000)

Male —— *Female* - - - -

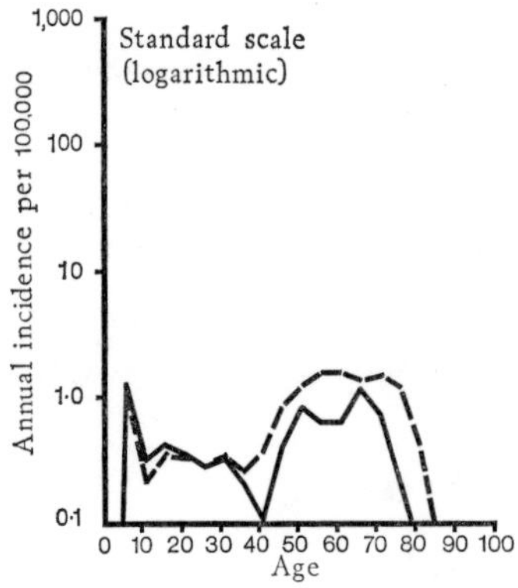

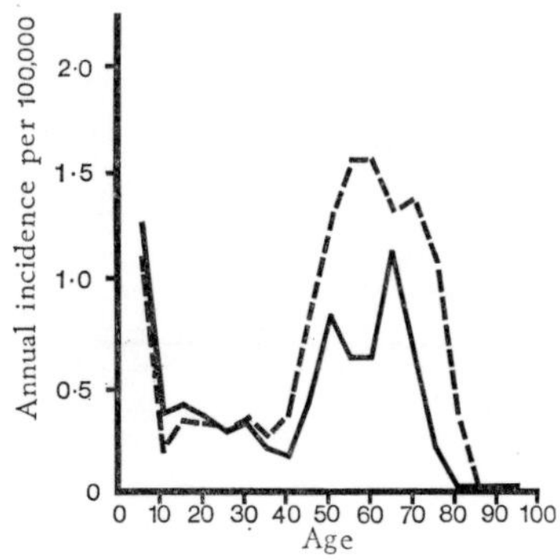

INCIDENCE RATES (per 100,000) by Age

Total cases 78 *males*; 111 *females* (of which age not stated for 0 *males* and 0 *females*)

Age	M	F	Age	M	F	Age	M	F
0–4	2·0	2·0	*35–39*	0·1	0·2	*70–74*	0·3	1·4
5–9	0·4	0·1	*40–44*	0·2	0·5	*75–79*	0·0	0·6
10–14	0·3	0·3	*45–49*	0·6	1·1	*80–84*	0·0	0·0
15–19	0·5	0·4	*50–54*	1·0	1·4	*85–89*	0·0	0·0
20–24	0·2	0·2	*55–59*	0·1	1·7	*90–94*	0·0	0·0
25–29	0·3	0·3	*60–64*	1·3	1·3	*95+*	0·0	0·0
30–34	0·3	0·3	*65–69*	0·9	1·3	*All ages*	0·6	0·8

SEX AND AGE DISTRIBUTION

	Male	*Female*
Mean age (*years*)	29·3	41·2
95% between ages	0 & 69	1 & 74
Children under 15 (%)	41·0	23·4
Median age (*years*)	25·0	49·8
Proportion by sex (%)	41·2	58·8
Proportion of all cancers by sex (%)	0·2	0·3
Trend over 10 years	(−)	(+)

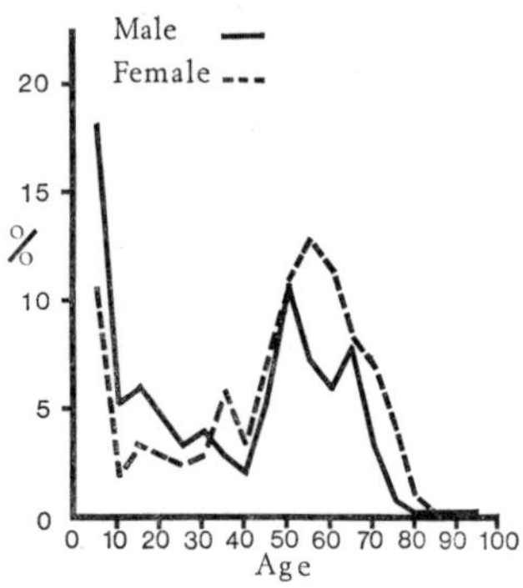

NOTES

Includes: Cranial nerves, including optic nerve.

Excludes: Cerebral meninges (192·1 in 8th revision; 193·2 in 7th), which are classified with BRAIN.

5-YEAR SURVIVAL RATES BY AGE

Crude ——— *Corrected* - - - -

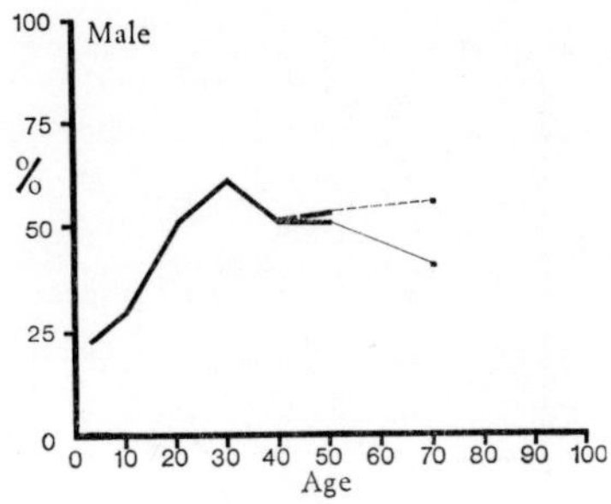

ALL CASES

Total	90
Male	48
Female	42

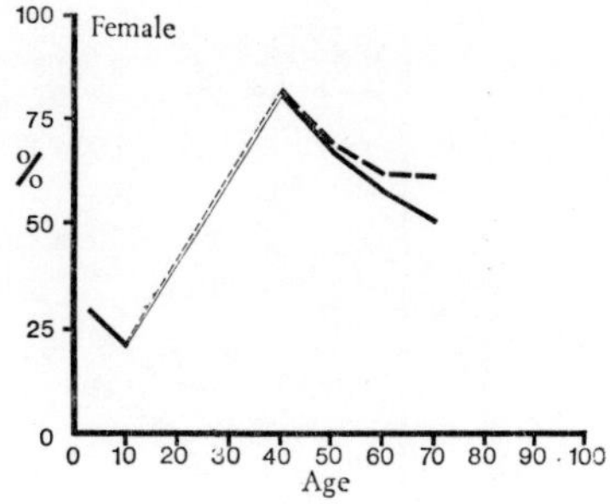

RADICAL TREATMENT

(56·7% of total)
50·0% *male*
64·3% *female*

INDICES OF SURVIVAL

	All cases *Male*	All cases *Female*	Radical Treatment *Male*	Radical Treatment *Female*
FIVE YEAR SURVIVAL RATE (%)				
Crude	35·4	47·6	45·8	66·7
Corrected	*37·6*	*50·0*	*48·8*	*69·8*
Total cases†	48	42	24	27
TEN YEAR SURVIVAL RATE (%)				
Crude	47·6	50·3	58·6	68·1
Corrected	*52·9*	*58·1*	*66·6*	*79·2*
Total cases†	42	94	29	69
SURVIVAL TIME (*months*)				
First quartile (75% S.R.)	2·2	1·9	8·8	9·5
Median (50% S.R.)	**12·5**	**36·0**	**26·5**	**>60**
Third quartile (25% S.R.)	>60	>60	>60	>60

† Number of cases on which survival rate is based

ANNUAL SURVIVAL RATES

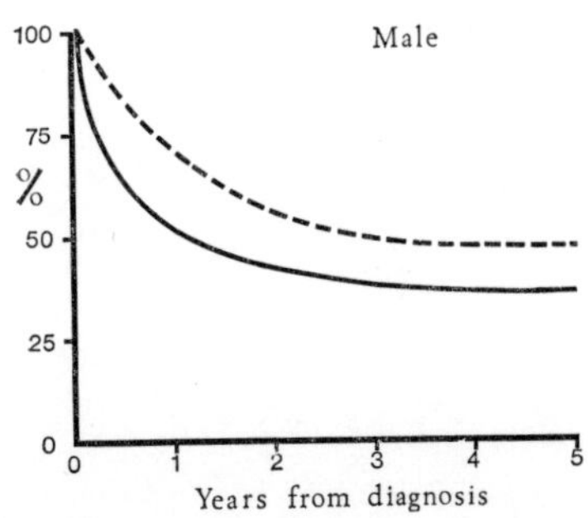

All cases ———
Radical treatment - - - -

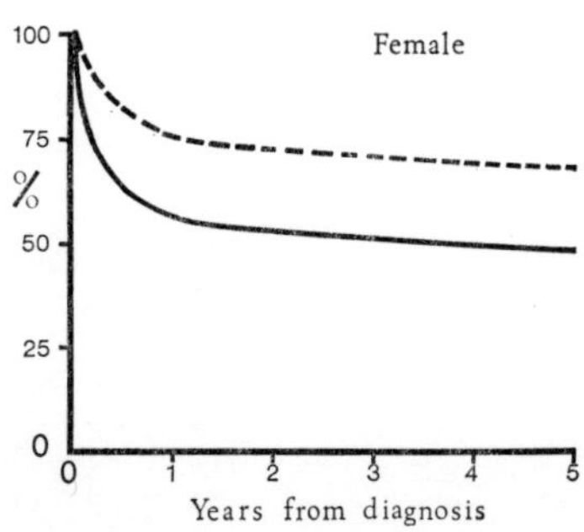

INCIDENCE RATE (per 100,000)

Male —— *Female* - - - -

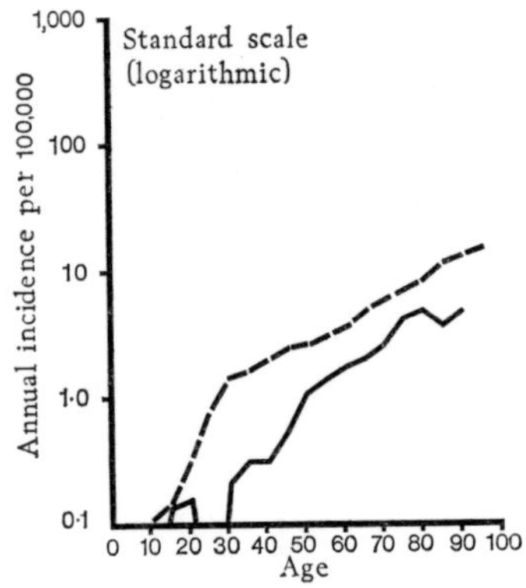

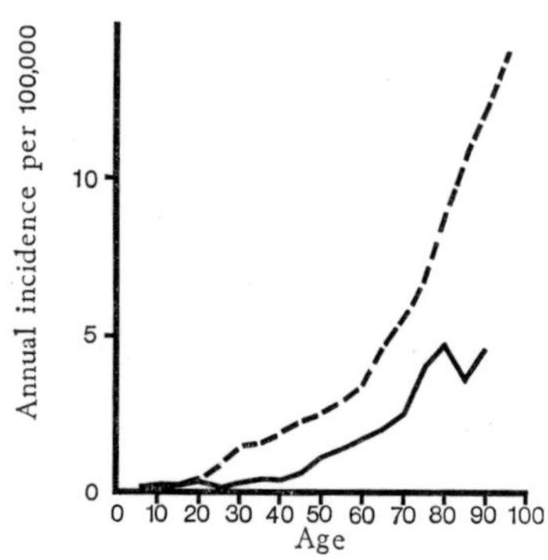

INCIDENCE RATES (per 100,000) by Age

Total cases 88 *males*; 290 *females* (of which age not stated for 0 *males* and 0 *females*)

Age	M	F	Age	M	F	Age	M	F
0–4	0·0	0·0	*35–39*	0·3	1·4	*70–74*	2·8	6·0
5–9	0·0	0·0	*40–44*	0·3	2·2	*75–79*	5·5	7·8
10–14	0·0	0·2	*45–49*	0·7	2·1	*80–84*	2·8	10·4
15–19	0·3	0·1	*50–54*	1·2	2·7	*85–89*	5·3	11·2
20–24	0·0	0·4	*55–59*	1·3	2·8	*90–94*	0·0	16·4
25–29	0·0	1·1	*60–64*	1·9	4·0	*95+*	0·0	0·0
30–34	0·3	1·6	*65–69*	2·0	5·2	*All ages*	0·6	2·0

SEX AND AGE DISTRIBUTION

	Male	*Female*
Mean age (*years*)	59·9	59·1
95% between ages	19 & 85	25 & 88
Children under 15 (%)	0·0	0·7
Median age (*years*)	60·8	61·0
Proportion by sex (%)	23·2	76·8
Proportion of all cancers by sex (%)	0·2	0·7
Trend over 10 years	(+)	+

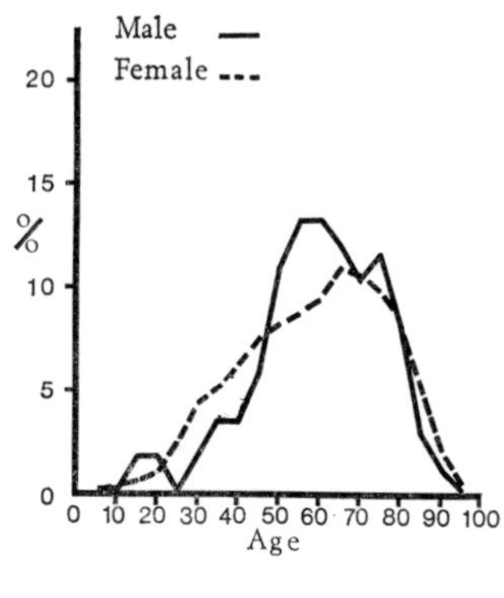

5-YEAR SURVIVAL RATES BY AGE

Crude —— *Corrected* ----

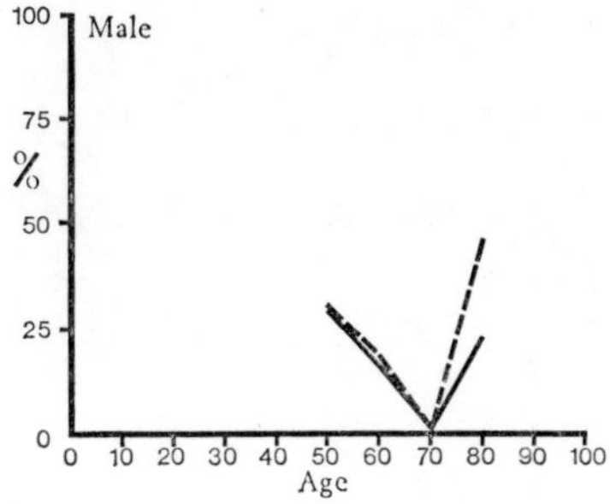

ALL CASES

Total 179
Male 46
Female 133

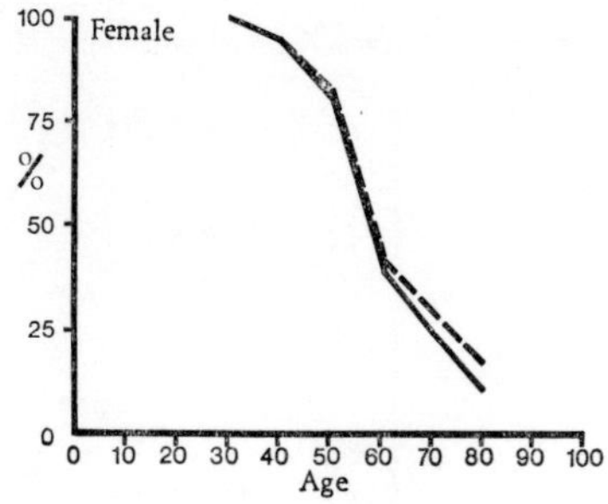

RADICAL TREATMENT

(65·9% of total)
56·5% *male*
69·2% *female*

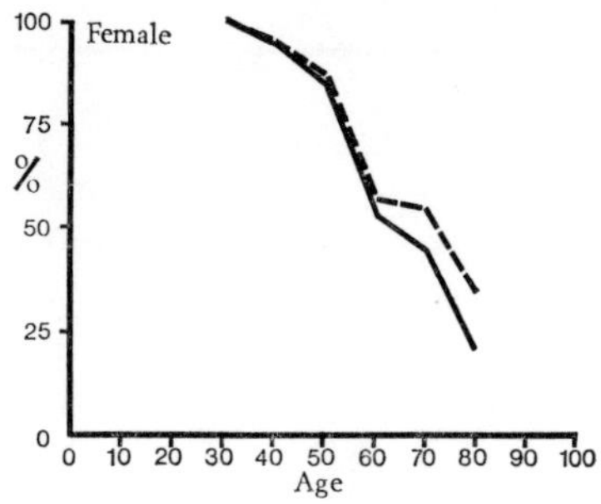

INDICES OF SURVIVAL

	All cases *Male*	All cases *Female*	Radical Treatment *Male*	Radical Treatment *Female*
FIVE YEAR SURVIVAL RATE (%)				
Crude	23·9	48·9	42·3	69·6
Corrected	*30·0*	*56·8*	*50·4*	*75·8*
Total cases†	46	133	26	92
TEN YEAR SURVIVAL RATE (%)				
Crude	20·0	38·5	34·8	60·0
Corrected	*30·4*	*53·1*	*46·5*	*73·5*
Total cases†	40	96	23	60
SURVIVAL TIME (*months*)				
First quartile (75% S.R.)	1·0	2·6	6·1	33·8
Median (50% S.R.)	**7·0**	**47·5**	**36·0**	**>60**
Third quartile (25% S.R.)	40·8	>60	>60	>60

† Number of cases on which survival rate is based

ANNUAL SURVIVAL RATES

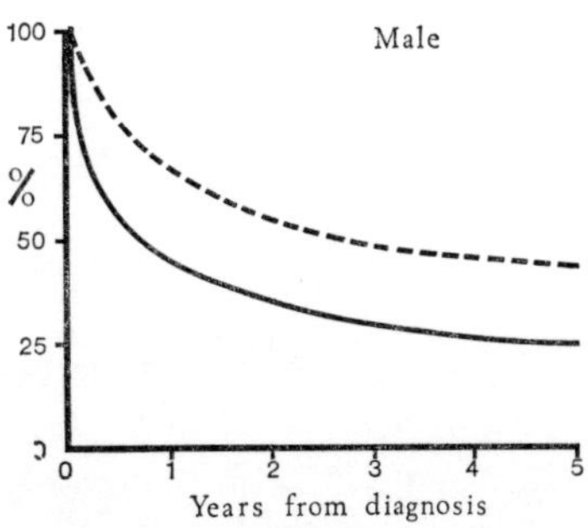

All cases ——
Radical treatment ----

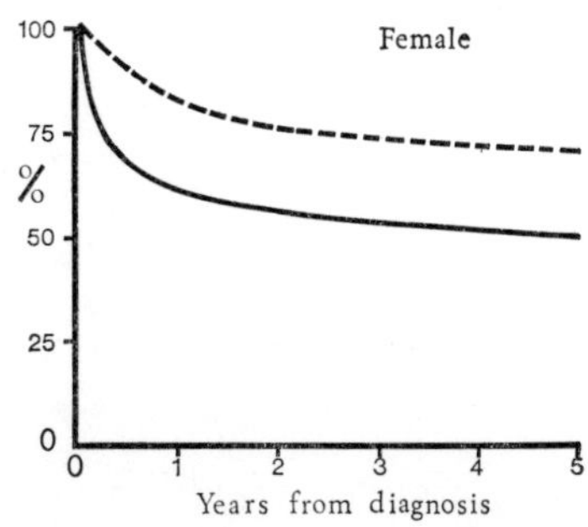

OTHER ENDOCRINE GLANDS

INCIDENCE RATE (per 100,000)

Male ——— *Female* - - - -

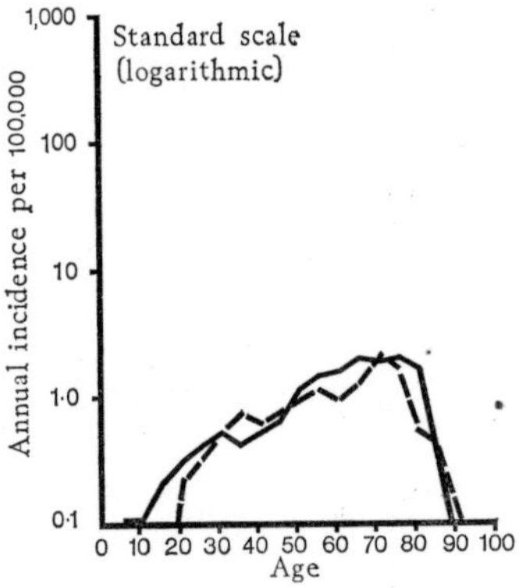

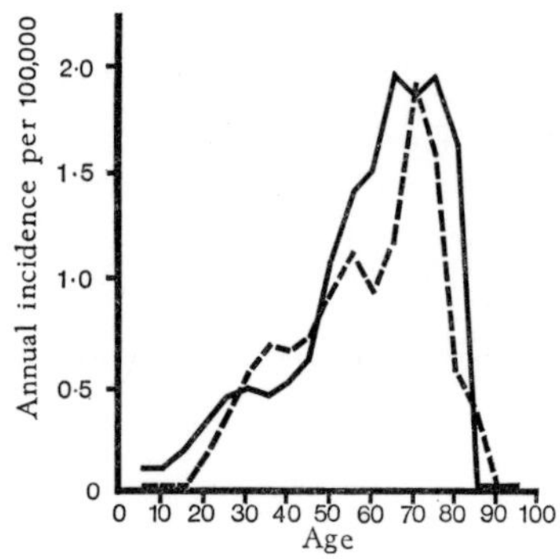

INCIDENCE RATES (per 100,000) by Age

Total cases 92 *males*; 84 *females* (of which age not stated for 1 *male* and 1 *female*)

Age	M	F	Age	M	F	Age	M	F
0–4	0·2	0·0	*35–39*	0·4	0·6	*70–74*	1·6	2·3
5–9	0·0	0·0	*40–44*	0·6	0·7	*75–79*	2·5	0·6
10–14	0·2	0·0	*45–49*	0·6	0·7	*80–84*	0·0	0·5
15–19	0·2	0·0	*50–54*	1·6	1·2	*85–89*	0·0	0·0
20–24	0·4	0·3	*55–59*	1·2	1·0	*90–94*	0·0	0·0
25–29	0·4	0·3	*60–64*	1·9	0·8	*95+*	0·0	0·0
30–34	0·5	0·7	*65–69*	2·0	1·6	*All ages*	0·7	0·6

SEX AND AGE DISTRIBUTION

	Male	*Female*
Mean age (*years*)	50·4	53·2
95% between ages	11 & 78	23 & 77
Children under 15 (%)	4·4	0·0
Median age (*years*)	53·5	53·9
Proportion by sex (%)	52·2	47·8
Proportion of all cancers by sex (%)	0·2	0·2
Trend over 10 years	(–)	(–)

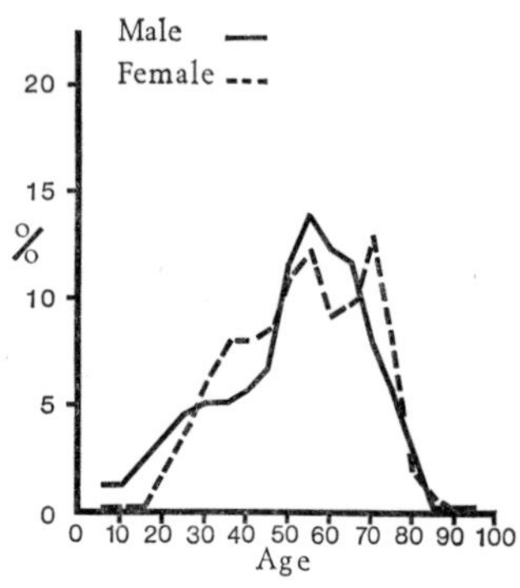

NOTES

Includes: Spleen (other than reticuloses).

Excludes: Pancreas, ovary, testis.
Sympatheticoblastoma of adrenal, which is classified with OTHER NERVOUS TISSUE.
Craniopharyngioma, which is classified with extra-gonadal developmental tumours (see ENDOCRINE GLANDS, ETC., p. 72).

5-YEAR SURVIVAL RATES BY AGE

Crude ——— *Corrected* - - - -

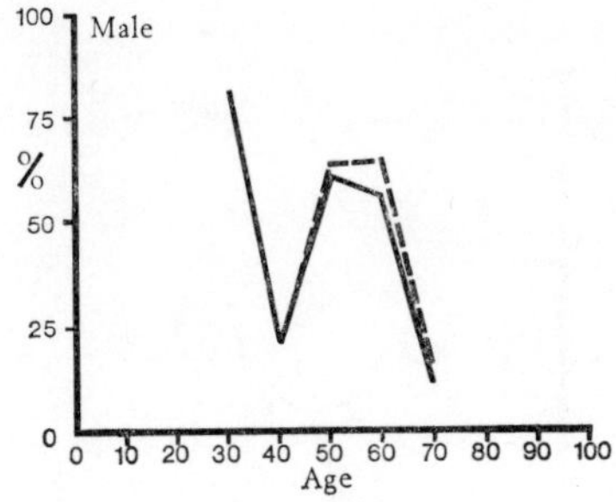

ALL CASES

Total	87
Male	53
Female	34

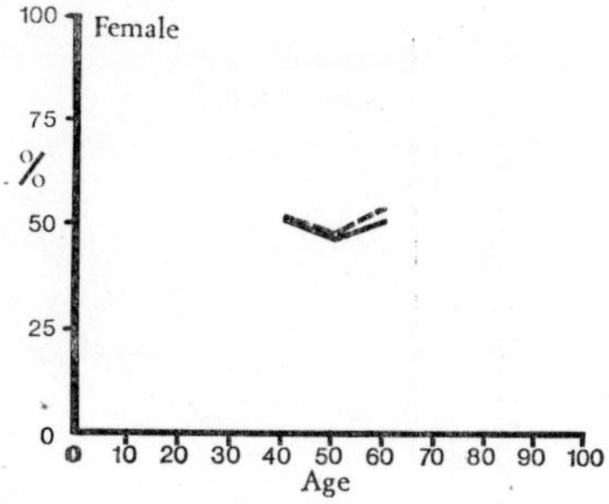

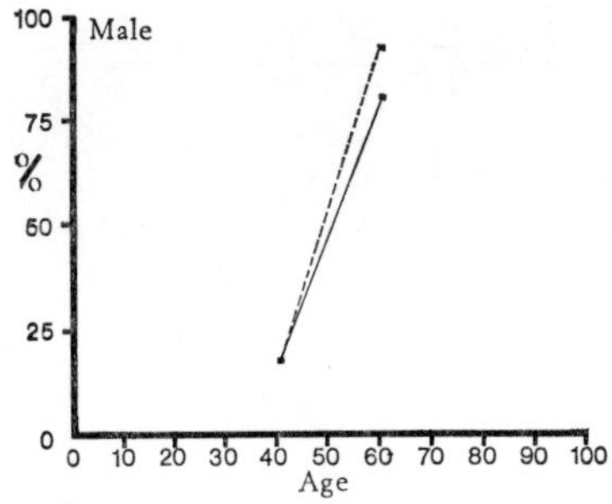

RADICAL TREATMENT

(52·9% of total)
50·9% *male*
55·9% *female*

INDICES OF SURVIVAL

	All cases *Male*	All cases *Female*	Radical Treatment *Male*	Radical Treatment *Female*
FIVE YEAR SURVIVAL RATE (%)				
Crude	39·6	47·1	59·3	73·7
Corrected	*44·5*	*49·2*	*63·9*	*76·3*
Total cases†	53	34	27	19
TEN YEAR SURVIVAL RATE (%)				
Crude	39·5	35·1	60·9	55·6
Corrected	*44·8*	*39·2*	*68·8*	*60·8*
Total cases†	43	37	23	18
SURVIVAL TIME (*months*)				
First quartile (75% S.R.)	0·8	0·8	19·5	28·5
Median (50% S.R.)	**17·8**	**54·0**	**>60**	**>60**
Third quartile (25% S.R.)	>60	>60	>60	>60

† Number of cases on which survival rate is based

ANNUAL SURVIVAL RATES

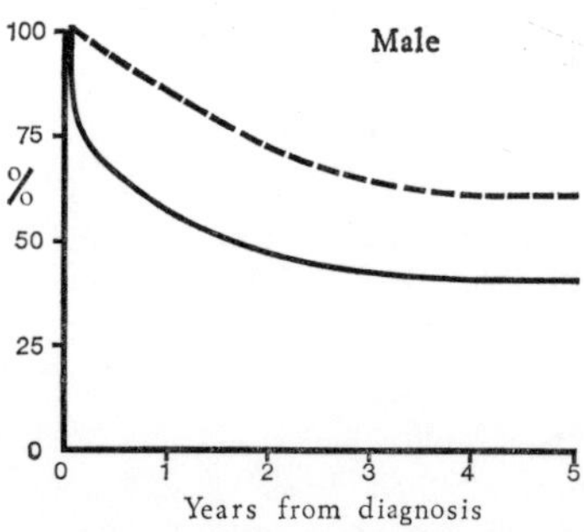

All cases ———
Radical treatment - - - -

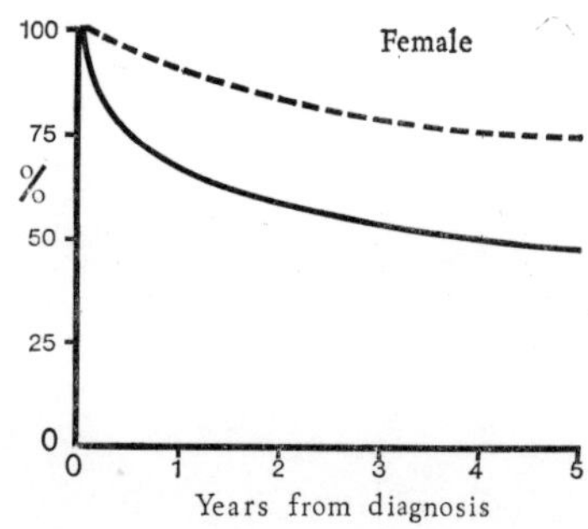

RETICULOSARCOMA ICD (8th) **200.0**

INCIDENCE RATE (per 100,000)

Male —— *Female* - - - -

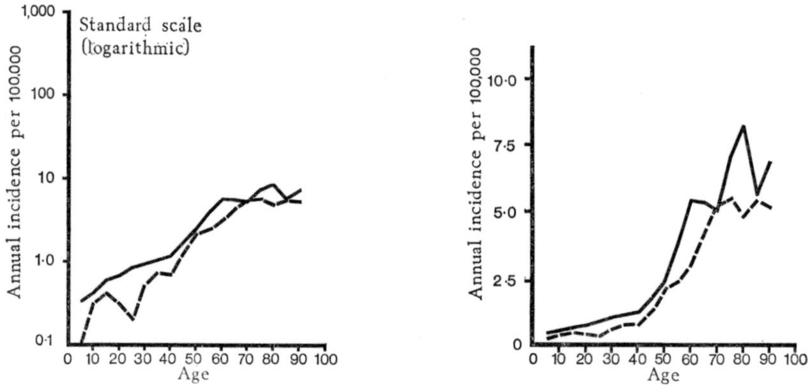

INCIDENCE RATES (per 100,000) by Age

Total cases 258 *males*; 213 *females* (of which age not stated for 0 *males* and 1 *female*)

Age	M	F	Age	M	F	Age	M	F
0–4	0·3	0·1	*35–39*	1·1	0·6	*70–74*	5·1	6·0
5–9	0·4	0·2	*40–44*	1·1	0·8	*75–79*	10·0	4·6
10–14	0·5	0·3	*45–49*	2·2	1·5	*80–84*	4·7	5·0
15–19	0·6	0·4	*50–54*	2·4	2·5	*85–89*	8·0	6·2
20–24	0·6	0·2	*55–59*	5·2	2·1	*90–94*	0·0	0·0
25–29	1·0	0·2	*60–64*	5·5	4·0	*95+*	0·0	0·0
30–34	0·9	0·8	*65–69*	4·9	4·5	*All ages*	1·8	1·5

SEX AND AGE DISTRIBUTION

	Male	*Female*
Mean age (*years*)	53·0	58·7
95% between ages	8 & 82	13 & 85
Children under 15 (%)	5·5	3·3
Median age (*years*)	56·8	62·0
Proportion by sex (%)	54·8	45·2
Proportion of all cancers by sex (%)	0·6	0·5
Trend over 10 years	(+)	(−)

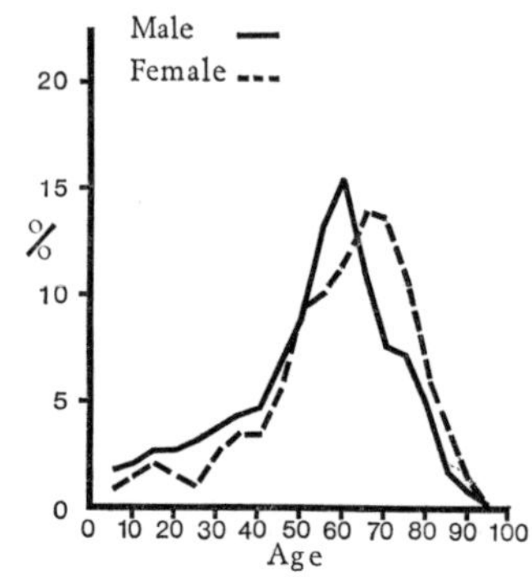

NOTES

A unifocal tumour of the lympho-reticular system is included with the type of reticulosis, not by the site of the focus. Thus reticulosarcoma of stomach is classified as a reticulosarcoma, not as a tumour of the stomach. Such tumours can be subsequently distinguished by means of a specific localisation coding.

5-YEAR SURVIVAL RATES BY AGE

Crude —— *Corrected* ----

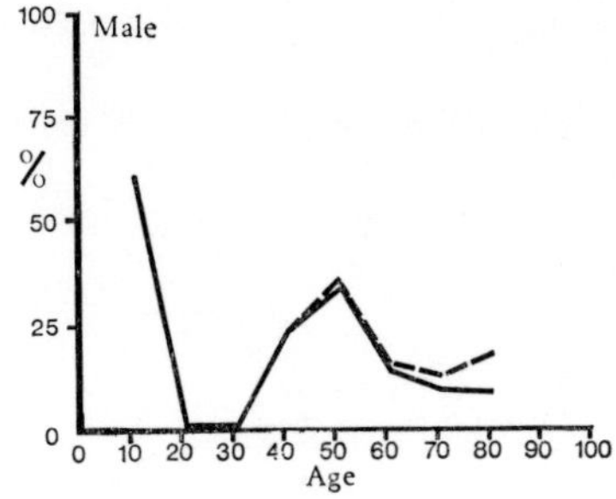

ALL CASES

Total 281

Male 144

Female 137

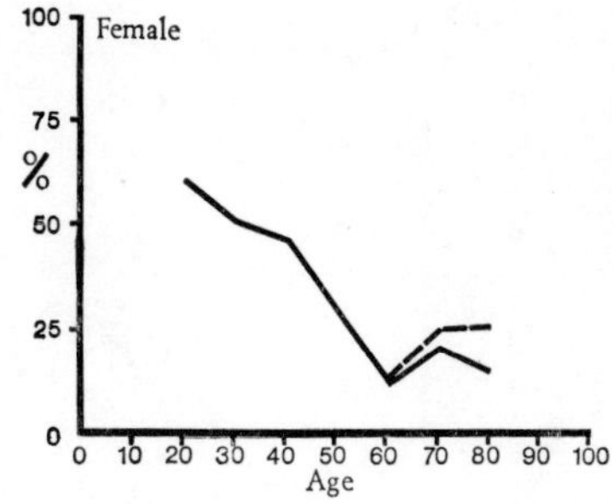

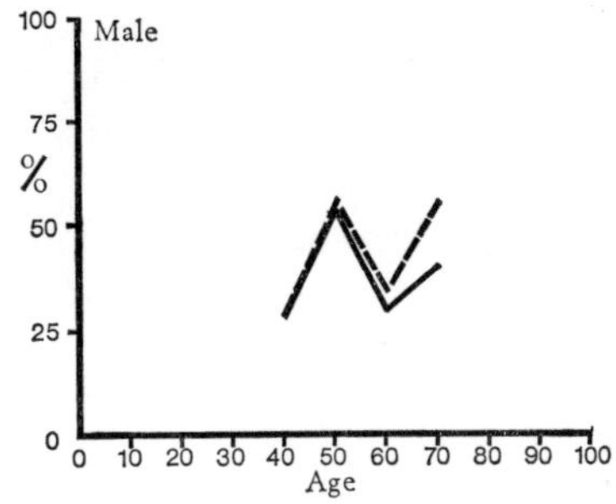

RADICAL TREATMENT

(43·1% of total)

43·8% *male*

42·3% *female*

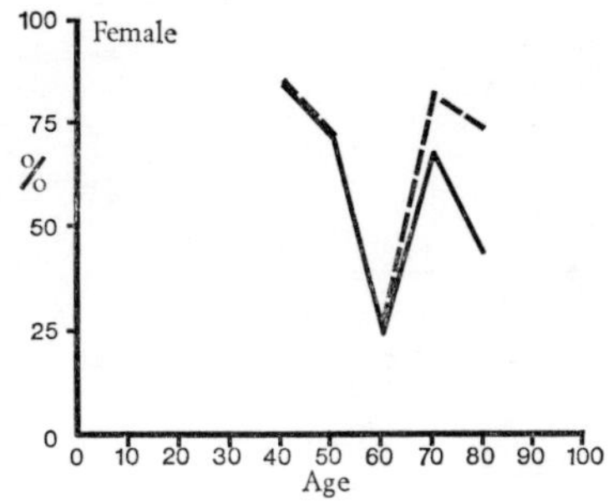

INDICES OF SURVIVAL

	All cases *Male*	All cases *Female*	Radical Treatment *Male*	Radical Treatment *Female*
FIVE YEAR SURVIVAL RATE (%)				
Crude	18·1	22·6	36·5	48·3
Corrected	*20·9*	*26·8*	*40·6*	*54·8*
Total cases†	144	137	63	58
TEN YEAR SURVIVAL RATE (%)				
Crude	16·1	10·6	43·8	25·7
Corrected	*22·0*	*14·0*	*56·4*	*33·7*
Total cases†	93	85	32	35

† Number of cases on which survival rate is based

SURVIVAL TIME (*months*)				
First quartile (75% S.R.)	1·4	2·1	5·9	8·4
Median (50% S.R.)	**5·5**	**8·4**	**31·5**	**55·0**
Third quartile (25% S.R.)	33·3	48·0	>60	>60

ANNUAL SURVIVAL RATES

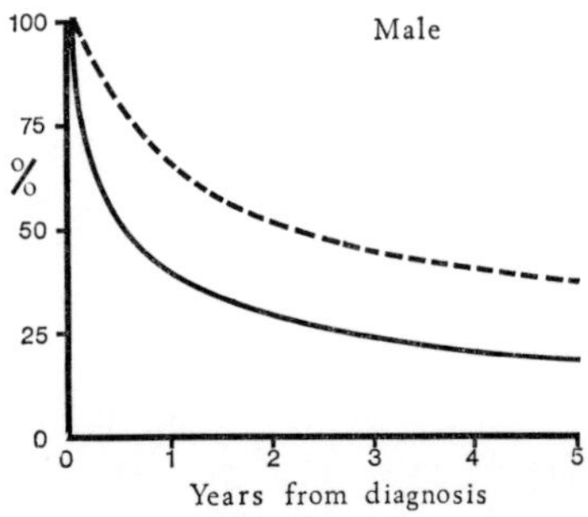

All cases ——

Radical treatment ----

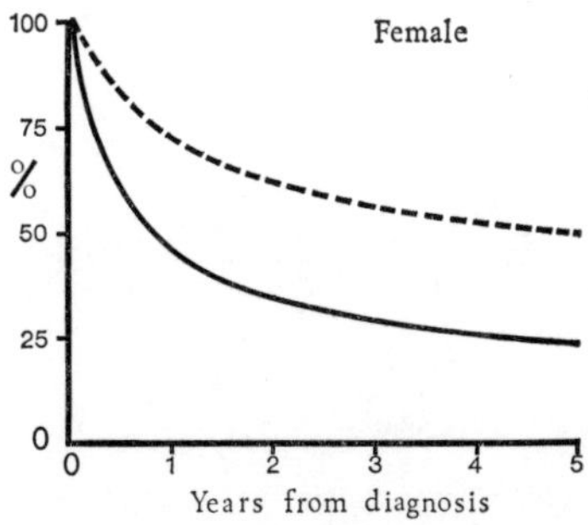

LYMPHOSARCOMA ICD (8th) **200.1**

INCIDENCE RATE (per 100,000)

Male —— *Female* ----

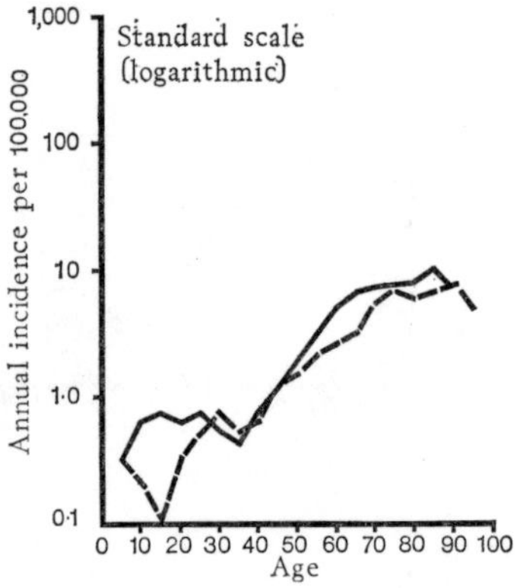

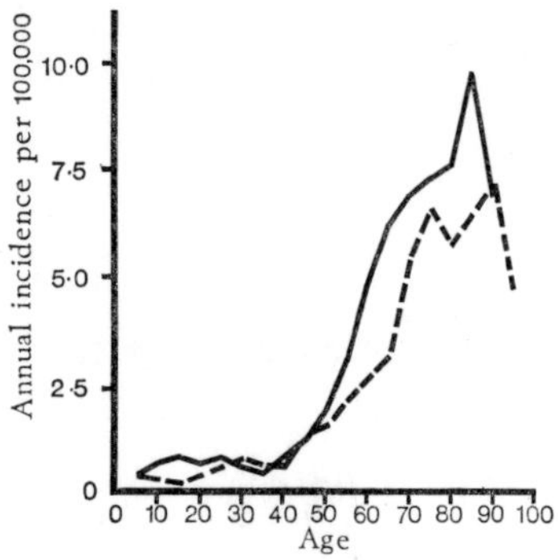

INCIDENCE RATES (per 100,000) by Age

Total cases 239 *males*; 202 *females* (of which age not stated for 0 *males* and 0 *females*)

Age	M	F	Age	M	F	Age	M	F
0–4	0·4	0·2	*35–39*	0·5	0·3	*70–74*	7·9	7·2
5–9	0·2	0·5	*40–44*	1·0	0·9	*75–79*	6·0	5·5
10–14	0·9	0·0	*45–49*	1·3	1·5	*80–84*	10·3	6·0
15–19	0·5	0·3	*50–54*	2·4	1·4	*85–89*	8·0	7·5
20–24	0·7	0·3	*55–59*	3·7	2·7	*90–94*	0·0	5·5
25–29	0·6	0·7	*60–64*	6·2	2·2	*95+*	0·0	0·0
30–34	0·4	0·6	*65–69*	6·0	3·9	*All ages*	1·7	1·4

SEX AND AGE DISTRIBUTION

	Male	*Female*
Mean age (*years*)	54·8	59·6
95% between ages	7 & 84	8 & 87
Children under 15 (%)	7·5	3·5
Median age (*years*)	59·6	63·8
Proportion by sex (%)	54·2	45·8
Proportion of all cancers by sex (%)	0·6	0·5
Trend over 10 years	(–)	(–)

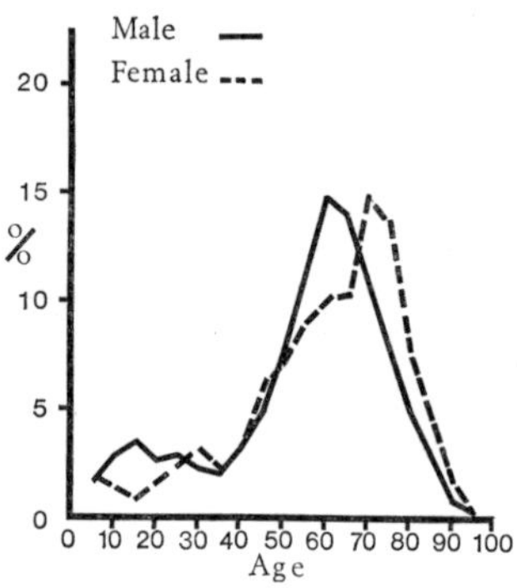

NOTES

A unifocal tumour of the lympho-reticular system is included with the type of reticulosis, not by the site of the focus. Thus reticulosarcoma of stomach is classified as a reticulosarcoma, not as a tumour of the stomach. Such tumours can be subsequently distinguished by means of a specific localisation coding.

5-YEAR SURVIVAL RATES BY AGE

Crude —— *Corrected* ----

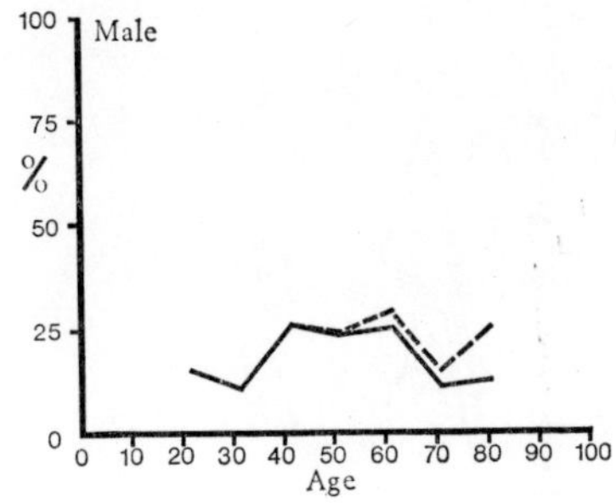

ALL CASES

Total 247
Male 157
Female 90

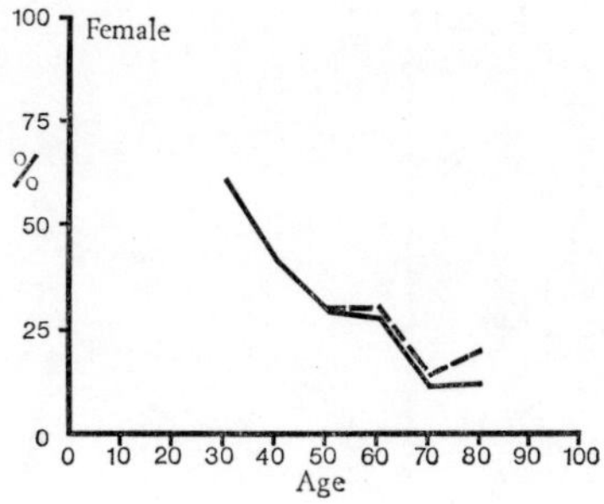

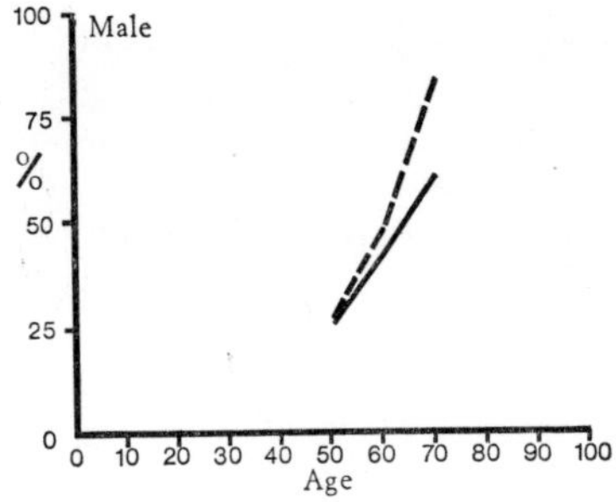

RADICAL TREATMENT

(22·7% of total)
24·2% *male*
20·0% *female*

INDICES OF SURVIVAL

	All cases		Radical Treatment	
	Male	*Female*	*Male*	*Female*
FIVE YEAR SURVIVAL RATE (%)				
Crude	17·8	20·0	39·5	0·0
Corrected	*20·6*	*23·8*	*44·1*	*0·0*
Total cases†	157	90	38	18
TEN YEAR SURVIVAL RATE (%)				
Crude	11·5	11·8	36·0	24·0
Corrected	*16·1*	*17·1*	*48·4*	*31·5*
Total cases†	104	69	25	26
SURVIVAL TIME (*months*)				
First quartile (75% S.R.)	1·7	2·5	3·6	5·3
Median (50% S.R.)	**7·7**	**10·0**	**29·0**	**16·0**
Third quartile (25% S.R.)	31·0	38·8	>60	24·8

† Number of cases on which survival rate is based

ANNUAL SURVIVAL RATES

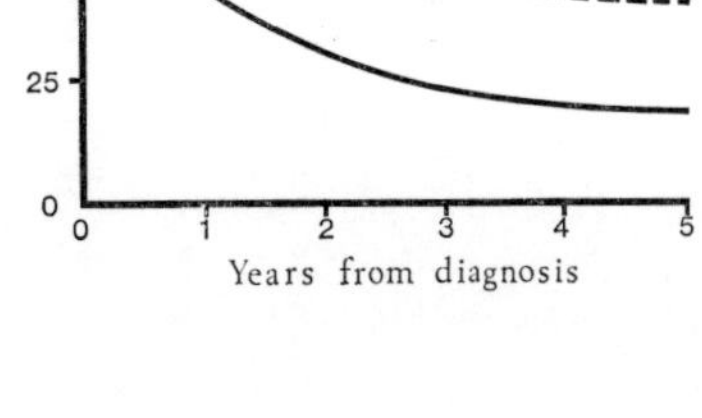

All cases ——
Radical treatment ----

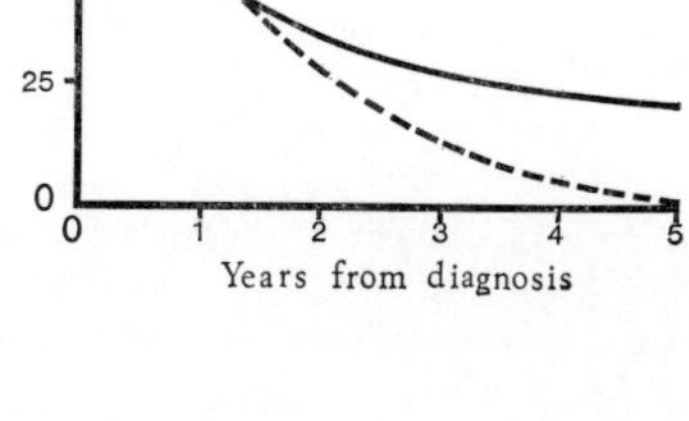

HODGKIN'S DISEASE ICD (8th) **201**

INCIDENCE RATE (per 100,000)

Male —— *Female* ----

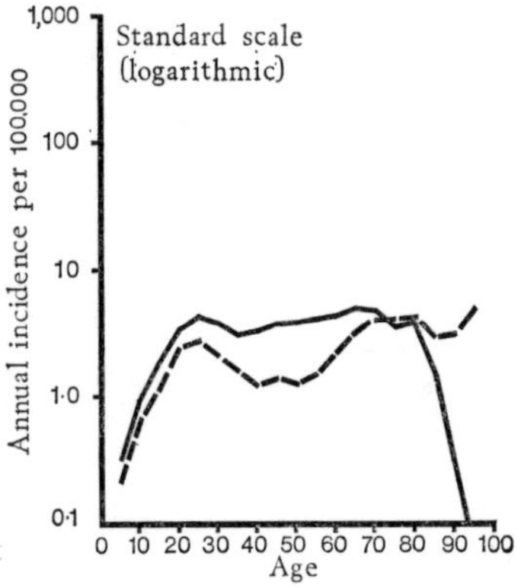

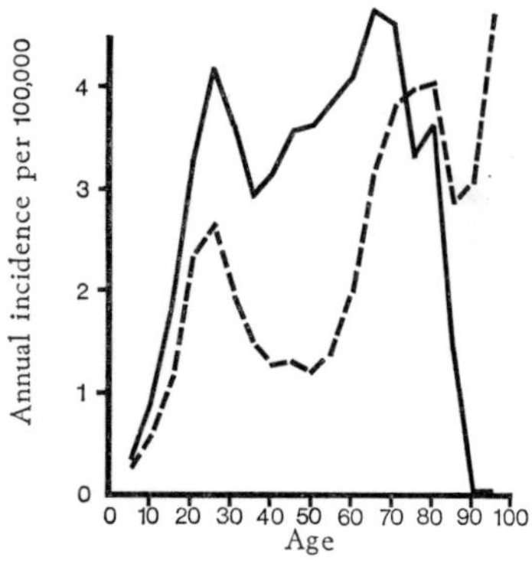

INCIDENCE RATES (per 100,000) by Age

Total cases 397 *males*; 240 *females* (of which age not stated for 0 *males* and 0 *females*)

Age	M	F	Age	M	F	Age	M	F
0–4	0·0	0·0	*35–39*	2·9	1·2	*70–74*	2·5	3·5
5–9	0·7	0·5	*40–44*	3·3	1·3	*75–79*	4·5	4·6
10–14	1·1	0·6	*45–49*	3·7	1·2	*80–84*	1·9	3·0
15–19	2·6	1·6	*50–54*	3·4	1·2	*85–89*	0·0	2·5
20–24	3·9	3·0	*55–59*	4·3	1·6	*90–94*	0·0	5·5
25–29	4·3	2·1	*60–64*	3·8	2·4	*95+*	0·0	0·0
30–34	2·9	1·8	*65–69*	6·0	4·0	*All ages*	2·8	1·7

SEX AND AGE DISTRIBUTION

	Male	*Female*
Mean age (*years*)	41·7	46·4
95% between ages	11 & 76	11 & 83
Children under 15 (%)	5·1	5·0
Median age (*years*)	41·7	45·8
Proportion by sex (%)	62·3	37·7
Proportion of all cancers by sex (%)	0·9	0·6
Trend over 10 years	(+)	(–)

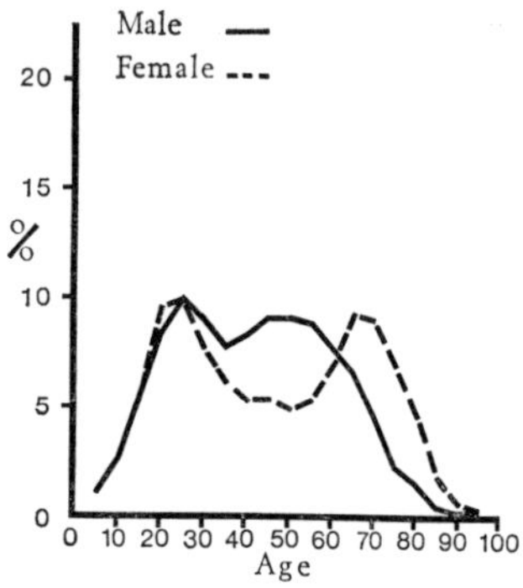

NOTES

A unifocal tumour of the lympho-reticular system is included with the type of reticulosis, not by the site of the focus. Thus reticulosarcoma of stomach is classified as a reticulosarcoma, not as a tumour of the stomach. Such tumours can be subsequently distinguished by means of a specific localisation coding.

5-YEAR SURVIVAL RATES BY AGE

Crude —— *Corrected* ----

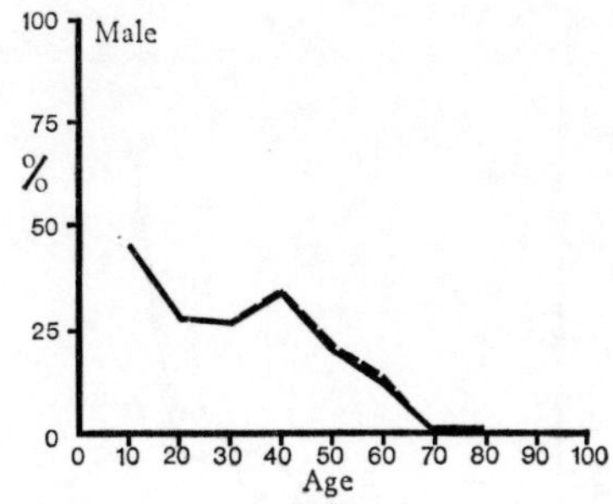

ALL CASES

Total 347
Male 207
Female 140

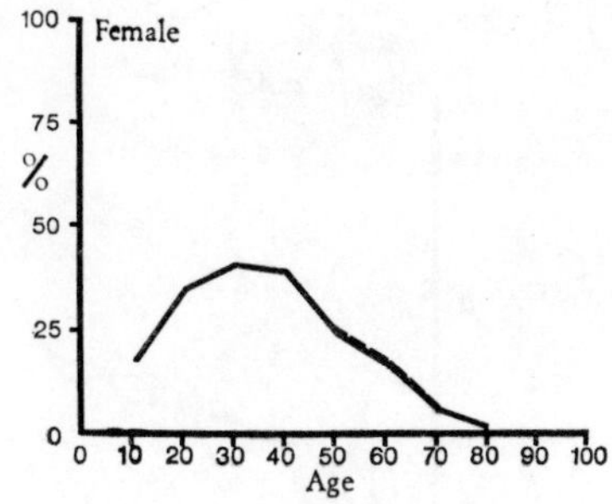

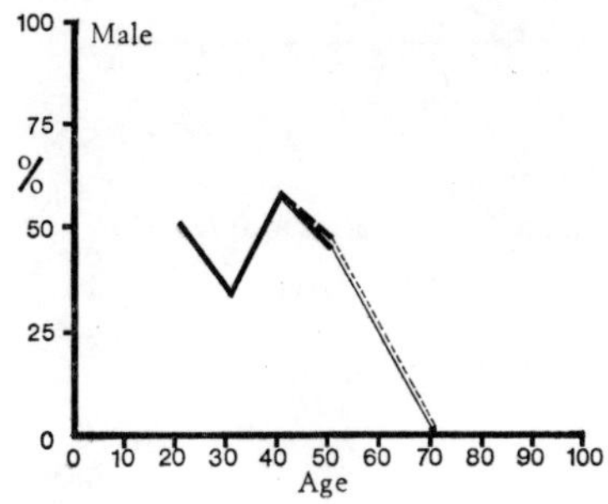

RADICAL TREATMENT

(28·5% of total)
28·0% *male*
29·3% *female*

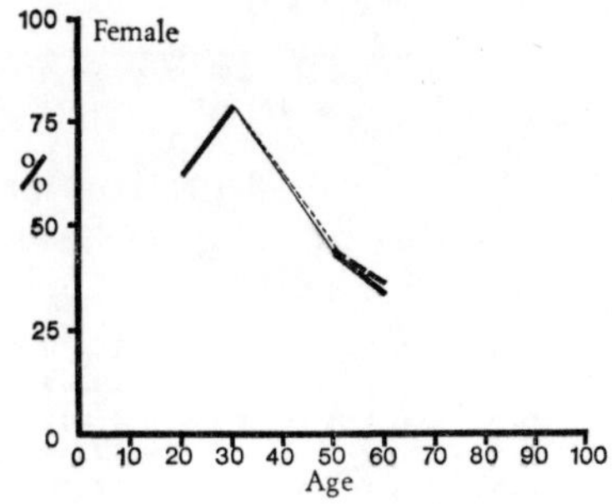

INDICES OF SURVIVAL

	All cases *Male*	All cases *Female*	Radical Treatment *Male*	Radical Treatment *Female*
FIVE YEAR SURVIVAL RATE (%)				
Crude	20·8	23·6	41·4	51·2
Corrected	*22·5*	*25·5*	*44·5*	*52·6*
Total cases†	207	140	58	41
TEN YEAR SURVIVAL RATE (%)				
Crude	11·0	15·6	13·0	26·9
Corrected	*12·9*	*17·0*	*14·6*	*28·9*
Total cases†	100	77	23	26
SURVIVAL TIME (*months*)				
First quartile (75% S.R.)	3·0	4·6	15·3	31·0
Median (50% S.R.)	**14·3**	**21·0**	**42·0**	**>60**
Third quartile (25% S.R.)	50·5	57·3	>60	>60

† Number of cases on which survival rate is based

ANNUAL SURVIVAL RATES

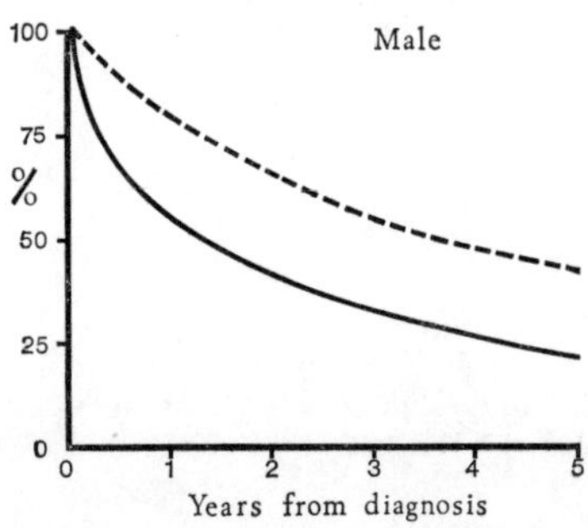

All cases ——
Radical treatment ----

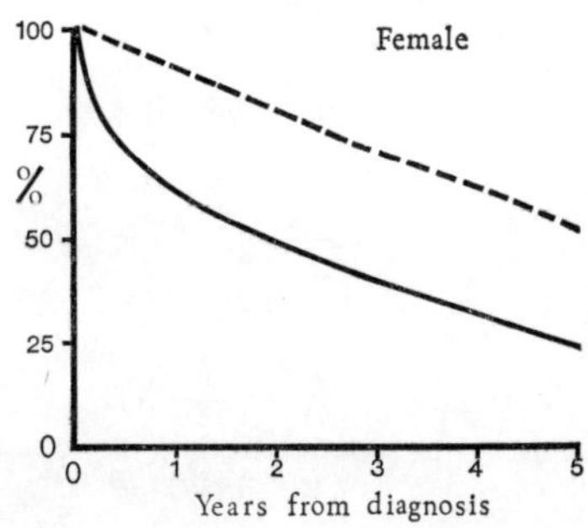

OTHER RETICULOSES | ICD (8th) **202**

INCIDENCE RATE (per 100,000)

Male —— *Female* ----

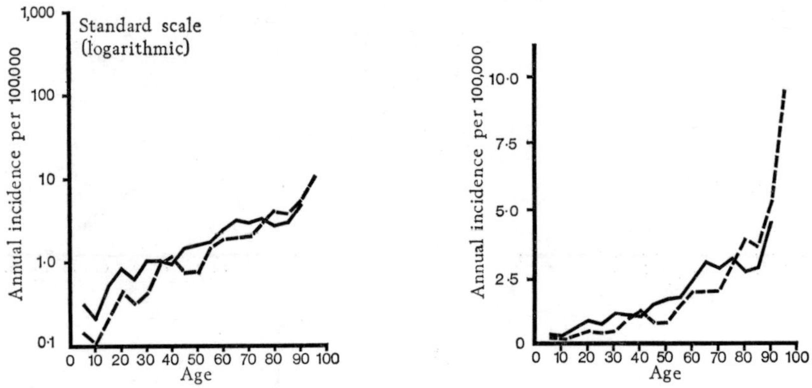

INCIDENCE RATES (per 100,000) by Age

Total cases 160 *males*; 132 *females* (of which age not stated for 0 *males* and 0 *females*)

Age	M	F	Age	M	F	Age	M	F
0–4	0·3	0·2	*35–39*	0·6	1·3	*70–74*	3·2	2·1
5–9	0·2	0·1	*40–44*	1·3	1·0	*75–79*	3·0	4·0
10–14	0·2	0·1	*45–49*	1·5	0·4	*80–84*	1·9	3·5
15–19	0·8	0·4	*50–54*	1·7	1·0	*85–89*	5·3	3·7
20–24	0·7	0·3	*55–59*	1·5	1·7	*90–94*	0·0	10·9
25–29	0·5	0·3	*60–64*	3·3	2·0	*95+*	0·0	0·0
30–34	1·5	0·4	*65–69*	2·5	1·8	*All ages*	1·1	0·9

SEX AND AGE DISTRIBUTION

	Male	*Female*
Mean age (*years*)	47·9	55·9
95% between ages	5 & 80	11 & 88
Children under 15 (%)	5·7	3·1
Median age (*years*)	50·3	58·7
Proportion by sex (%)	54·8	45·2
Proportion of all cancers by sex (%)	0·4	0·3
Trend over 10 years	(−)	(+)

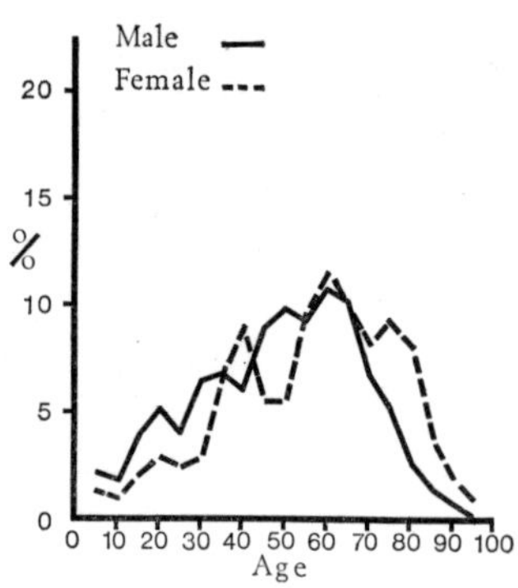

NOTES

Includes: Brill-Symmers' disease (giant follicular lymphoma); mycosis fungoides.

A unifocal tumour of the lympho-reticular system is included with the type of reticulosis, not by the site of the focus. Thus reticulosarcoma of stomach is classified as a reticulosarcoma, not as a tumour of the stomach. Such tumours can be subsequently distinguished by means of a specific localisation coding.

5-YEAR SURVIVAL RATES BY AGE

Crude —— *Corrected* ----

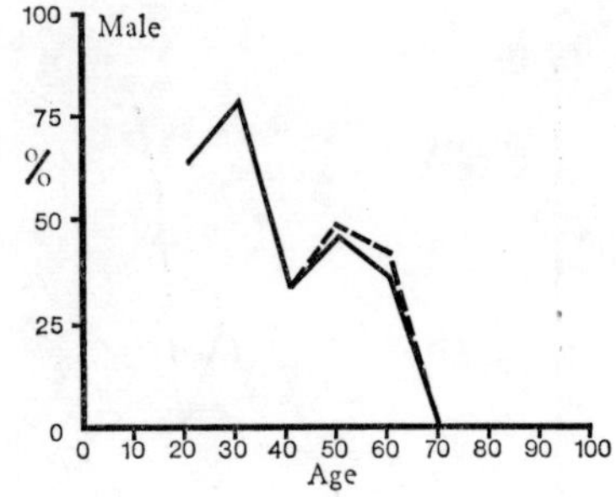

ALL CASES

Total 159
Male 87
Female 72

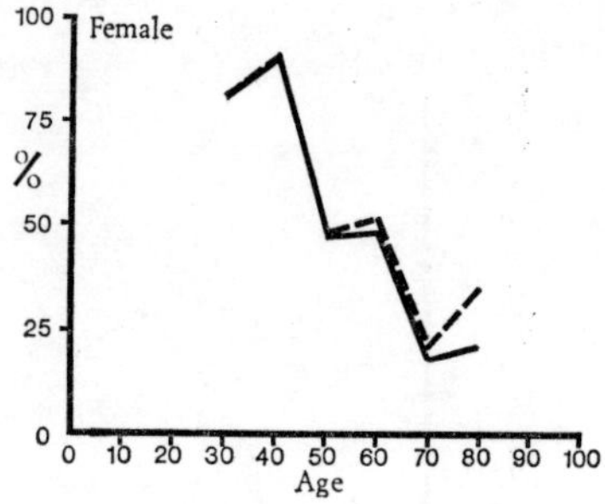

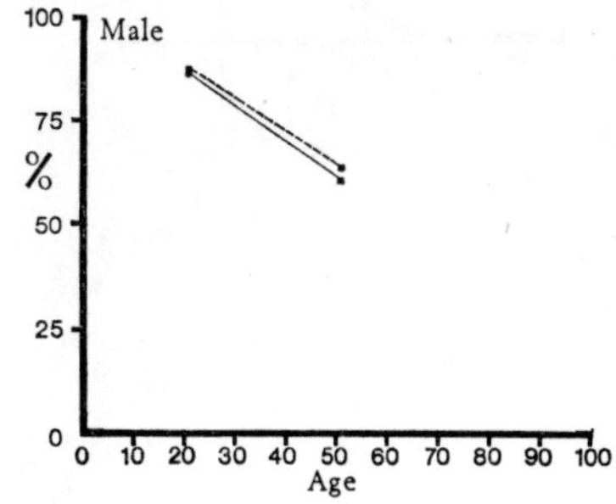

RADICAL TREATMENT

(28·3% of total)
32·2% *male*
23·6% *female*

INDICES OF SURVIVAL

	All cases		Radical Treatment	
	Male	*Female*	*Male*	*Female*
FIVE YEAR SURVIVAL RATE (%)				
Crude	40·2	45·8	57·1	70·6
Corrected	*44·5*	*51·5*	*60·0*	*73·8*
Total cases†	87	72	28	17
TEN YEAR SURVIVAL RATE (%)				
Crude	29·6	37·3	47·2	60·0
Corrected	*35·7*	*46·9*	*53·9*	*69·3*
Total cases†	81	67	36	25
SURVIVAL TIME (*months*)				
First quartile (75% S.R.)	5·8	7·8	33·8	53·0
Median (50% S.R.)	**40·5**	**45·0**	**>60**	**>60**
Third quartile (25% S.R.)	>60	>60	>60	>60

† Number of cases on which survival rate is based

ANNUAL SURVIVAL RATES

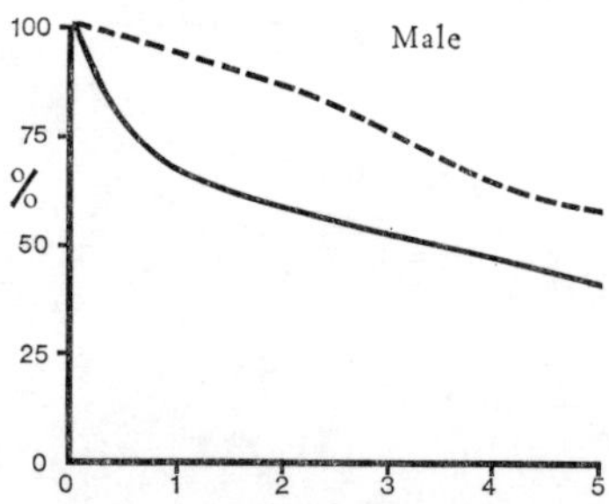

All cases ——

Radical treatment ----

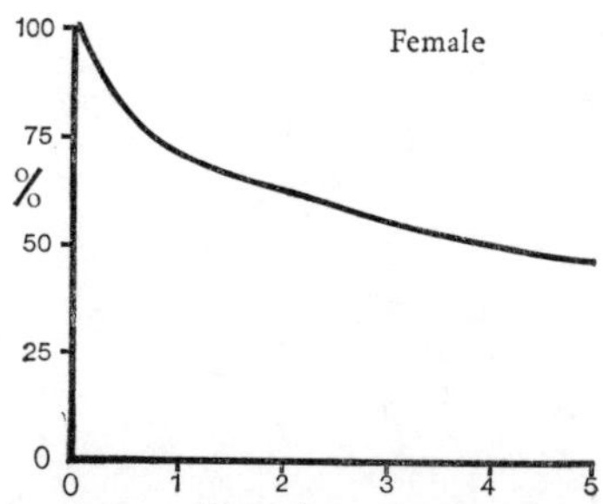

MYELOMATOSIS **ICD (8th) 203**

INCIDENCE RATE (per 100,000)

Male —— *Female* ----

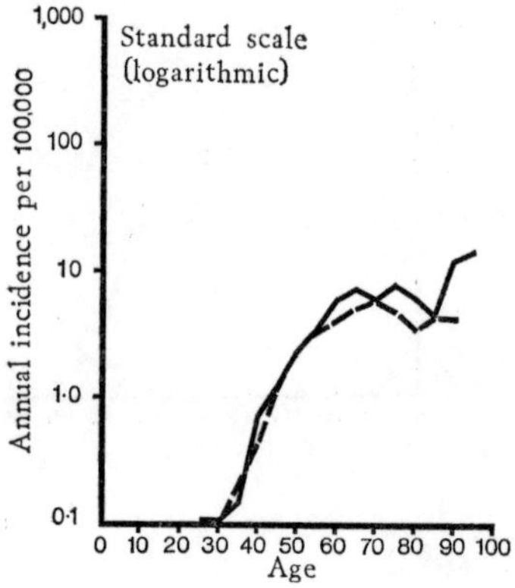

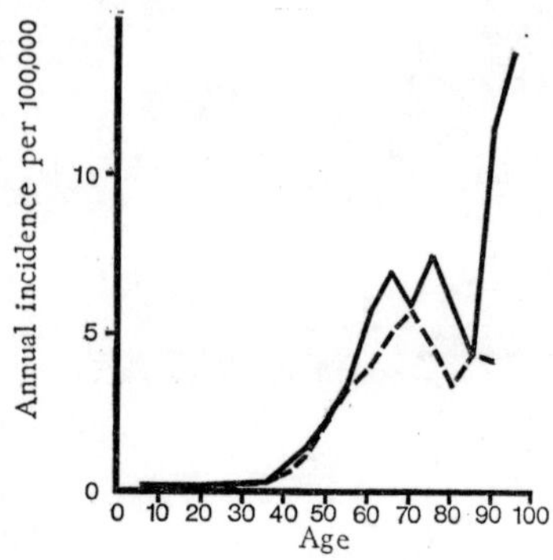

INCIDENCE RATES (per 100,000) by Age

Total cases 208 *males*; 198 *females* (of which age not stated for 0 *males* and 0 *females*)

Age	M	F	Age	M	F	Age	M	F
0–4	0·0	0·0	*35–39*	0·2	0·2	*70–74*	7·0	5·8
5–9	0·0	0·0	*40–44*	1·2	0·7	*75–79*	8·0	2·9
10–14	0·0	0·0	*45–49*	1·3	1·4	*80–84*	1·9	4·0
15–19	0·0	0·0	*50–54*	3·1	2·9	*85–89*	10·7	5·0
20–24	0·0	0·0	*55–59*	3·6	3·4	*90–94*	15·4	0·0
25–29	0·1	0·0	*60–64*	8·2	4·3	*95+*	0·0	0·0
30–34	0·1	0·1	*65–69*	4·9	5·5	*All ages*	1·5	1·4

SEX AND AGE DISTRIBUTION

	Male	*Female*
Mean age (*years*)	61·3	62·5
95% between ages	41 & 84	41 & 84
Children under 15 (%)	0·0	0·0
Median age (*years*)	61·4	62·7
Proportion by sex (%)	51·2	48·8
Proportion of all cancers by sex (%)	0·5	0·6
Trend over 10 years	(+)	(+)

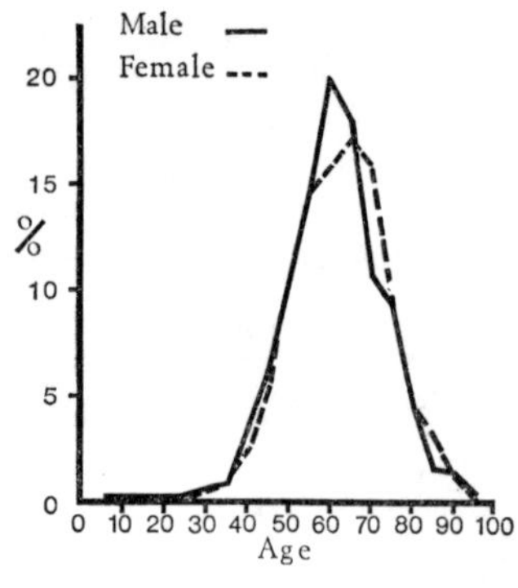

5-YEAR SURVIVAL RATES BY AGE

Crude ——— *Corrected* - - - -

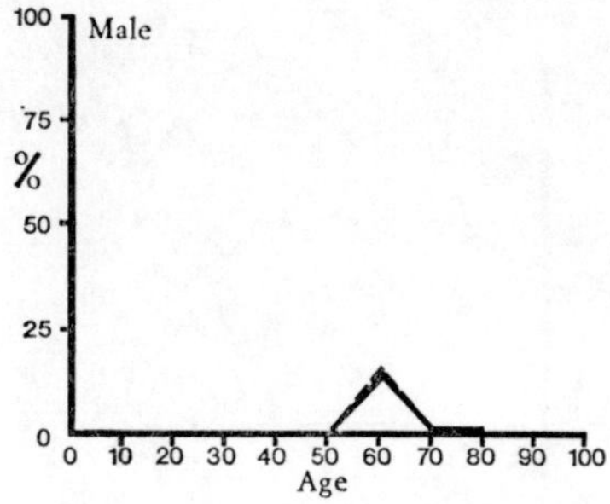

ALL CASES

Total 179
Male 90
Female 89

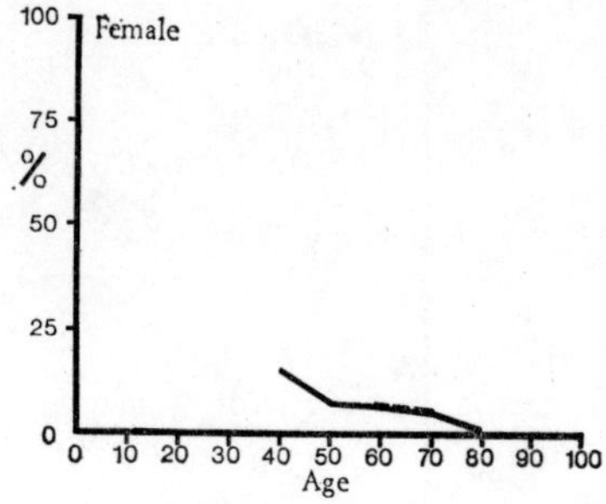

RADICAL TREATMENT

(6·1% of total)
6·7% *male*
5·6% *female*

INDICES OF SURVIVAL

	All cases		Radical Treatment	
	Male	*Female*	*Male*	*Female*
FIVE YEAR SURVIVAL RATE (%)				
Crude	6·7	5·6	66·7	60·0
Corrected	*8·0*	*6·3*	*73·5*	*66·9*
Total cases†	90	89	6	5
TEN YEAR SURVIVAL RATE (%)				
Crude	6·9	0·0	20·0	0·0
Corrected	*10·3*	*0·0*	*26·9*	*0·0*
Total cases†	29	38	5	4
SURVIVAL TIME (*months*)				
First quartile (75% S.R.)	1·0	1·3	54·3	36·0
Median (50% S.R.)	**3·9**	**6·7**	**>60**	**>60**
Third quartile (25% S.R.)	12·4	18·0	>60	>60

† Number of cases on which survival rate is based

ANNUAL SURVIVAL RATES

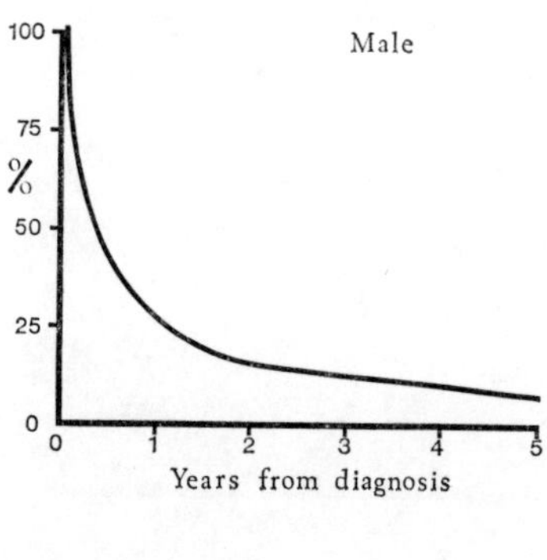

All cases ———
Radical treatment - - - -

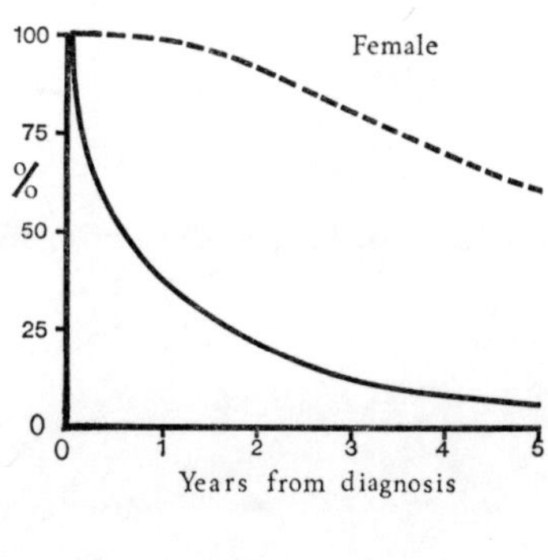

LEUKAEMIA, ACUTE ICD (8th) **204.0, 205.0, 206.0, 207.0**

INCIDENCE RATE (per 100,000)

Male —— *Female* - - - -

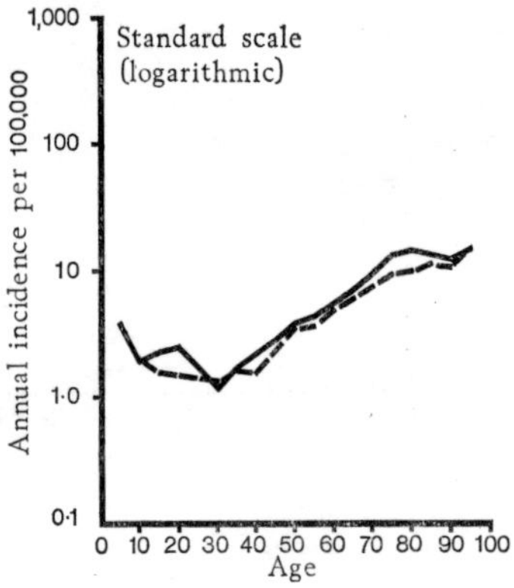

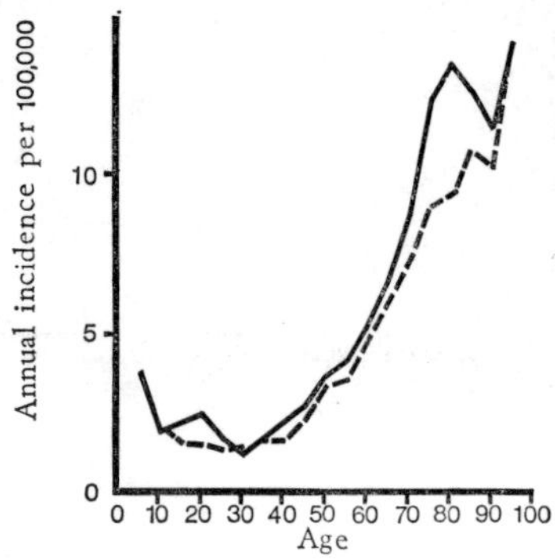

INCIDENCE RATES (per 100,000) by Age

Total cases 470 *males*; 454 *females* (of which age not stated for 1 *male* and 1 *female*)

Age	M	F	Age	M	F	Age	M	F
0–4	4·8	4·5	*35–39*	2·2	1·6	*70–74*	11·4	9·3
5–9	2·3	2·4	*40–44*	1·9	1·3	*75–79*	13·5	8·4
10–14	1·4	1·6	*45–49*	3·2	3·0	*80–84*	13·1	10·9
15–19	2·8	1·5	*50–54*	3·8	3·3	*85–89*	10·7	10·0
20–24	1·8	1·3	*55–59*	4·2	3·5	*90–94*	15·4	10·9
25–29	1·4	1·2	*60–64*	6·3	5·9	*95+*	0·0	32·2
30–34	0·9	1·4	*65–69*	6·7	5·6	*All ages*	3·3	3·1

SEX AND AGE DISTRIBUTION

	Male	*Female*
Mean age (*years*)	43·0	47·0
95% between ages	1 & 83	1 & 85
Children under 15 (%)	21·1	20·3
Median age (*years*)	48·4	53·5
Proportion by sex (%)	50·9	49·1
Proportion of all cancers by sex (%)	1·1	1·1
Trend over 10 years	(+)	(+)

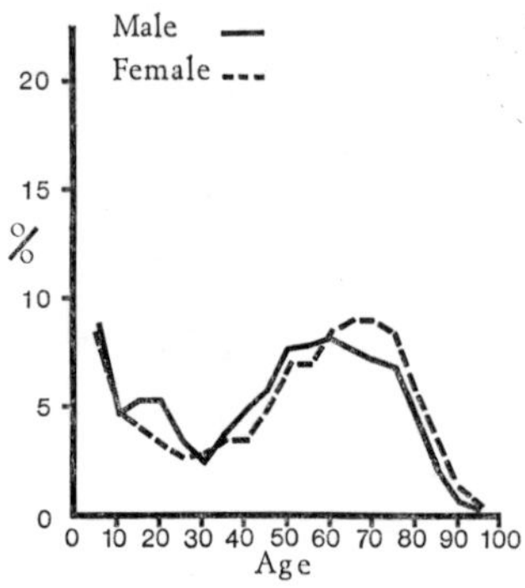

NOTES

Includes: All forms of leukaemia specified as acute.

5-YEAR SURVIVAL RATES BY AGE

Crude —— *Corrected* ----

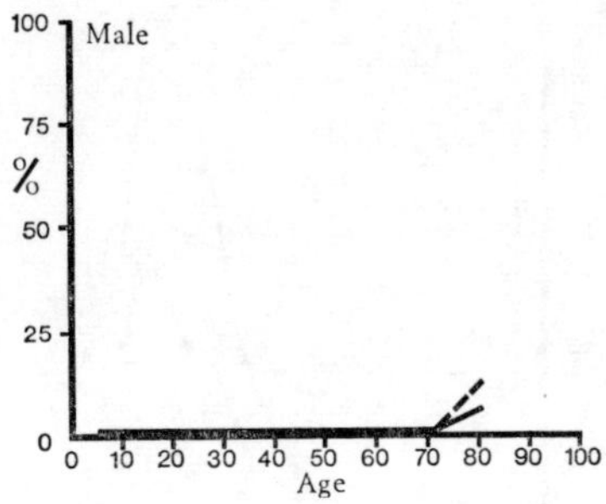

ALL CASES

Total	364
Male	192
Female	172

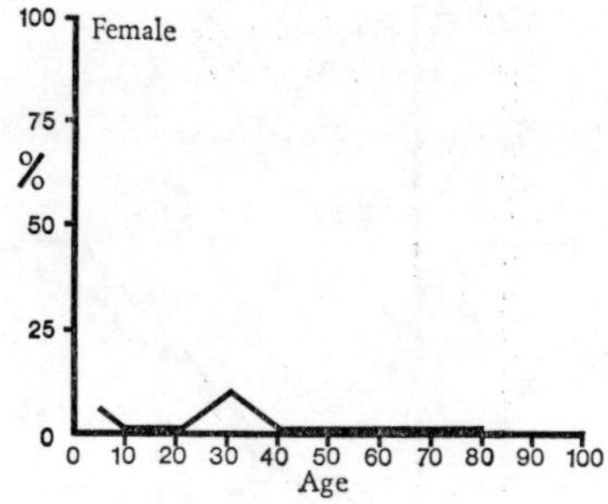

RADICAL TREATMENT

(0·0% of total)
0·0% *male*
0·0% *female*

INDICES OF SURVIVAL

	All cases *Male*	All cases *Female*	Radical Treatment *Male*	Radical Treatment *Female*
FIVE YEAR SURVIVAL RATE (%)				
Crude	0·5	1·2	—	—
Corrected	*0·6*	*1·3*	—	—
Total cases†	192	172	0	0
TEN YEAR SURVIVAL RATE (%)				
Crude	0·0	0·0	—	—
Corrected	*0·0*	*0·0*	—	—
Total cases†	108	81	0	0
SURVIVAL TIME (*months*)				
First quartile (75% S.R.)	0·6	0·5	—	—
Median (50% S.R.)	**1·8**	**1·4**	—	—
Third quartile (25% S.R.)	4·8	5·3	—	—

† Number of cases on which survival rates is based

ANNUAL SURVIVAL RATES

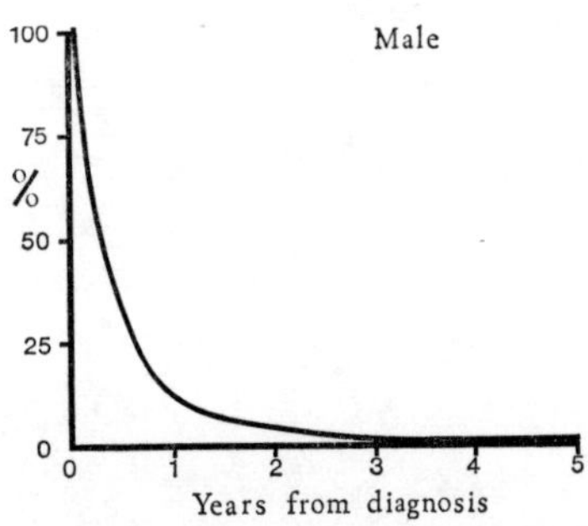

All cases ————
Radical treatment - - - -

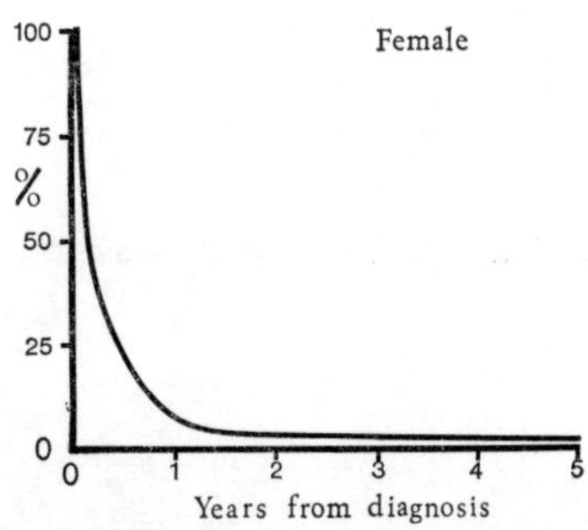

LEUKAEMIA, OTHER ICD (8th) **204, 205, 206, 207 (rem.)**

INCIDENCE RATE (per 100,000)

Male —— *Female* - - - -

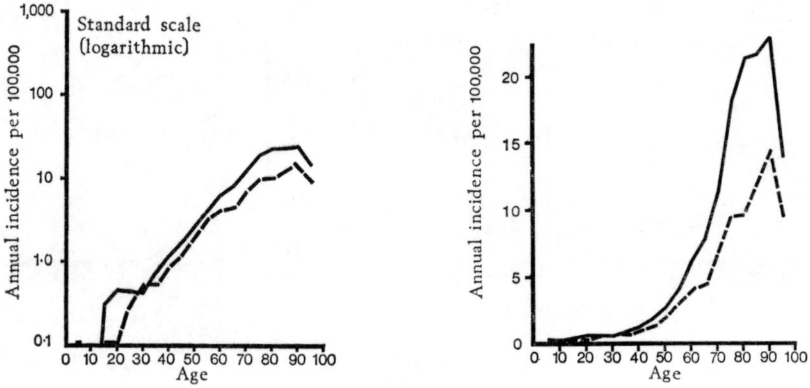

INCIDENCE RATES (per 100,000) by Age

Total cases 343 *males*; 266 *females* (of which age not stated for 1 *male* and 1 *female*)

Age	M	F	Age	M	F	Age	M	F
0–4	0·3	0·2	*35–39*	1·0	0·6	*70–74*	15·8	9·7
5–9	0·0	0·0	*40–44*	1·1	1·0	*75–79*	21·5	8·9
10–14	0·1	0·1	*45–49*	2·2	1·2	*80–84*	20·6	10·4
15–19	0·5	0·1	*50–54*	2·8	2·4	*85–89*	24·0	15·0
20–24	0·4	0·1	*55–59*	5·0	3·4	*90–94*	15·4	10·9
25–29	0·4	0·6	*60–64*	7·4	4·2	*95+*	0·0	0·0
30–34	0·4	0·4	*65–69*	8·1	4·2	*All ages*	2·4	1·8

SEX AND AGE DISTRIBUTION

	Male	*Female*
Mean age (*years*)	62·0	64·0
95% between ages	20 & 86	27 & 88
Children under 15 (%)	1·2	1·2
Median age (*years*)	63·9	66·3
Proportion by sex (%)	56·3	43·7
Proportion of all cancers by sex (%)	0·9	0·7
Trend over 10 years	(–)	–

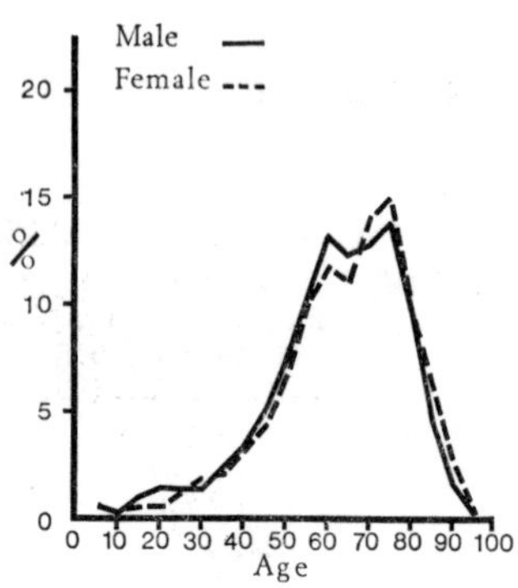

NOTES

Includes: All forms of leukaemia specified as chronic, or not further specified.

5-YEAR SURVIVAL RATES BY AGE

Crude —— *Corrected* ----

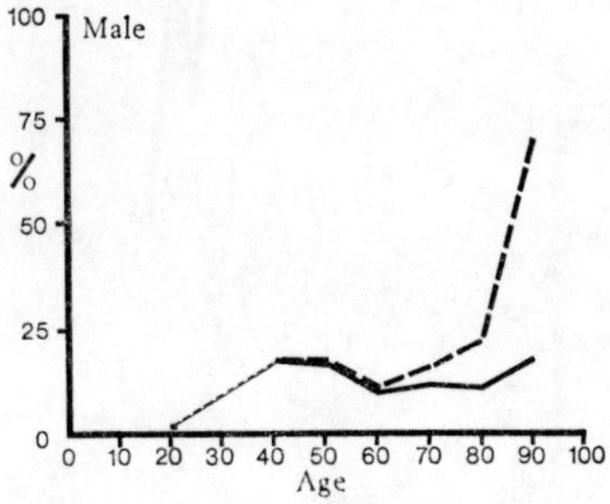

ALL CASES

Total 445

Male 225
Female 220

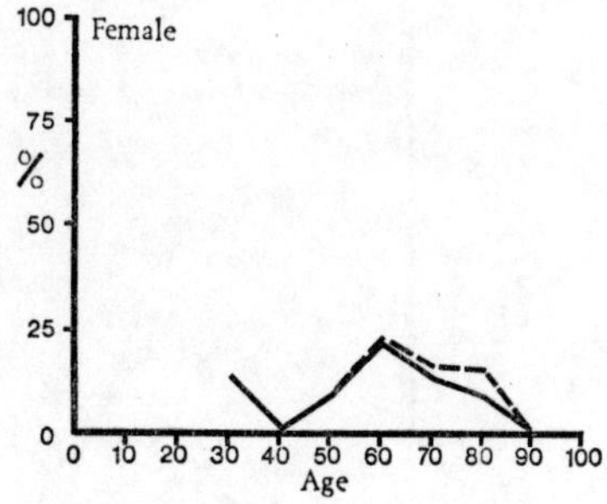

RADICAL TREATMENT

(0·7% of total)
0·4% *male*
0·9% *female*

INDICES OF SURVIVAL

	All cases *Male*	All cases *Female*	Radical Treatment *Male*	Radical Treatment *Female*
FIVE YEAR SURVIVAL RATE (%)				
Crude	11·1	12·7	100·0	0·0
Corrected	*14·1*	*15·2*	*100·0*	*0·0*
Total cases†	225	220	1	2
TEN YEAR SURVIVAL RATE (%)				
Crude	1·7	3·5	50·0	0·0
Corrected	*2·6*	*4·6*	*100·0*	*0·0*
Total cases†	117	114	2	1

† Number of cases on which survival is based

	All cases *Male*	All cases *Female*	Radical Treatment *Male*	Radical Treatment *Female*
SURVIVAL TIME (*months*)				
First quartile (75% S.R.)	2·5	3·9	>60	4·3
Median (50% S.R.)	**10·8**	**14·8**	**>60**	**15·0**
Third quartile (25% S.R.)	35·5	36·9	>60	15·8

ANNUAL SURVIVAL RATES

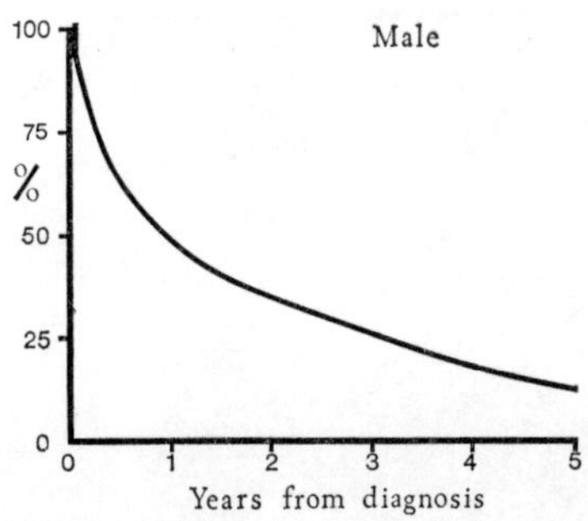

All cases ——
Radical treatment ----

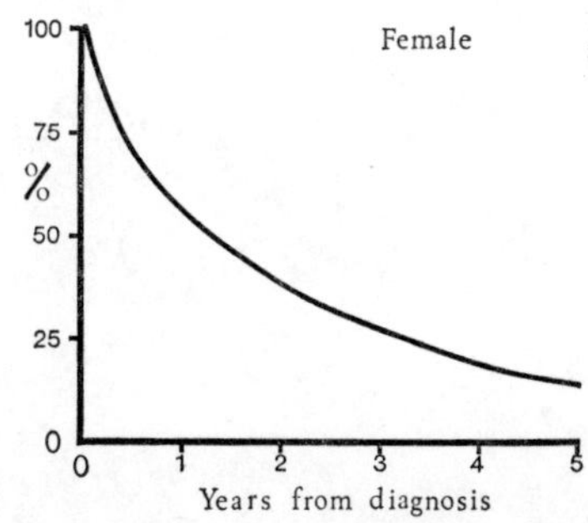

POLYCYTHAEMIA ICD (8th) **208**

INCIDENCE RATE (per 100,000)

Male —— *Female* - - - -

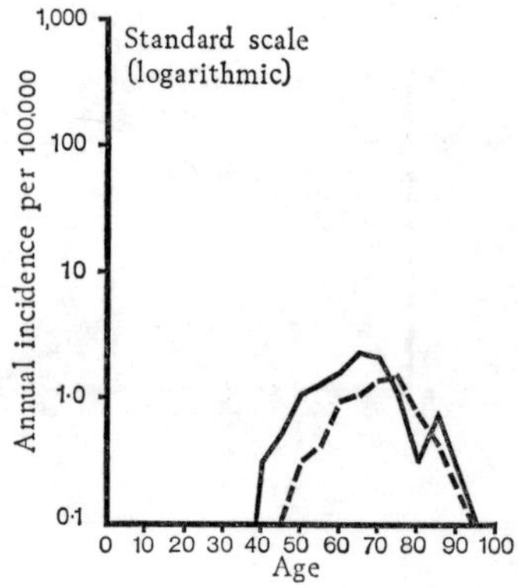

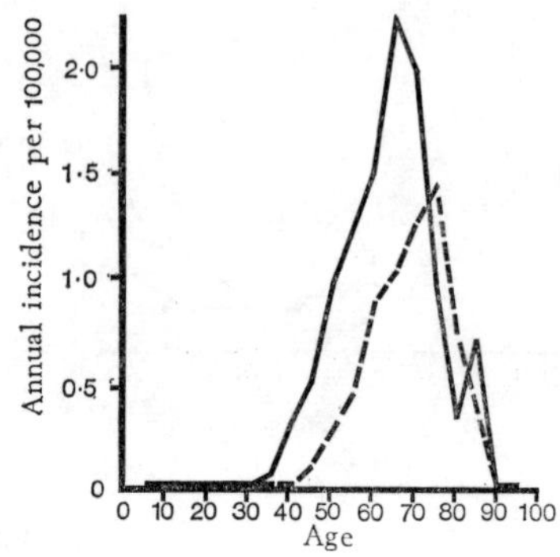

INCIDENCE RATES (per 100,000) by Age

Total cases 63 *males*; 37 *females* (of which age not stated for 0 *males* and 0 *females*)

Age	M	F	Age	M	F	Age	M	F
0–4	0·0	0·0	*35–39*	0·1	0·0	*70–74*	1·6	1·9
5–9	0·0	0·0	*40–44*	0·5	0·0	*75–79*	0·0	0·9
10–14	0·0	0·0	*45–49*	0·5	0·2	*80–84*	0·9	0·5
15–19	0·0	0·0	*50–54*	1·5	0·3	*85–89*	0·0	0·0
20–24	0·0	0·0	*55–59*	1·0	0·6	*90–94*	0·0	0·0
25–29	0·0	0·0	*60–64*	2·2	1·2	*95+*	0·0	0·0
30–34	0·0	0·0	*65–69*	2·2	0·8	*All ages*	0·4	0·3

SEX AND AGE DISTRIBUTION

	Male	*Female*
Mean age (*years*)	58·4	65·1
95% between ages	41 & 74	47 & 80
Children under 15 (%)	0·0	0·0
Median age (*years*)	59·1	64·7
Proportion by sex (%)	63·0	37·0
Proportion of all cancers by sex (%)	0·1	0·1
Trend over 10 years	(+)	(+)

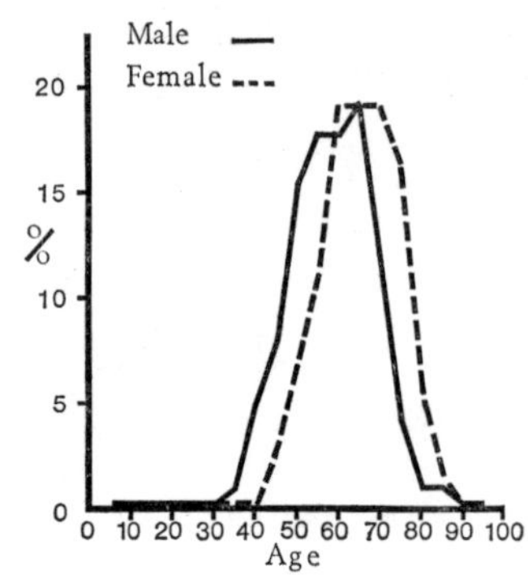

5-YEAR SURVIVAL RATES BY AGE

Crude ——— *Corrected* - - - -

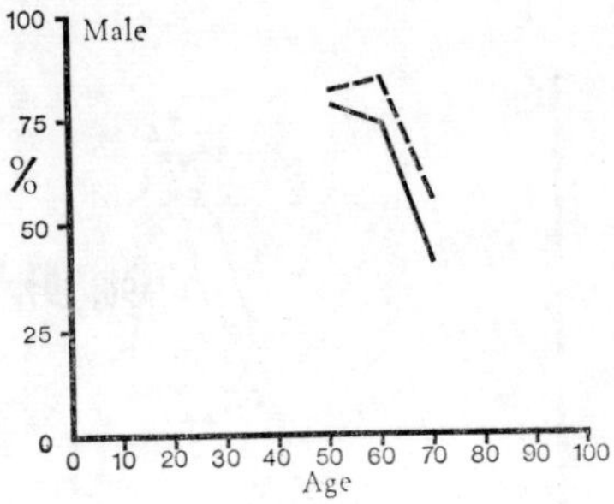

ALL CASES

Total	51
Male	36
Female	15

RADICAL TREATMENT

(2·0% of total)
0·0% *male*
6·7% *female*

INDICES OF SURVIVAL

	All cases *Male*	All cases *Female*	Radical Treatment *Male*	Radical Treatment *Female*
FIVE YEAR SURVIVAL RATE (%)				
Crude	63·9	80·0	—	0·0
Corrected	*74·8*	*91·8*	—	*0·0*
Total cases†	36	15	0	1
TEN YEAR SURVIVAL RATE (%)				
Crude	40·0	50·0	—	—
Corrected	*46·6*	*63·8*	—	—
Total cases†	20	12	0	0

† Number of cases on which survival rate is based

SURVIVAL TIME (*months*)				
First quartile (75% S.R.)	43·8	> 60	—	34·0
Median (50% S.R.)	**> 60**	**> 60**	—	**34·5**
Third quartile (25% S.R.)	> 60	> 60	—	35·0

ANNUAL SURVIVAL RATES

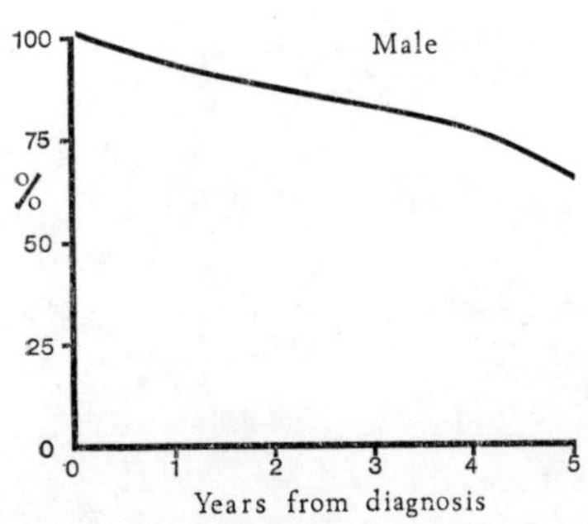

All cases ———
Radical treatment - - - -

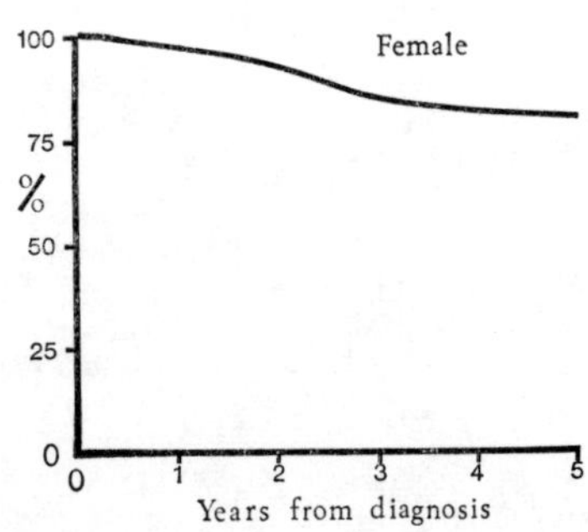

UNKNOWN PRIMARY ICD (8th) **159, 163.9, 195, 196, 197, 198, 199**

INCIDENCE RATE (per 100,000)

Male —— *Female* ----

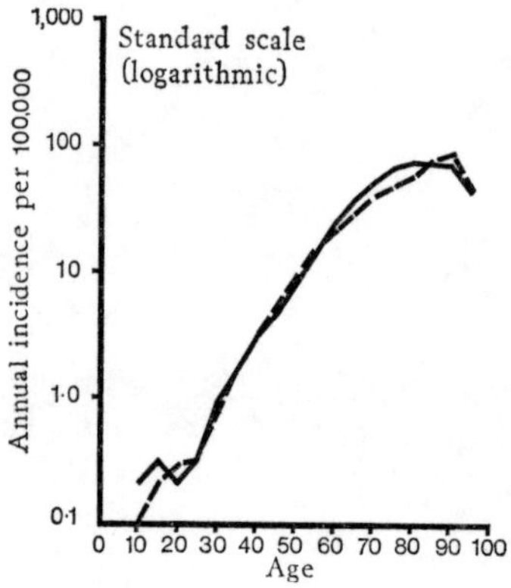

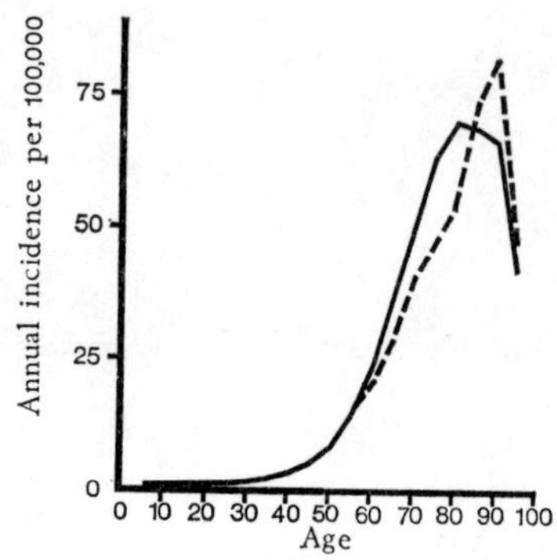

INCIDENCE RATES (per 100,000) by Age

Total cases 1181 *males*; 1395 *females* (of which age not stated for 0 *males* and 1 *female*)

Age	M	F	Age	M	F	Age	M	F
0–4	0·0	0·0	*35–39*	2·0	2·2	*70–74*	58·5	45·7
5–9	0·1	0·1	*40–44*	3·9	4·1	*75–79*	69·6	47·3
10–14	0·2	0·2	*45–49*	4·8	6·1	*80–84*	68·4	66·5
15–19	0·3	0·3	*50–54*	10·5	11·5	*85–89*	69·3	89·7
20–24	0·1	0·1	*55–59*	16·9	16·5	*90–94*	46·1	49·3
25–29	0·5	0·5	*60–64*	29·8	23·3	*95+*	0·0	32·2
30–34	1·2	0·8	*65–69*	42·3	35·2	*All ages*	8·4	9·7

SEX AND AGE DISTRIBUTION

	Male	*Female*
Mean age (*years*)	64·5	66·6
95% between ages	36 & 85	38 & 88
Children under 15 (%)	0·4	0·2
Median age (*years*)	65·6	67·8
Proportion by sex (%)	45·9	54·1
Proportion of all cancers by sex (%)	2·7	3·4
Trend over 10 years	(+)	(+)

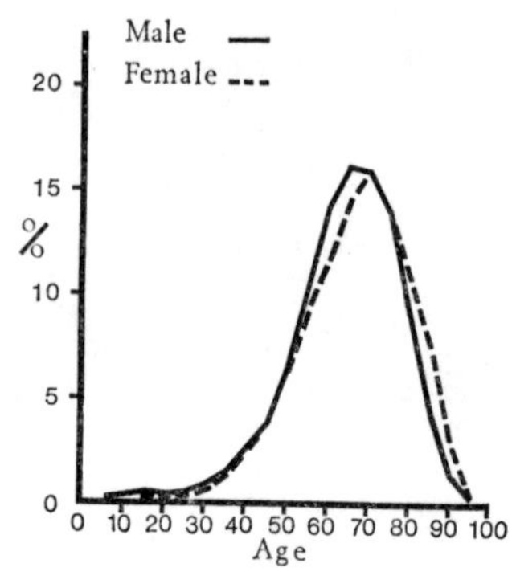

NOTES

Includes: All cases of malignant disease in which it has not been possible to identify the site of the primary tumour. They have been classified in relation to the sites of secondaries on p. 84.

ICD (7th) 156, 159, 163, 165, 198, 199 **UNKNOWN PRIMARY**

5-YEAR SURVIVAL RATES BY AGE

Crude —— *Corrected* - - - -

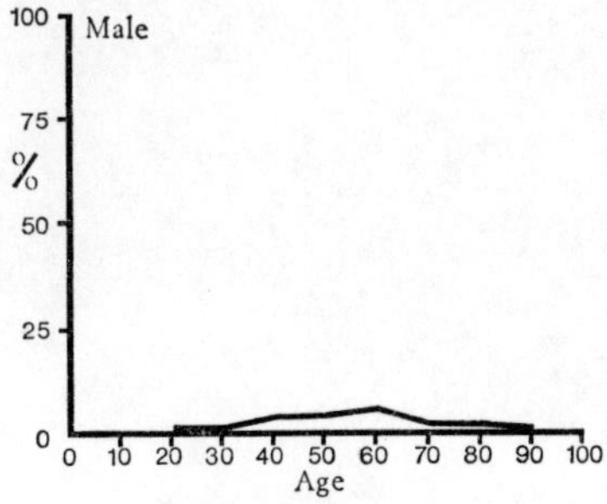

ALL CASES

Total 1283

Male 579
Female 704

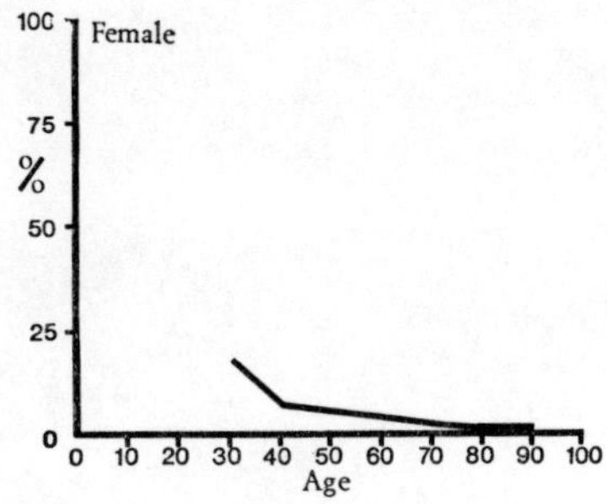

RADICAL TREATMENT

(1·0% of total)
0·7% *male*
1·3% *female*

INDICES OF SURVIVAL

	All cases *Male*	All cases *Female*	Radical Treatment *Male*	Radical Treatment *Female*
FIVE YEAR SURVIVAL RATE (%)				
Crude	2·8	2·1	0·0	11·1
Corrected	*3·6*	*2·5*	*0·0*	*12·4*
Total cases†	579	704	4	9
TEN YEAR SURVIVAL RATE (%)				
Crude	1·9	3·4	25·0	16·7
Corrected	*3·2*	*5·1*	*44·4*	*23·4*
Total cases†	303	322	4	6
SURVIVAL TIME (*months*)				
First quartile (75% S.R.)	0·8	0·9	4·8	1·5
Median (50% S.R.)	**1·8**	**2·3**	**7·0**	**6·5**
Third quartile (25% S.R.)	4·6	5·5	9·3	23·0

† Number of cases on which survival rate is based

ANNUAL SURVIVAL RATES

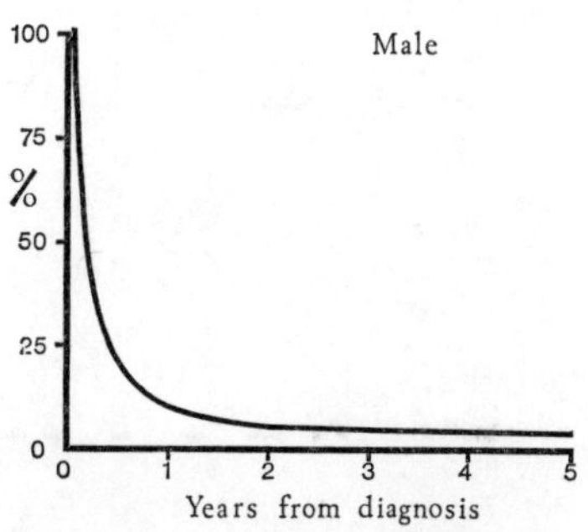

All cases ————

Radical treatment - - - -

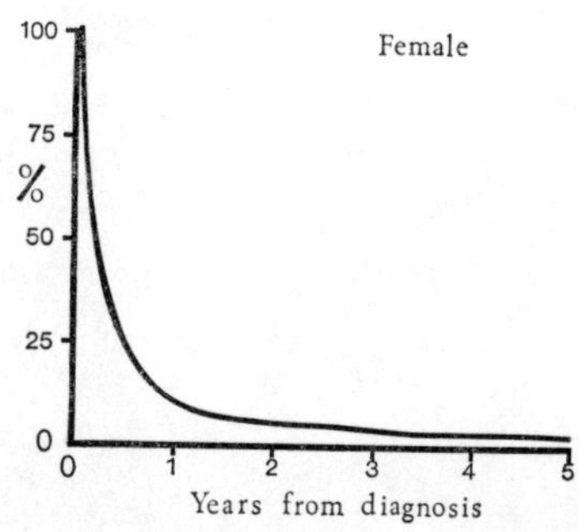

Printed in Great Britain by
T. & A. Constable Ltd., Hopetoun Street
Printers to the University of Edinburgh